Ward-based Critical Care
A Guide for Health Professionals

Edited by
Ann M. Price, Sally A. Smith and Alistair Challiner

Full the full range of M&K Publishing books please visit our website:

www.mkupdate.co.uk

Ward-based Critical Care
A Guide for Health Professionals

Edited by

Ann M. Price RGN BSc (Hons) ENB 100 PGCE MSc MA
Senior Lecturer, Canterbury Christ Church University,
Canterbury, Kent, UK

Sally A. Smith DN, MSc, DipHE, ENB 100, ENB 998, ENB 934
Chief Nurse & Director of Quality, East Kent Hospitals University
NHS Foundation Trust.

Alistair Challiner MBA FFICM FRCA FIMC EDIC
Consultant Intensivist and Anaesthetist, Maidstone Hospital,
Maidstone and Tunbridge Wells NHS Trust, Kent.

Ward-based Critical Care: a guide for health professionals 2nd edition

Edited by:
Ann M Price
Sally A Smith
Alistair Challiner

ISBN: 9781905539-92-5

First published 2010. This revised edition 2016

British Library Cataloguing in Publication Data

A catalogue record for this book is available from the British Library

Notice

Clinical practice and medical knowledge constantly evolve. Standard safety precautions must be followed, but, as knowledge is broadened by research, changes in practice, treatment and drug therapy may become necessary or appropriate. Readers must check the most current product information provided by the manufacturer of each drug to be administered and verify the dosages and correct administration, as well as contraindications. It is the responsibility of the practitioner, utilising the experience and knowledge of the patient, to determine dosages and the best treatment for each individual patient. Any brands mentioned in this book are as examples only and are not endorsed by the publisher. Neither the publisher nor the authors assume any liability for any injury and/or damage to persons or property arising from this publication.

Disclaimer

M&K Publishing cannot accept responsibility for the contents of any linked website or online resource. The existence of a link does not imply any endorsement or recommendation of the organisation or the information or views which may be expressed in any linked website or online resource. We cannot guarantee that these links will operate consistently and we have no control over the availability of linked pages.

To contact M&K Publishing write to:
M&K Update Ltd · The Old Bakery · St. John's Street
Keswick · Cumbria CA12 5AS
Tel: 01768 773030 · Fax: 01768 781099
publishing@mkupdate.co.uk
www.mkupdate.co.uk

Designed and typeset by Mary Blood
Printed in Scotland by Bell & Bain, Glasgow.

Contents

Contents

Cardiovascular   159

Disability   **269**

Contents

About the contributors

Dr Gaurav Agarwal *MBBS, MRCP (UK); Consultant Physician in Acute and General Medicine at Tunbridge Wells Hospital, Maidstone and Tunbridge Wells NHS Trust*

Diane Blake *RGN, Dip HE, RM, BSc(Hons), MSc, PGCELT; Supervisor of Midwives, Senior Midwifery Lecturer, Canterbury Christ Church University, Kent*

Dr Kuno Budack *FRCP; Associate Specialist in Cardiology, Tunbridge Wells Hospital, Maidstone and Tunbridge Wells NHS Trust*

Dr Russell E. M. Canavan *Consultant Gastroenterologist and Associate Medical Director, Bronglais Hospital, Aberystwyth, Wales*

Dr Alistair Challiner *MBA, PgDip (Systems Prac), EDIC, FFICM, FRCA, FIMCRCSEd; Consultant in Intensive Care Medicine and Anaesthesia. Maidstone and Tunbridge Wells NHS Trust.*

Dr Tim Collins *EdD, MSc, PGCLT(HE), BSc(Hons) ENB100, RN; Consultant Nurse, Acute Care, East Kent Hospitals University NHS Foundation Trust*

Julie Cook *Acute Pain Nurse Specialist, Kent and Sussex Hospital, Maidstone and Tunbridge Wells NHS Trust, Kent, UK*

Jo Cotton *RGN, RM, MTD, MA (Education); formerly Senior Lecturer, Canterbury Christ Church University, Kent*

Jane Donn *RGN, DipN, ENB N53, BSc(Hons), Nurse Independent Prescriber (NIP), MSc; Clinical Nurse Specialist Acute Pain, Maidstone and Tunbridge Wells NHS Trust*

Sarah Elliot *MA, PGCert, PGCert, BSc(Hons), MCSP; Physiotherapy Practitioner in Critical Care, Medway Maritime Hospital, Medway NHS Foundation Trust*

Dr Jorge da Fonseca *BA, MBChB, DA(UK), FRCA, FFICM, PgCert (Medical Education), MSc (Patient Safety); Consultant Intensivist and Anaesthetist, Maidstone and Tunbridge Wells NHS Trust*

Jayne Fraser *Senior Outreach Sister, Maidstone and Tunbridge Wells NHS Trust*

Deborah Higgs *Consultant Nurse in Critical Care, East Kent Hospitals University NHS Foundation Trust*

Debbie King *RGN, DipN, BSc, MA, PGCLT; Senior Lecturer, Canterbury Christ Church University, Kent*

Karen E. Lumsden *PGCert (Critical Care), BSc (Hons), PGCLT, RN; Senior Lecturer, Canterbury Christ Church University, Kent*

Dr Julie Macinnes *PhD, MSc, BSc (Hons), PGCE, Dip (HE), RN, RNT; Senior Lecturer Cardiac Care, Canterbury Christ Church University, Kent*

Dr Simon Merritt *Consultant Sleep and Respiratory Medicine, Conquest Hospital, Hastings*

Victor Nebbiolo *Resuscitation Consultant, Victor Nebbiolo Ltd, East Sussex*

About the contributors

Catherine Plowright RN, BSc Nursing, MSc Nursing, MA in Applied Professional Research, Diploma in Management Studies, ENB 100; Consultant Nurse Critical Care, Medway NHS Foundation Trust, Medway Maritime Hospital, Gillingham, Kent

Ann M. Price RGN, BSc(Hons), ENB 100, PGCE, MSc, MA; Senior Lecturer, Canterbury Christ Church University, Kent

Wendy-Ling Relph RGN, MSc in Care Policy and Management, ENB 100; Matron for Nutrition and Quality Improvement, East Kent Hospitals University NHS Foundation Trust

Ian Setchfield MSc, BSc (Open), RN, Critical Care Matron, East Kent Hospitals University NHS Foundation Trust

Dr Sally A. Smith DN, MSc, DipHE, ENB 100, ENB 998, ENB 934; Chief Nurse & Director of Quality, East Kent Hospitals University NHS Foundation Trust.

Amanda Sudan RGN, BSc(Hons), MBPsS; Staff Nurse, Immunisation Service, Kent Community NHS Foundation Trust

Dr Angus Turner Consultant in Anaesthesia and Intensive Care, Maidstone and Tunbridge Wells NHS Trust, Kent

Dr Michelle C. Webb MB, BChir, MD, FRCP; Consultant Nephrologist, East Kent Hospitals University NHS Foundation Trust

Philip Woodrow MA, RGN, DipN, Grad Cert Ed, ENB 100; Practice Development Nurse, Critical Care, East Kent Hospitals University NHS Trust

Preface to the second edition

Ann M. Price, Sally A. Smith and Alistair Challiner

Like the original *Ward-based Critical Care,* this second edition aims to guide practitioners in the initial management of critically ill adult patients within the ward setting. It should be of value to a wide range of healthcare professionals, including junior doctors, nurses, physiotherapists and students. It will also be relevant to practitioners who are moving into any setting that cares for acutely ill patients.

This volume has been slightly reorganised since the first edition to ensure that practical aspects are incorporated within the relevant sections. The book is still structured around the ABCDE approach to assessing and managing patients, as this is promoted in critical care and resuscitation care training. The focus on practical examples and 'hot tips' to aid memory of key points continues.

All the chapters have been updated with the most recent guidance, as available at the time of writing. This has meant that some chapters have required major revisions, while others have remained relatively unchanged. Some new chapters have been included, such those on anaphylactic shock, patient safety, dealing with pregnant women in the ward setting, and massive blood transfusion. In addition, each section now starts with a chapter giving an overview of the A–E approach in order to provide more detail about assessing and managing those aspects of patient care.

As the editors, we hope you will find this book informative and useful in the practical setting. We hope it will inform your practice and improve initial management of acutely ill patients.

Acknowledgements

The Editors wish to thank all the contributors who updated chapters and the new authors who helped fill gaps from the previous edition.

Thanks to the Canterbury Christ Church University Clinical Skills Laboratory staff who helped prepare equipment to update some of the photographs.

Thanks to the various organisations and people who have given permission to reproduce aspects of their work to ensure that this edition is current and draws on best practice guidance.

We would also like to thank Mike Roberts at M&K publishing for his patience when preparing the manuscript and to Kelly Davis and Mary Blood for their work on producing the final book.

Finally, thanks to our families and friends who have encouraged and supported us whilst updating the text for this second edition.

Ann M. Price, Sally A. Smith and Alistair Challiner

Introduction

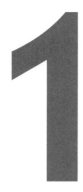

Critical care outreach

Deborah Higgs

I n recent years, the term 'critical care outreach' has become synonymous with the management and care of acutely ill patients on general wards within acute Trusts across the UK. Outreach teams have become a popular choice for organisations managing an increasingly complex group of patients with a higher acuity of illness. This chapter explores the role of outreach teams in the context of today's healthcare.

Background

Access to critical care facilities is crucial for effective management of sick patients. However, capacity issues are affecting the provision of these services. Factors such as the increasing complexity of medical and surgical interventions, an ageing inpatient population, and a continuing reduction in the number of hospital beds, have led to an increased acuity of hospital inpatients. The situation has been further compounded by the continuing debate over the management of acutely ill patients outside designated critical care areas.

There is growing evidence that patients who become – or who are at risk of becoming – acutely unwell on general wards may receive suboptimal care (McQuillan *et al.* 1998). Significantly, early recognition and management of the premonitory symptoms of serious deterioration, including cardiac arrest, might improve outcomes for these patients (Franklin & Mathew 1994; McQuillan *et al.* 1998; Buist *et al.* 1999; Goldhill *et al.* 1999; McGloin *et al.* 1999). There has been an international acknowledgement of the need to improve identification and management of the clinically unstable patient. The UK National Health Service (NHS) has developed clinical services to recognise and manage the onset of deteriorating health in the form of critical care outreach teams (CCOTs), based on the Medical Emergency Team (MET) initiative (Lee *et al.* 1995). Latterly, in the United States, Rapid Response Teams (RRTs) have been advocated as a means to ensure that the healthcare system responds to the sick patient more quickly and effectively (Berwick *et al.* 2006).

The early MET work influenced the recommendations made in *Comprehensive Critical Care* (DOH 2000). This report reviewed adult critical care services and recognised the need to modernise them. It promoted a hospital-wide approach, with services that extended beyond the physical boundaries of the Intensive Care Unit (ICU). Critical care was to be driven by patient need, not by location or specialty. The deployment of outreach services was one of the key recommendations.

Critical care outreach teams

Critical care and acute Trusts enthusiastically embraced the concept of outreach, with many NHS acute hospitals in England that routinely provided level 1 care appointing a formal outreach team. Level 1 care is the level of care a patient requires that can be delivered on the ward, although they may need extra help from critical care teams. The main aims of the critical care outreach service were:

- To prevent admission to critical care or ensure admission was appropriate
- To enable patients to be discharged from critical care
- To share skills with ward and community staff.

Since 2000, outreach services have continued to evolve, primarily to meet local Trust requirements. Whilst the rapid devolvement of teams across the NHS led to wide variation in service models (from a single nurse-led service to a multidisciplinary team with allied health professionals and medical input), improving care for acutely ill patients remained the common aim and a key priority. Working collaboratively, the National Outreach Forum and the Critical Care Stakeholders' Forum produced a document that described the role of outreach in supporting patient care and provided indicators of effectiveness for outreach services (Critical Care Stakeholders' Forum 2007).
This document noted that the objectives of any service should be:

- To improve the quality of acute patient care and patient experience and reduce adverse clinical events
- To enhance clinical staff confidence, competence and experience through training and the sharing of skills
- To improve organisational agility and resilience by delivering comprehensive care across organisational and professional boundaries, directorates or locations.

The pathway of care can conveniently be divided into three phases:

- The recognition and management of the acutely unwell patient on the general wards
- Clinical involvement on the general wards in the care of patients after a period of critical illness
- Outpatient support to the patient following discharge from hospital.

As service provision varies, teams may in fact deliver some or all of the above. In 2012, the National Outreach Forum responded to calls for a standardised approach to outreach services by setting out an operational framework of standards and competencies for outreach and acute care teams (NOrF 2012). This framework attempts to address the absence of national guidelines and provide a standardised operational framework that organisations can use as a benchmark.

However, what remains pivotal to the success of such interventions is the ability of staff to recognise critical illness. Clinical deterioration can happen at any point in a patient's illness or care pathway, but patients are particularly vulnerable following an emergency admission to hospital, after surgery and during recovery from a critical illness. It is important for nursing and medical staff to be competent in recognising and responding to signs of critical illness.

Unfortunately, for a variety of reasons (many of which are poorly understood), ward-based teams often do not recognise patients who deteriorate. Articulating the reasons for substandard care is difficult as many factors may contribute – organisational problems, inadequate supervision, failure to seek advice from senior staff and poor communication, among others. The National Confidential Enquiry into Patient Outcomes and Death (NCEPOD 2005) found that delayed recognition of the acutely unwell, poor communication between teams and the institution of inappropriate therapy led to poor outcomes. The National Patient Safety Agency's 2007 report, *Safer Care for the Acutely Ill Patient: Learning from Serious Incidents* (NPSA 2007), identified deterioration as a key theme. Over a period of a year, it was found that 11% of reports related to the subject of deterioration that was not recognised or acted upon. This was attributed to three key factors:

1. No observations were made for a prolonged period so changes in the patient's condition and vital signs were not detected.
2. There was no recognition of the importance of the deterioration and/or no action was taken, other than recording of observations.
3. There was a delay in the patient receiving medical attention, even when their deterioration had been detected and recognised.

The aim is to develop strategies to equip healthcare providers with the right skills and knowledge to begin treating acutely ill patients at the earliest stage of their deterioration. Outreach plays an important role in supporting ward staff to identify sick patients. A key aspect of the work is about sharing critical care skills by being clinically available at the bedside. Nursing staff often claim that they know intuitively when the patient 'is not right'; although intuition is a useful aid, it is important to use a systematic physiology-based approach when assessing critically ill patients (Subbe 2006). Outreach services are aware that effective assessment of patients at risk is a prerequisite for early recognition of critical illness, and they use a variety of strategies to educate ward teams.

Early recognition of critical illness improves outcomes

Physiological track and trigger systems

Physiological track and trigger systems are designed to help ward staff quickly identify patients at risk of developing critical illness. Scores are allocated to each abnormal vital sign parameter, resulting in a total score, which may (or may not) indicate a need to call for assistance. The majority of acute Trusts in the UK adopted such a system in an effort to reduce serious adverse events relating to the deteriorating patient.

Vital sign measurement is an important aspect of inpatient care, and efficient and thorough recording of vital signs can reveal trends in the patient's progress. However, this approach was not standardised, and this lack of consistency across the NHS posed a risk. For instance, there was wide variation in the physiological variables used in different settings, as well as variation in the triggers set to 'call' for help. These inconsistencies reduced staff members' confidence in the ability of response teams to identify all patients at risk (Smith *et al.* 2008).

In response, the Royal College of Physicians commissioned a working party to develop a national scoring system. The National Early Warning Score (NEWS) is designed to enable clinical staff to recognise and respond to acute illness/deterioration and to trigger varying levels of clinical response, proportionate to illness severity (RCP 2012). Based on the 2007 National Institute for Health and Clinical Excellence guidance, it was agreed that the frequency of monitoring should be dictated by a patient's clinical condition, with a minimum of 12-hourly monitoring for the most stable patients (NICE 2007).

The NICE guideline makes evidence-based recommendations on recognising and managing acute illness in hospital, provides key priorities for implementation by acute Trusts, and emphasises the importance of physiological observations. A key recommendation was that track and trigger systems should be used to monitor all adult patients in acute hospital settings (NICE 2007). The adoption of a national scoring system has provided a standardised approach to the recording of abnormal vital signs and the response to those signs. The NEWS system recommends a locally agreed response to score around three graded triggers (low, medium and high). Each NEWS trigger level should define:

- The speed/urgency of response – including an escalation process to ensure that a response always occurs
- Who responds – the seniority and clinical competencies of the responder/s
- The appropriate clinical setting for ongoing acute care
- The frequency of subsequent monitoring of the patient.

The national score has been widely adopted across the UK and is proving to be an effective tool in identifying and managing clinically unstable patients. Many healthcare organisations are also benefiting from innovative systems based on hand-held devices that enable the user to capture observations at the bedside, triggering immediate action based on the agreed response.

Box 1.1 National Early Warning Score (NEWS)

This national tool was developed in 2012 and it is available via the Royal College of Physicians website:

https://www.rcplondon.ac.uk/sites/default/files/documents/news-observation-chart-a3-size-_0.pdf

It is recommended that all acute settings should have an early warning system based on this guideline.

An effective and thorough assessment is always crucial. Staff in an acute setting should have the skills needed to identify patients at risk of deterioration, intervening in a timely and appropriate manner. Many clinicians use a systematic physiology-based approach when assessing patients. However, the evidence of suboptimal care found by McQuillan and colleagues (1998), mentioned earlier, led to the development of the Acute Life-Threatening Events Recognition and Treatment course, otherwise known as ALERT®.

The ALERT® course is based on other life-support training programmes (such as ALS, ATLS and BLS) and uses a structured and prioritised system of patient assessment and management. This approach assists healthcare professionals because it uses Airway, Breathing, Circulation, Disability and Exposure (ABCDE) as a fundamental assessment tool, therefore ensuring that they perform to a safe, consistent standard.

Many outreach services use this approach in conjunction with their local resuscitation team. Once the initial 'ABC' assessment is completed, a more thorough assessment should be undertaken, including a review of the patient's past medical history and drug history. Many outreach personnel, via extended roles, have the ability to take arterial blood gases, order x-rays and prescribe drugs. Such extensions in practice enable a timely response to any deterioration in a patient's clinical condition.

Sharing skills

Effective sharing of critical care skills is vital, and outreach teams play a key role in the planning and delivery of Trust-wide education in critical care (DH & NHS Modernisation Agency 2003). Education and training courses on acute clinical interventions (such as non-invasive ventilation, care of the tracheotomy and chest auscultation) have been delivered both in local hospitals and nationally. The goal is that ward-based teams will eventually need less support from outside organisations.

The success of any system that promotes the early recognition of critical illness (in terms of improved patient outcomes) depends on the effectiveness of the response strategy (Subbe 2006). The support of critically ill ward patients via outreach services is achieved through the knowledge, expertise and experience of the staff who make up the team. Outreach nurses appear to develop clear and focused action plans, and contribute to clinical decision-making by co-coordinating medical and nursing care and facilitating communication (Coad & Haines 2002, Chellel *et al.* 2006).

More recently, there have been some innovative developments, such as 'Call 4 concern' (Odell *et al.* 2010), an outreach service that is activated by patients and relatives. This service was piloted and introduced by an outreach team to demonstrate a patient-focused approach to improving care for this group of vulnerable patients. The follow-up of patients who have had a critical care stay also ensures that they receive continued care. Work continues to develop around the rehabilitation of patients who have experienced profound critical illness.

Conclusion

It appears that critical care outreach services remain a key resource for ward-based staff. However, concerns regarding the endorsement of a service introduced on the basis of set objectives, rather than clear evidence, have meant that outreach continues to attract attention in the literature. The variation in service models makes it difficult for researchers to evaluate the impact of outreach teams in practice (McDonnell *et al.* 2007).

These complexities were illustrated by the 2005 Medical Early Response Intervention and Therapy (MERIT) study – the only multicentre cluster randomised controlled trial of a similar service with wide variability in models of provision. Numbers of cardiac arrests, unexpected deaths and unplanned admissions to intensive care were not significantly reduced (MERIT Study Investigators 2005). A few years later, a cohort study evaluated the effect of visits from the critical care outreach teams before admission to and following discharge from critical care. The results suggested that the follow-up visits were beneficial but evidence for pre-critical care visits was inconclusive (Harrison *et al.* 2010).

However, outreach provision remains at the forefront of patient safety improvement initiatives around the UK, particularly regarding such conditions as sepsis and acute kidney injury and the reduction of adverse clinical incidents. Outreach teams use their skill and knowledge to improve the care of acutely ill patients, supporting junior doctors and inexperienced nursing staff in complex clinical situations. Outreach teams can also provide valuable support for ward staff, facilitating the early recognition of deteriorating patients and triggering early intervention (Coad & Haines 2002, Chellel *et al.* 2006).

Any change in service provision requires organisations to evaluate and review the impact of the intervention. Critical care provision is continually evolving, responding to the ever-changing environment of the NHS. It is important for the service to use audit and research to shape the future of critical care outreach.

References and further reading

Berwick, D.M., Calkins, D.R., McCannon, C.J. & Hackbarth, A.D. (2006). The 100,000 lives campaign: Setting a goal and a deadline for improving health care quality. *JAMA: The Journal of the American Medical Association.* **295** (3), 324–27.

Buist, M.D., Jarmolowski, E., Burton, P.R., Bernard, S.A., Waxman, B.P. & Anderson, J. (1999). Recognising clinical instability in hospital patients before cardiac arrest or unplanned admission to intensive care. A pilot study in a tertiary-care hospital. *Medical Journal of Australia.* **171**, 22–25.

Chellel, A., Higgs, D. & Scholes, J. (2006). An evaluation of the contribution of critical care outreach to the clinical management of the critically ill ward patient in two acute NHS Trusts. *Nursing in Critical Care.* **11** (1), 42–51.

Coad, S. & Haines, S. (2002). Supporting staff caring for critically ill patients in acute areas. *Nursing in Critical Care.* **4**, 245–48.

Critical Care Stakeholders' Forum, National Outreach Forum (2007). *Clinical Indicators for Critical Care Outreach Services; Clinical document.* London. Department of Health.

Department of Health (2000). *Comprehensive Critical Care – A Review of Adult Critical Care Services.* London: DH.

Department of Health & NHS Modernisation Agency (2003). *Critical Care Outreach: Progress in Developing Services.* London: DH and NHS Modernisation Agency.

Franklin, C. & Mathew, J. (1994). Developing strategies to prevent in hospital cardiac arrest: analyzing responses of physicians and nurses in the hours before the event. *Critical Care Medicine.* **22**, 244–47.

Goldhill, D.R., White, S.A. & Sumner, A. (1999). Physiological values and procedures in the 24 hours before intensive care unit admission from the ward. *Anaesthesia.* **54**, 529–34

Harrison, D.A., Gao, H., Welch, C. & Rowan K.M. (2010). The effects of Critical Care Outreach Services before and after critical care. A matched-cohort analysis. *Journal of Critical Care.* **25**, 196–204.

Lee, A., Bishop, G., Hilman, K. & Daffurn, K. (1995). The medical emergency team. *Anesthetic Intensive Care.* **23**, 183.

McDonnell, A., Esmonde, L., Morgan, R., Brown, R., Bray, K., Parry, G., Adam, S., Sinclair, R., Harvey, S., Mays, N. & Rowan, K. (2007). The provision of critical care outreach services in England: findings from a national survey. *Journal of Critical Care.* **22**, 212–18.

McGloin, H., Adam, S. & Singer, M. (1999). Unexpected deaths and referrals to intensive care of patients on general wards. Are some cases potentially avoidable? *Journal of the Royal College of Physicians of London.* **33**, 255–59.

MERIT Study Investigators (2005). Introduction of the medical emergency team (MET) system: a cluster-randomised controlled trial. *Lancet.* **365**, 2091–97.

McQuillan, P., Pilkington, S., Allan, A., Taylor, B., Short, A., Morgan, G., Nielsen, M., Barrett, D. & Smith, G. (1998). Confidential inquiry into quality of care before admission to intensive care. *British Medical Journal.* **316**, 1853–58.

National Confidential Enquiry into Patient Outcome and Death (2005). *An Acute Problem?* London: NCEPOD.

National Institute for Health and Care Excellence (NICE) (2007). *Clinical Guideline 50: Acutely ill patients in hospital: Recognition of and response to acute illness in adults in hospital.* London: NICE.

National Outreach Forum (2012). *National Outreach Forum Operational Standards and Competencies for Critical Care Outreach Services.* NOrF.

National Patient Safety Agency (2007). *Safer care for the acutely ill patient: learning from serious incidents.* London: NPSA.

Odell, M., Gerber, K. & Gage, M. (December 2010). Call 4 Concern: patient and relative activated critical care outreach. *British Journal of Nursing.* **19**(22), 1390-5

Royal College of Physicians (2012). *National Early Warning Score (NEWS): Standardising the assessment of acute-illness severity in the NHS.* Report of a working party. London: RCP.

Smith, G.B., Prytherch, D.R., Schmidt, P.E., Featherstone, P.I. & Higgins, B. (2008). A review, and performance evaluation, of single-parameter 'track and trigger' systems. *Resuscitation.* **79**, 11–21.

Subbe, C. (2006). Recognition and assessment of critical illness. *Anaesthesia and Intensive Care Medicine.* **8** (1), 21–23.

Useful websites

National Institute for Health and Care Excellence (NICE)
http://www.nice.org.uk/ (Accessed 3 June 2015)

National Outreach Forum
http://www.norf.org.uk/ (Accessed 3 June 2015)

National Patient Safety Agency
http://www.npsa.nhs.uk/ (Accessed 3 June 2015)

Patient Safety First Campaign
http://www.patientsafetyfirst.nhs.uk/ (Accessed 3 June 2015)

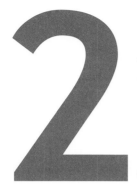

Assessing and monitoring the acutely ill ward patient

Alistair Challiner and Sally A. Smith

It is well recognised that the acuity of ward patients has increased (Audit Commission 1999, Department of Health 2000, National Institute for Health and Care Excellence (NICE) 2007). The patient population is ageing, with greater dependency and higher coexisting morbidity (NICE 2007). Technology is becoming more complex with regard to the management and monitoring of acutely ill ward patients.

Patients with tracheostomies, non-invasive ventilation and continuous positive airway pressure (CPAP) are now commonly cared for in the ward setting, rather than the intensive care unit (ICU). Due to the pressure on beds in high-dependency and intensive care units, acutely ill patients residing in ward beds inevitably require close assessment, observation and monitoring. This increased complexity has placed more pressure on ward staff, who need adequate critical care knowledge and expertise to ensure safe practice.

This chapter outlines how to assess a sick patient effectively and quickly, and then describes in more detail how to assess a patient at each point. At the end of this chapter you will be able to outline a systematic way of assessing an acutely ill patient and describe the required monitoring and observation.

Background

Detailed assessment of an acutely ill patient is essential, and attention to detail is imperative. A systematic and simple assessment protocol will ensure that a thorough assessment is undertaken. Always using the same systematic approach ensures that the whole team works towards the same therapeutic goals (Smith 2003). Many tools have been designed to aid appropriate examination and assessment of patients, and many of them use the ABC system. This prioritises the airway, then breathing, then circulation and then the neurological aspects. The same assessment system may be applied to trauma, impending cardiac arrest or paediatrics.

How to examine an acutely unwell patient

The first assessment performed by experienced clinicians is to look at the patient and gauge how sick they are. This is achieved by experience, but the three key observations to make are (Resuscitation Council 2011):

- Ask a simple question ('How are you?') to assess the level of consciousness
- Observe breathing pattern and rate for any distress
- Undertake vital signs monitoring early – BP, pulse, ECG, saturation.

Case scenario

A 58-year-old woman is admitted to a surgical ward with pancreatitis. Previously fit and well, she says she smokes 40 cigarettes per day and has a minimal alcohol intake, but reports having felt lethargic and in pain for the previous five days. She is admitted to a surgical ward. An intravenous infusion is commenced at 125ml per hour, and she is made nil by mouth. Antibiotics are commenced. Overnight her blood pressure remains low for several hours with a systolic of 70–90mmHg, and a urine output of 15–20ml per hour. Other observations are stable, although at 8 a.m. her respiratory rate is 20 breaths per minute, her SpO_2 is 92%, her heart rate is 120 beats per minute and her blood pressure is 90/40mmHg. The nursing staff called the surgical team to review. Her track and trigger score was 6, requiring an urgent review.

If you were the nurse caring for this patient, or the junior doctor asked to review, what assessment, observations and monitoring would you undertake or request?

A patient who is deteriorating, such as the woman in the above scenario, will require an immediate 'triage-type' assessment, to identify the immediate resuscitation or interventions required. A more detailed examination will follow once the patient is stabilised. This will largely be a physical assessment, commencing with the Airway, then Breathing, Circulation and Disability (neurological assessment), then Exposure examination – namely, the ABCDE approach.

The principle of this method is to deal with each aspect before moving on to the next. For example, if a patient's airway is compromised, this needs to be managed before breathing can be assessed.

Level of consciousness

The level of consciousness must be assessed quickly:

- Is the patient awake?
- Do they look at you and follow you with their eyes?
- If they look as if they are asleep, do they respond to speech, or are they unresponsive even to touch?

Answers to these questions give a rapid indication of how ill a patient is. Any decrease in consciousness indicates a very sick patient.
Think of the causes as:

1. Hypoxaemia
2. Hypercapnia from ventilatory failure
3. Shock or circulatory failure
4. Neurological impairment from metabolic or non-traumatic cerebral injury
5. Drug or alcohol intoxication

This pattern follows the ABCDE system.

Always consider the first four problems very seriously before diagnosing a patient as 'just drunk'.

Colour

The colour of the patient gives a rapid indication of sickness and underlying problems. For example:

- A blue patient is hypoxaemic until proved otherwise.
- A pale patient may have acute blood loss or shock.
- Skin mottling may indicate sepsis.
- The patient may be sweaty or dry-skinned.

Respiratory rate

The rate and pattern (particularly the depth of the breaths) are important.

- A *very rapid* respiratory rate, particularly if it is over 30 breaths per minute (with 2 seconds between breaths) may be due to severe compromise of the respiratory system or circulatory system.
- A *very slow* rate, of less than 10 breaths per minute, implies respiratory depression from exhaustion, carbon dioxide narcosis, or respiratory depressant drugs.
- Deep, rapid breaths are typical of the effects of metabolic acidosis or lung diseases such as acute pneumonia.

Does the patient look as if they have just run a marathon despite lying in a bed? If so, then there are severe respiratory or circulatory problems. The patient will not keep breathing like this forever because they will get tired and develop respiratory failure. Also, look at whether the respiratory pattern implies obstruction of the airway. What position have they placed themselves in? Partial upper airway obstruction usually causes a patient to sit up, drool and look very frightened. This rapid assessment takes just a few seconds with experience, but it tells the observer a great deal and reflects the real-life clinical situation.

Following the initial quick look, the healthcare practitioner should run through the ABCDE system to exclude acute life-threatening risks.

The ABCDE system is very good for teaching and using as a prioritised assessment and treatment algorithm, but *don't* wait until Step D to decide whether the patient is unconscious or not! Assess for this quickly, then get appropriate help and undertake appropriate treatment.

Assessing an acutely ill patient using the ABCDE system

The **ABCDE** system (**A**irway, **B**reathing, **C**irculation, **D**isability, **E**xposure/**E**nvironment/**E**verything **E**lse) will identify:

1. Whether the airway is clear, obstructed or potentially obstructed
2. Whether air is going in and out of each lung (exclude clinical pneumothorax and examine clinically the unventilated lung and the nature of breath sounds, particularly wheeze and crackles)
3. Respiratory rate and pulse oximetry
4. Heart rate, pulse volume (central and peripheral), skin temperature and blood pressure (gives the observer an overall idea of circulatory impairment or shock, and checks for any obvious blood loss)
5. Level of consciousness, Glasgow Coma Scale (see Chapter 34) or AVPU (see Box 2.1), pupils and posture
6. Any relevant factors in the environment and everything else, depending on the clinical situation (e.g. trauma or medical); as part of Step E also look at step 7 (below)
7. What has been done (e.g. oxygen mask and percentage of oxygen, intravenous lines and fluids, urinary catheterisation) and what is coming out (e.g. surgical drains and central venous catheters, if present).

Box 2.1 AVPU assessment

A – Patient is **Alert**

V – Patient responds to **Verbal** stimulation or command

P – Patient responds to **Painful** stimuli

U – Patient is **Unresponsive**

Each section of the system will now be discussed in more detail.

A-Airway

The goal is to ensure a patent airway. A simple question to the patient may be enough to assess it. If the patient is able to speak clearly, then they have a patent airway.

Look (inspect)

Look for chest and abdominal movements. A patient with an obstructed airway who is making respiratory effort will have paradoxical chest and abdominal movements. Tracheal tug may be noted, along with use of their accessory muscles. Tracheal tug is a rhythmic downward pull (Jarvis 2000). The patient may also be cyanosed or dusky in colour (remember that skin tone may mask these signs). The patient will clearly be distressed unless the obstruction has led to unconsciousness with possible respiratory arrest.

Feel (palpate)

If there is doubt at this stage regarding the airway, feel for airflow at the mouth and nose. An effective way is to moisten your cheek and feel for airflow against your cheek.

Listen (auscultate)

In partial airway obstruction, the entry of air is reduced, although breathing is noisy. Box 2.2 describes commonplace sounds.

Box 2.2 Sounds of partial airway obstruction

Expiratory wheeze – obstruction of lower airways, which tend to collapse and obstruct during expiration

Gurgling – suggests presence of liquid or semi-solid material in upper airways

Snoring – pharynx partially occluded by tongue or palate

Crowing – laryngeal obstruction or spasm

Stridor – obstruction above or at the level of the larynx.

If you have any doubt regarding the patency of a patient's airway, summon urgent help and commence basic life support manoeuvres. Please see Chapter 6 on airway management. The patient in this scenario had a patent airway and was able to answer questions from the surgical team.

B-Breathing

The assessment of breathing is an essential aspect of the monitoring and observation of the acutely ill ward patient. According to the National Confidential Enquiry into Patient Outcome and Death, changes in respiratory function are sensitive indicators of deterioration (NCEPOD 2005, NICE 2007). A change of 5 respirations per minute in a resting patient is very significant, but we know that respiratory rates are frequently not recorded on vital sign charts (National Patient Safety Agency 2007, NICE 2007). Using the 'look, listen, feel, measure' approach, breathing can be accurately assessed, with the goal of ensuring adequate oxygenation of vital organs.

Look (inspect)

When assessing an acutely ill, deteriorating patient, the way they look will give many clues as to their wellbeing. Observation and assessment of the following are necessary:

- What is the patient's colour like? If there is evidence of central cyanosis (bluish tinge on the lips and tongue), they are very seriously ill because this is a late sign of poor oxygenation.
- Does the patient look distressed? Are they sweating? Are they using accessory muscles to breathe? Routinely assess their respiratory rate (count for a full minute), the depth of each breath and whether the chest is moving equally on both sides. Any abnormalities need to be addressed immediately.

Feel (palpate)

Place your hands on the patient's chest wall to enable you to assess the bilateral chest movement, feel surgical emphysema, and possibly crepitus (crackling due to presence of secretions). Assessing the position of the trachea is vital because any deviation may indicate a pneumothorax or fluid in the chest (i.e. mediastinal shift requiring immediate treatment). If you are concerned about your findings, get senior help from a medical registrar or anaesthetist. See Chapter 3 on making a physical examination of the chest.

Feel (percuss)

Examination of the chest also involves percussing the lung fields. If trained to undertake this assessment, it will enable you to validate your palpation examination.

Listen (auscultate)

You will have already noted airway sounds when assessing the airway. Before using the stethoscope, listen to the patient's breathing and note what you can hear. You may hear rattling of secretions or wheeze. The stethoscope will allow you to evaluate the quality of breathing, and whether there is bilateral air entry throughout, or any fluid, secretions and wheeze. Note any abnormality and treat it.

Measure (monitoring and intervention)

You may at this stage consider it necessary to undertake an arterial blood gas, while monitoring is being established. Observation and monitoring of respiratory function can be via continuous pulse oximetry and increasing the vital sign observations to hourly, or more frequently if required. In our case scenario, oxygen was administered in order to maintain the patient's SpO_2 above 95%. She required 60% oxygen to meet this goal. A respiratory rate of 20 breaths per minute was high for her at rest, and her arterial blood gas showed a metabolic acidosis with a pH of 7.1 (see Chapter 10). She was clearly attempting to compensate by increasing her respiratory rate. Her chest sounded quiet, with crackles at the bases. She required close observation to monitor for any further deterioration in her condition. Continuous monitoring of her oxygen saturations was commenced.

All critically ill patients should receive oxygen in order to prevent further organ damage or sudden deterioration. The use of high-flow oxygen (15 litres/minute) via a reservoir oxygen mask will provide a high percentage of supplementary oxygen to a patient with low saturations and respiratory problems. If the rate or depth of breathing is deemed to be inadequate, artificial ventilation via a bag–valve mask should be commenced and urgent assistance sought.

C-Circulation

Assessment of this patient's airway shows that it is patent. Her breathing requires supplementary oxygen, and hourly respiratory rate and continuous monitoring of her oxygen saturations is in progress. Relevant tests have been undertaken and noted (these will vary with the suspected cause of the acute illness). Assessment of circulation is usually determined by taking the pulse and blood pressure. Temperature monitoring is also useful for obtaining supplementary information. Assessment of circulation can now take place; the goal is to ensure the patient is well perfused.

Look (inspect)

A patient who is compromised cardiovascularly will look pale and sometimes sweaty; observe for this. These patients may also appear drowsy. Look also for any evidence of external bleeding, but consider whether internal bleeding or fluid loss could be present. Assess the capillary refill time (Box 2.3), which is a quick and easy way of assessing perfusion.

Box 2.3 Capillary refill

Ensure the patient's hand is above the heart level, and press firmly on the nail bed of one finger (ideally on the first digit) for 5 seconds. Alternatively, if the patient's hands are cold, press the skin over the sternum.

Release the pressure and observe the nail bed or skin. The pallor should return to a pink colour within 2 seconds normally.

If there is a slow response, it may indicate poor perfusion.

Observe the patient's heart rhythm. Either undertake a 12-lead ECG or place the patient on a cardiac monitor for continuous monitoring. A knowledgeable person will need to assess any ECG findings, but consider if the rhythm is regular, fast or slow (over 100 or below 60 beats per minute). If a heart rhythm changes, first check how the patient feels and ensure it is not due to artefact. If the patient feels worse, call for assistance. If the patient does not respond, follow cardiac arrest procedures. If competent to do so, assess for jugular venous distension. Many hypotensive patients are also hypovolaemic. If their instability is cardiac, this will also help you make a clinical judgement in the absence of advanced monitoring techniques in ward areas.

Look at the patient's fluid chart, if they have one (if not, commence one). This particular patient had received 6 litres of crystalloid and colloid overnight. The fluid had no impact on her blood pressure or her urine output. Her daughter described her as boggy and swollen looking. Assessing how dry the patient's mouth is will give some indication of hydration needs. This can be done by looking at the mouth and lips, or asking the patient.

Feel (palpate)

More and more observations are being taken by non-registered personnel in the ward areas. It is common practice for medical devices to be used to take pulse and blood pressure recordings. The negative aspect of this is that it has now become less routine practice to feel a pulse on a patient, which means that vital information can be missed. Palpating peripheral and central pulses will give you an idea of perfusion. The pulse needs to be assessed for strength, rate, regularity and equality at each point. Thready pulses suggest a poor cardiac output and bounding pulses suggest sepsis. See Chapters 21, 22 and 23 on sepsis, hypovolaemia and cardiogenic shock, respectively. It is also necessary to feel limb temperature, which will give a good indication of perfusion. A warm limb usually means the patient is well perfused, and a cold limb usually means they are not. Note at which point on the limb the coolness begins.

Listen (auscultate)

Listening to the patient's blood pressure is the most common way of checking perfusion. If the blood pressure machine is unable to record a blood pressure, palpate one manually using a stethoscope and a manual blood pressure manometer. Remember to follow the manufacturer's instructions about frequency of observations when using monitoring devices, as they can be inaccurate in certain situations.

Shocked, poorly perfused patients will have low blood pressures. However, some patients may maintain an adequate blood pressure due to compensatory mechanisms, but will have other signs of compensation such as high heart rate or poor urine output. Consider this in the light of your other cardiovascular assessment findings.

Auscultation of the heart may also reveal valvular abnormalities, although it has limited value in the immediate assessment of an acutely unwell patient. Observe for the Portsmouth Sign (Smith 2003), whereby the heart rate is higher than the systolic blood pressure. This is a late sign of a seriously ill patient and needs urgent action.

Measure (monitoring and intervention)

The patient in our scenario presented with a low blood pressure that had not responded to fluid resuscitation. She was oliguric and looked puffy. We already know that she had a metabolic acidosis. A patient like this requires very close monitoring and observation. Many hypotensive patients are hypovolaemic and the administration of a fluid challenge may well reduce heart rate and increase blood pressure, enabling them to pass urine and perfuse vital organs more effectively. A mean arterial blood pressure of 70mmHg and a urine output of at least 0.5ml/kg per hour (use a urometer to measure hourly urine) are acceptable goals; they can be easily measured and monitored in the ward area. If the patient does not improve, consider the use of vasopressors (drugs that improve blood pressure). For this, the advice of critical care personnel and senior members of the multidisciplinary team will be required, and transfer to a specialist area is usually necessary.

In acutely ill patients who have not responded to initial resuscitative treatment, and whose cardiovascular system remains a concern, monitoring the central venous pressure via a central venous catheter will be necessary (see Chapter 20 on monitoring central venous pressure). This can be continuously monitored via a transduced line and monitor, and is becoming more common in ward areas.

The observation and monitoring of this patient includes continuous monitoring of respiratory rate, oxygen saturations, heart rate and rhythm, blood pressure, central venous pressure, and hourly recording of vital signs, urine output and fluid input, with four-hourly fluid balance measurements. Bloods for urea and electrolytes and other tests need to be considered at this point.

D-Disability

Assessment of the patient's conscious level is undertaken once airway, breathing and circulation are stabilised. With the acutely ill patient this can be undertaken swiftly and crudely using the AVPU system (Alert, Verbal, Pain, Unconscious; see Box 2.1 above). Blood glucose should be measured and treated, if low, with 50% glucose intravenously (according to local hospital policy). In the meantime, position the patient with altered conscious level in the lateral recovery position to maintain their safety while the cause of the change is investigated, and more in-depth neurological examination is carried out. The patient in our scenario was alert and orientated, and able to cooperate with the care she was receiving. See Chapter 34 on how to undertake a Glasgow Coma Score properly.

E-Exposure, Environment and Examination

Once the initial assessment of vital signs and interventions to stabilise the patient have been carried out, a closer examination of the patient should be undertaken. This will ensure that no detail is missed and will involve careful and systematic exposure of the patient. This is where you can check drips and drains, observe abdominal distension, check patency of lines and tubes, observe fluid loss or bowel actions and note anything else of relevance.

At this point you should have a good idea of how sick the patient is. Are they getting worse or are they stable? And what are you going to do next? Now is a good time to look at the patient's chart to check the temperature, and any trends in blood pressure and heart rate, respiratory rate, GCS, if recorded, blood glucose and fluid balance.

In an acutely unwell patient, if the blood tests have not been recently done (i.e. during the previous 6 hours) and if the patient has deteriorated, then take a full set of blood tests. These include:

- Full blood count; haemoglobin, white cell count, platelets
- Clotting, prothrombin time, activated partial APTT
- Urea and electrolytes, sodium, potassium, urea, creatinine

- Blood sugar
- Liver function tests
- Arterial blood gas
- Blood cultures if infection is suspected or signs of sepsis
- Lactate level (especially if sepsis is possible)
- Amylase to exclude pancreatitis (in cases of abdominal pain)
- Troponin (if there is chest pain).

This is an appropriate time to look at the notes if the patient is new to you. Look at existing blood tests, ECGs and radiology. Look at the latest blood results, ideally noting the trends. Check the potassium. Is it dangerously high or low? Compare a low potassium with the magnesium, as this is usually concurrently low. The sodium value is commonly related to intravenous fluid infusions. The urea and creatinine may be increased due to renal impairment. Ideally, compare with an earlier result to identify chronic renal failure. The haemoglobin level not only identifies blood loss or anaemia but is also related to the fluid status. Excess intravenous fluids can cause an apparent anaemia, and dehydration can haemoconcentrate and make the haemoglobin look higher.

The white blood count (WBC) is usually raised due to infection or other cause of stress. A very low WBC or high WBC can be caused by sepsis. The platelet count may be decreased due to disseminated intravascular coagulation (DIC). If so, look at the clotting results. A prolonged prothrombin time (PT) or INR (international normalised ratio) and a prolonged activated partial thromboplastin time (APTT) give a good indication of this in a very sick patient. The INR may be deranged due to warfarin treatment or liver impairment and this can be confirmed by review of the liver function tests.

A blood gas is very valuable for assessing lung function regarding ventilation and oxygenation. The base excess and bicarbonate identify acid–base abnormalities. In acutely ill patients, the most common of these will be a metabolic acidosis. Take the blood samples at the same time that a cannula is sited, except for the blood gas and blood culture.

An ECG is essential in any patient with chest pain, any arrhythmia or hypotension. Previous ECGs are useful for comparison to identify acute changes. Look at the most recent chest x-rays and obtain one if the patient is acutely unwell because the chest is commonly involved as a primary cause or complication.

When reviewing the notes, look at the last entries to see what the last clinician was thinking about, diagnosing and treating. Then look at the original admission notes to get a full history. Also, look at the letters section of the notes. Previous admissions or specialist consultations should have a letter or electronic discharge notification (EDN) with important information on pre-existing diseases. It is also very important to review the nursing notes. Their documentation of events is usually very detailed and may tell you what happened during any gaps in the medical notes. At this point you should have:

- Identified how sick the patient is, with the intention of knowing what to do next or who to call
- Initiated life-saving treatment based on the ABC principles
- Have a good idea why the patient is in hospital, their past medical history and what has happened to them.

With acutely ill patients, the priority is to keep them alive and stable by correcting the physiology as much as possible. A precise diagnosis may not be possible; for example, a patient may be identified as being in septic shock.

Life-saving treatment includes oxygen, intravenous access and fluids and broad-spectrum antibiotics. The patient should have a central line inserted and a urinary catheter, and one-to-one nursing. The blood pressure may not respond to fluids; therefore urgent referral to intensive care is required for invasive, intensive monitoring, for vasopressor therapy and possibly for ventilation. Finding the source of sepsis may not be a priority compared to urgent treatment and referral; the C-reactive protein and CT scan can wait.

Continuing assessment

It is very difficult for ward staff to provide the level of care that is available in high dependency units (HDUs) and intensive care units (ICUs). However, patients who are unstable and acutely unwell must not be left unattended for long periods. From a nursing perspective, they will require continuous input. From a medical perspective, they must be reviewed (at the very least) twice during the day and again by the Night Team, or team that is working out of hours.

The use of a track and trigger scoring system may help staff detect trends and changes in the patient's condition. Handover to other teams at the end of the shift must be succinct and clear, with the management plan agreed and documented to maintain continuity (NICE 2007, NPSA 2007). Many Trusts now have a critical care outreach team, who need to be made aware of potentially critical patients, and can support ward staff with monitoring and management.

Imaging

In addition to portable chest X-rays, bedside ultrasound technology is now sufficiently advanced to allow rapid echocardiology to assess for contractility, cardiac output, valve function and evidence of pericardial effusions. Ultrasound can also be used to identify pleural effusions and allow safe drainage, as well as assessing the abdomen to identify kidney size, intestinal obstruction, any abnormalities in the liver and gall bladder, and identify free fluid in the abdomen. In addition, ultrasound can be used to assess vessels (for safer vascular access) and to assess for intravascular clots.

CT scanning has advanced in resolution, but – perhaps more importantly – in speed. What used to take over half an hour can now be achieved in 1–2 minutes, making the process safer for acutely ill patients.

Conclusion

The patient in this scenario was successfully managed by the ward teams, with support and input from the critical care outreach team. She required physiotherapy for her chest, and humidified oxygen. Her acidosis and renal failure improved as her blood pressure increased. She was treated for fluid overload with diuretics and began to pass urine. Her pancreatitis slowly resolved. She did not require inotropic support or high-dependency facilities.

The full monitoring of this patient, with the use of a central line, made it possible to manage her fluids, respiratory and cardiovascular systems effectively. Eventually she was discharged home.

Use the ABCDE approach for assessment, addressing each aspect before moving on:

- Get help quickly.
- Instigate non-invasive monitoring of heart rate, rhythm, pulse oximetry and non-invasive blood pressure on all acutely ill patients.
- Increase frequency of vital sign recording to hourly.
- Start a fluid chart and maintain it.
- Document your actions and findings.

References and further reading

Audit Commission (1999). *Critical to Success: The Place of Efficient and Effective Critical Care Services within the Acute Hospital.* London: The Audit Commission.

Department of Health (2000). *Comprehensive Critical Care: A Review of Adult Critical Care Services.* London: The Stationery Office.

Jarvis, C. (2000). *Physical Examination and Health Assessment.* 3rd edn. Philadelphia: WB Saunders.

National Confidential Enquiry into Patient Outcome and Death (2005). *An Acute Problem?* London: NCEPOD.

National Institute for Health and Care Excellence (2007). *Acutely Ill Patients in Hospital: Recognition of and Response to Acute Illness in Adults in Hospital.* https://www.nice.org.uk/guidance/cg50 (Accessed 3 June 2015).

National Patient Safety Agency (2007). *Safer Care for the Acutely Ill Patient: Learning from Serious Incidents. Fifth Report from the Patient Safety Observatory.* London: NPSA.

Resuscitation Council (2011). *A Systematic Approach to the Acutely Ill Patient (ABCDE approach).* https://www.resus.org.uk/resuscitation-guidelines/a-systematic-approach-to-the-acutely-ill-patient-abcde/#principles (Accessed 19 June 2015).

Smith, G. (2003). *Acute Life-Threatening Events Recognition and Treatment: A Multiprofessional Course in the Care of the Acutely Ill Patient.* Portsmouth: University of Portsmouth.

Useful websites

National Outreach Forum
http://www.norf.org.uk
(Accessed 3 June 2015)

Resuscitation Council
https://www.resus.org.uk
(Accessed 3 June 2015)

ALERT Course
http://www.alert-course.com
(Accessed 3 June 2015)

National Patient Safety Agency
http://www.npsa.nhs.uk
(Accessed 3 June 2015)

3 Examination of the sick ward patient

Alistair Challiner

This chapter assumes that the patient has already been admitted and fully clerked, with a full history, and that examination has already taken place. Assume this is an unwell patient who has deteriorated. The basic examination system described here will quickly help you ascertain why the patient is deteriorating and what you need to do to manage the situation straight away.

First, you need to assess for life-threatening problems by assessing and treating (using ABCDE), as already described in initial assessment (see Chapter 2), and review the patient's medical notes (Resuscitation Council 2005).

An effective assessment of breathing and circulation requires examination skills. Medically qualified staff are trained in clinical examination. Nursing staff do not always have this full training during their qualifying training but the skills can be learned and are particularly relevant initially in detecting abnormality. There are many texts on the technique of clinical examination (such as Bickley & Bates 2013), which should also be consulted, but the best way is through observation of an expert and practice. This chapter explains how to determine if something has changed from the normal or from how it was previously.

Starting the examination

Always follow the order:

1. Inspection
2. Palpation
3. Percussion
4. Auscultation.

For further details and diagrams of the techniques outlined below, it is recommended that you consult a physical assessment textbook or seek advice from a senior clinician.

Examine from the patient's right, and, ideally, have the patient sitting up at a 30° angle.

Clinical examination should be supported by bedside monitoring. This should include reviewing the observation chart to check:

- Temperature
- Pulse rate
- Respiratory rate
- Blood pressure
- Pulse oximetry
- Urine output
- Fluid input
- Blood sugar.

The results of any existing investigations should also be reviewed, including laboratory blood tests and imaging (such as chest x-rays and CT scans), to gain further information and possibly focus the physical examination.

Examining the respiratory system

The key signs to look for are described below.

1 Inspection

Initially, check the patient's colour, particularly looking for cyanosis, pallor or mottling. Also look for recent or old scars that imply previous surgery, such as cardiac surgery if the scar is down the middle of the sternum or lung surgery if it is running between the ribs.

Check the sputum pot or ask either the nurses or the patient what the patient's sputum is like. For instance, is it clear or thick and yellowy brown? And is there any blood in it?

Abnormal chest movement

Stand at the foot of the bed and observe the patient's chest movements. You may find that one side of the chest does not move as much as the other, as may occur with a pneumothorax.

Abnormal rate of breathing

This is covered in the initial assessment (see Chapter 2). You may observe increased effort when breathing, and use of accessory muscles in the neck due to the patient working hard to breathe. This can be caused by obstruction in the upper or lower airways or it may occur because the patient is getting tired due to prolonged difficulty in breathing, as in pneumonia, pulmonary oedema or respiratory compensation in acidosis.

Movement of the chest may be very shallow, as in the case of an underlying chest infection, an exhausted patient or muscular weakness.

2 Palpation

Decreased chest movement on one side or both can be checked for by placing the hands flat on each side of the chest, with the thumbs meeting in the middle.

Check the position of the trachea. It should be in the middle. If it is deviated to one side, it is abnormal.

- **Lung collapse** pulls the trachea towards the affected side. This occurs when there is an obstruction to one of the lung airways such as a mucous plug.
- **Tension pneumothorax** pushes the trachea towards the non-affected side.

3 Percussion

The technique of percussion is done using both hands. The left hand is placed flat over the chest, with the fingers apart. With the right hand tap, over one of your left fingers with the tip of your right middle finger. Do this as if tapping out morse code, extending your right wrist fully and then flexing it quickly. The aim of this technique is to detect if the space under the body wall is hollow or solid. It is similar to tapping on a wall to find a door that has been wallpapered over.

Percussing over the rib cage should produce a hollow sound if there is lung underneath. Compare both sides. It should sound dull over the heart if you tap over the lower sternum, and dull over the lower right chest where there is liver under the ribs. The upper part of the rib cage on each side should sound resonant (hollow). If there is *consolidation* of lung (as in a lobar pneumonia), it should sound dull. If there is an *effusion* then the dullness is pronounced and termed 'stony' dull. A *pneumothorax* should sound more resonant than the opposite side of the chest.

This technique should be demonstrated by a doctor and practised. It will help to determine effusion and consolidation if dullness is where it shouldn't be, and a pneumothorax if it is more resonant.

4 Auscultation (listening with a stethoscope)

Listen over all areas of the chest at the front and the back, using the diaphragm of the stethoscope. Normally you will hear quiet sounds of air moving in and out.

Listen over each zone, comparing the right with the left. If breath sounds are absent, the underlying lung is not being ventilated (as in collapse, consolidation or a large effusion). A pneumothorax may be quiet or it may sound like quiet or distant breath sounds.

Revise the lung lobes and zones, and identify where the stethoscope should be placed when auscultating lung sounds.

Refer to a website such as 'Easy Auscultation Lung Sounds':

http://www.easyauscultation.com/lung-sounds

(There are many other similar websites available.)

At the edge of a consolidated area there may be loud hissing-like sounds called bronchial breathing, which helps diagnosis.

Listen for added sounds. Wheezing, particularly on expiration, means lower respiratory obstruction (as in asthma). Louder added sounds on inspiration are usually caused by upper airway obstruction, termed stridor.

Expiratory wheeze can be caused by bronchospasm as in asthma, COPD and anaphylaxis. It can also be caused by left ventricular failure (LVF) due to pulmonary oedema.

Crackles in the chest can be caused by pneumonia, due to increased secretions. Also classic signs of pulmonary oedema are crackles in the lung bases when listening to the lower part of the back over the lower ribs. Asking the patient to cough may clear crackles due to secretions. However, crackles in pulmonary oedema do not clear.

There is often confusion between a chest infection and left ventricular failure (LVF), especially in the elderly, who may have difficult-to-determine symptoms. Look for other signs of chest infection (such as temperature, sputum, white cell count) and history of pre-existing lung disease. For LVF, ask if this is sudden onset and whether there are cardiovascular signs, ECG abnormalities or a history of poor cardiac function. If it is still unclear, get senior medical help because treatment is completely different for each of these conditions.

HOT TIP

The key point of the examination is to determine if something has *changed*. Patients should be examined every day and the results recorded in the notes. This gives a baseline to determine an acute change.

Examining the cardiovascular system

The same systematic method is used to examine the cardiovascular system in a patient who is deteriorating, commencing with inspection.

1 Inspection

Look at the colour of the patient, as you did in the respiratory examination.

Look at the patient's observations, and particularly check the blood pressure (BP), pulse rate and ECG monitor if present. Ask for a recent 12-lead ECG to look at.

Examine the patient's neck. Can the pulse be seen over the carotid or the jugular vein? Are the veins in the neck distended, showing either a well-filled patient or raised pressure in the thorax (as in severe asthma or tension pneumothorax)? Remember that the respiratory and cardiac systems are very closely related.

Check for oedema. The ankles are usually swollen in right heart failure but may not be obvious in bed-bound patients (check the sacral area instead). The oedema is typically pitting, meaning that direct thumb pressure will cause a dent (as with pastry dough). Remember other causes of oedema, such as fluid overload or low serum proteins, in debilitated patients.

2 Palpation

Feel the pulse at the radius. Is it strong or weak? Is it regular, irregular or irregularly irregular (as in atrial fibrillation)? Also feel the character of the pulse to determine whether it is weak but slowly rising, or bounding. If the pulse is weak, how does it compare with the carotid? The radial pulse is very difficult to feel if the blood pressure is around 80mmHg systolic or less.

Check the BP. If the diastolic pressure is low, this may be due to vasodilation (as in early sepsis). A high BP may be due to pain or stress. Compare with that obtained earlier on admission and with those recorded on the observation charts.

It may be useful to check other peripheral pulses (such as the femoral and dorsalis pedis on the top of the foot, between the first and second metatarsals), particularly in vascular patients.

Palpation over the heart is useful to feel the apex beat, which can be displaced further left with an enlarged heart.

It is *essential* that blood pressures are recorded in the notes.

Knowing the patient's normal BP is essential in order to determine whether their BP is currently abnormal.

A BP of 111/65mmHg may be considered good for most people, but if their normal is 170/94mmHg it is a significant drop. This may indicate shock, could explain a poor urine output, and will need addressing.

3 Auscultation

Listen over the heart. The apex is the easiest to listen to. Practise listening to the sounds made by a normal heart. Most people can hear two sounds of *lub* (systolic) and *dub* (diastolic). The initial *lub* is the atrioventricular valves closing and the *dub* is the pulmonary and aortic valves closing. Hearing other specific sounds takes lots of practice and practical teaching, but most people are able to hear murmurs. Some murmurs are not harmful, but some can be serious.

Murmurs due to **congenital heart disease** will have been present for life and the patient may well be aware of them, and have to take antibiotics for dental work or surgery to prevent endocarditis. Serious valve disorders produce murmurs (such as the systolic murmur of aortic stenosis). If severe, the patient may have a slow rising pulse and a low BP.

Remember that the patient will have already been clerked. Has the murmur been recorded in the notes? If not, check with the doctor. It may have been missed or something may have changed.

In endocarditis a changing murmur is significant and *must* be reported to the medical team. A sudden-onset murmur in a post myocardial infarction patient could be due to papillary muscle rupture and onset of a valve regurgitation. In most other cases, murmurs do not change. The lung fields need to be checked (as above) to determine signs of pulmonary oedema.

Examining the abdomen

A patient may become unwell if there is an acute abdominal problem so a basic knowledge of examination is required.

1 Inspection

Examine the patient lying flat, with their arms by their side and relaxed. If there are any dressings over the abdomen due to recent surgery, the abdomen will be tender and difficult to examine.

Check the patient's colour, looking particularly for jaundice or for pallor (as in anaemia).

Are there old scars? Ask the patient what caused them or check the notes.

Is there a colostomy or ileostomy? Does it work? If it has recently been formed, does it look healthy and pink? If it looks dusky or black, get the surgical team to check it. This does not necessarily mean it has failed but it should be checked.

Does the abdomen look distended? This could be due to fat or pregnancy. Otherwise it could be due to gaseous distension from obstruction, ascites or blood. Blood lying free in the abdomen could be due to catastrophic haemorrhage (several litres in the abdomen may show few signs except severe hypovolaemic shock and possibly pain). Measuring girth circumferences is pointless in this case.

Are there signs of bruising? If along the posterior of the abdomen and back (Grey–Turner's sign) this may be due to pancreatitis or extraperitoneal bleeding. Bruising around the umbilicus (Cullen's sign) is another possibility with pancreatitis.

2 Palpation

Ask the patient if there is any pain before touching them and ask where it is. Initially, gently palpate over the whole abdomen, watching the patient's face. The point is to detect tenderness, not to hurt them. Remember, a patient who has had abdominal surgery will have a tender abdomen for a few days afterwards.

If tenderness is found, isolate where it is worse or find out if it is generalised. This could be peritonitis. Typically, there may be 'guarding', which means the patient tenses their abdominal muscles and looks very anxious because the pain is severe. Confirm this by eliciting release tenderness (sometimes called 'rebound'). Warn the patient and press *slowly* over the site of tenderness. Then suddenly lift your hand. If this causes a sudden worsening of the pain, peritonitis is likely.

At this point, call for medical help or a surgeon to confirm peritonitis. Do not examine the abdomen further. Make sure bloods have been recently taken for full blood count, white cells, urea and electrolytes, liver function tests and amylase (test for pancreatitis). Keep the patient 'nil by mouth' until they have been seen by the specialist team.

If there are no signs of peritonitis, further examination may not be necessary. A full abdominal examination requires a detailed knowledge of the underlying anatomy. At initial clerking, an enlarged liver should have been detected.

- **Pancreatitis** causes an acute abdomen, with pain radiating through to the back. There may also be signs of septic shock and the amylase may be raised.
- **Acute ruptured aortic aneurysm** presents with abdominal pain and shock. Usually the aneurysm has already been found.
- **Acute appendicitis** usually presents with nausea and vomiting. The patient will have lost their appetite and will have acute abdominal pain starting in the middle, over the umbilicus, and moving to the right iliac fossa. There is usually guarding and release tenderness. Similar pain on the left side is usually due to a gynaecological condition.
- **Generalised peritonitis** can be caused by perforations of the bowel (such as diverticular abscess or tumour). Upper abdominal pain may be from a perforated gastric ulcer or duodenal ulcer. Perforations cause gas under the diaphragm which shows up on an erect chest x-ray.

Remember, any of these conditions can occur with an adult inpatient admitted for any other reason.

3 Percussion

This is especially useful for detecting ascites, where there is increased dullness in the flanks. It can also be used to detect an enlarged liver. Usually the front and middle of the abdomen are resonant due to an air-filled gut.

4 Auscultation

Bowel sounds are normally heard as occasional gurgling sounds when listening over the abdomen. No sound at all is usually caused by a paralytic ileus, which means there is no peristalsis in the gut. This is common after abdominal surgery and can delay feeding, as the stomach may not empty. It usually resolves with time.

Loud tinkling bowel sounds may be caused by obstruction of the bowel. The classic signs of obstruction with loud tinkling sounds are vomiting, distension of the abdomen and constipation with an empty rectum. If this is a new finding, call for medical/surgical help to confirm this.

Neurological examination

A neurological examination is required in order to determine acute changes and call for medical help if necessary. It is vital to assess the patient's level of consciousness as well as the pupil signs described elsewhere (see Chapter 34 on assessing and managing aspects of consciousness and disability). What is most important is to determine whether anything has changed due to an acute stroke so that it can be dealt with urgently.

Firstly, loss of motor function down one side of the body needs to be detected. The simplest way of doing this is to look at the patient and see if there are any differences on either side (such as drooping of one eye or one side of the mouth) or if the limbs look different.

- Ask the patient to smile. Is their smile even?
- Ask them to stick their tongue out. Does it deviate to one side?
- Get them to lift their arms up. Do they move evenly?
- Check their grip simultaneously.

As a further check, test their strength. Get them to bend and straighten their arms as you resist them. Compare on both sides and record the strength on a scale of 0 to 5:

- No movement – **score 0**
- Flicker of muscle movement – **score 1**
- Moves sideways but cannot lift against gravity – **score 2**
- Can lift against gravity but not against gentle downward pressure – **score 3**
- Weak against your resistance – **score 4**
- Normal power – **score 5**.

Ask the patient to flex their legs at the hip, bringing the knee up against you as you push down.

Also check the foot, bending up and down. Run your nail firmly along the sole, from the heel to the ball of the foot. Do not cause scratch marks. This is to check for the Babinski sign. Normally the big toe will bend. The result is considered abnormal (indicating a possible stroke) when the big toe extends.

If you find any new signs of a weakness on one side, consider the possibility of a stroke and call for urgent medical/specialist input. There may be a full neurological examination in the notes to compare with.

If you have any concerns that there are neurological changes, call for medical assistance because early treatment can reduce disability.

Immediate follow-up investigations

Changes in the respiratory system (including changes in respiratory rate and abnormal air entry or crackles) can be investigated with a portable chest x-ray.

If there is a decrease in oxygenation or you detect respiratory insufficiency, particularly with depressed consciousness level, then you should also consider arterial blood gases.

Cardiovascular changes indicate the need for an ECG and possibly a chest x-ray.

Signs of acute abdominal pain should be followed up with blood tests, including full blood count, urea and electrolytes, liver function tests, and amylase (to exclude pancreatitis). Further follow-up investigations may indicate the need for a CT scan or ultrasound or an erect chest x-ray (to detect air under the diaphragm if perforation is suspected).

Acute neurological deterioration, with depressed consciousness not due to hypoxaemia or shock, may require an urgent CT scan of the head.

Conclusion

With all examinations and assessments, record your findings. If the patient was normal this morning and there is something different now, then that is significant. If you think there is a problem with the patient, call a member of the outreach team and/or the medical team. See if they agree with you, watch what they do and ask questions. If their findings are different from yours, ask them why and get them to show you. After all, that's how they learned.

References and further reading

Bickley, L.S. & Bates, B. (2013). *Bates' Guide to Physical Examination and History Taking.* 11th edn. Philadelphia: Lippincott, Williams & Wilkins.

Cox, C. (2009). *Physical Assessment for Nurses.* 2nd edn. Oxford: Blackwell Publishing.

Douglas, G., Nicol, F. & Robertson, C. (2013). *Macleod's Clinical Examination: With STUDENT CONSULT Online Access.* 13th edn. Edinburgh: Churchill Livingstone.

Epstein, O., Perkin, G.D., Cookson, J. (2009). *Pocket Guide to Clinical Examination.* 4th edn. Edinburgh: Mosby.

Rawles, Z., Griffiths, B. & Alexander, T. (2009). *Physical Examination Procedures for Advanced Nurses and Independent Prescribers: Evidence and Rationale.* London: CRC Press, Taylor & Francis.

Resuscitation Council UK (2005). *A systematic approach to acutely ill patients.* http://www.resus.org.uk/pages/alsABCDE.htm (accessed 29 April 2015).

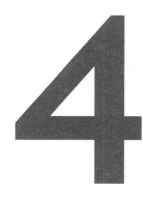

Respiratory physiotherapy and rehabilitation

Sarah Elliott

Physiotherapy is used in all areas of healthcare and is primarily concerned with human function, movement and maximising potential. Critical care is just one branch of physiotherapy. It mainly involves respiratory care in the acute phase and then the rehabilitation of these patients throughout their recovery.

Physiotherapists may also identify potential problems, implement preventative measures and act as educators on disease management or smoking cessation. Many physiotherapy departments now offer a seven-day service, supported by an 'out of hours' emergency respiratory service for patients who would deteriorate without respiratory physiotherapy when full active management is being planned. Please refer to your local physiotherapy service and on-call provision for guidance.

This chapter provides a brief overview of physiotherapy assessment, respiratory physiotherapy treatment interventions, and rehabilitation for critically ill patients.

Physiotherapy whole systems approach to patient assessment

Physiotherapists offer a whole systems (holistic) assessment, and begin by obtaining consent from the patient. Both objective and subjective assessments are then undertaken, and a problem list is drawn up in order to guide the decision-making process regarding the most appropriate treatment. The main aims of respiratory physiotherapy are:

- To increase lung volume
- To improve gas exchange
- To decrease the work of breathing
- To clear secretions.

Other physiotherapy-related problems affecting the patient's rehabilitation may also be identified. These may include issues such as:

- Decreased mobility and function
- Decreased range of motion (ROM)

- Decreased strength
- Decreased stamina or tolerance of exercise
- Decreased confidence
- Altered muscle tone.

A treatment plan is then established. This is agreed with the patient and its effectiveness is evaluated. Referrals may also be made to other professionals such as the occupational therapy team, speech and language therapists, dieticians, the critical care outreach team, the community physiotherapy team and/or social services.

Choosing the most appropriate respiratory physiotherapy intervention

Table 4.1 (below) offers an easy-to-use, quick-reference guide to the physiotherapy techniques that can be utilised to improve the respiratory status of critically ill patients. The appropriate treatment technique should be selected according to the patient's individual needs, problems and goals. Relevant considerations may include oxygen demand, level of fatigue, strength, level of patient compliance and other medical issues.

Table 4.1 An A–Z guide to physiotherapy treatment options

Technique	Problem			
	Sputum clearance	Increase lung volume	Decrease work of breathing	Improve gas exchange
Active cycle of breathing	√			
Autogenic drainage	√			
Breathing control (including pacing)			√	
Breathing exercises	√	√		
Cough assist (Mechanical insufflator–exsufflator)	√	√		√
Exercise/Mobilisation	√	√		√
EZPAP® positive airway pressure system	√	√	√	√
Humidification	√			
Hydration	√			
Incentive spirometry	√	√		

Intermittent positive pressure breathing (IPPB)	√	√		√
Manual techniques (percussion)	√			
Positive expiratory pressure (PEP)	√	√		
Positioning	√	√	√	√
Relaxation			√	
Suction	√			
Vibratory therapy	√			√

These treatments will now be described in more detail.

Active cycle of breathing

This a cycle of breathing exercises, including thoracic expansion exercises, breathing control (relaxed tidal breathing) and forced expiratory technique (FET) (Pryor & Prasad 2002). FET is described by Draper & Ritson (2004) as a gentle but forced breath out through an open mouth, following a breath in. Care should be taken not to invoke bronchospasm (Hough 2001).

Autogenic drainage (AD)

This technique utilises breathing control. The patient adjusts the rate, depth and location of respiration within the thoracic cavity in order to clear the chest of secretions, with minimal coughing. It is carried out in a seated or standing position, and is an extremely popular technique for chronic sputum disorders such as cystic fibrosis. However, the patient may require several sessions to learn the new breathing pattern (Agostini & Knowles 2007).

Breathing control

This is controlled tidal breathing, with the upper chest and shoulders relaxed. It is best taught as a coping strategy, as part of pulmonary rehabilitation, when the patient is feeling well.

Breathing exercises

With these exercises, the aim is to achieve maximal inspiration so as to recruit collateral ventilation. Patients are asked to carry out a few exercises at a time (three to five) to ensure that maximum effort is achieved. These exercises should be repeated hourly (Hough 2001).

Cough assist

This device delivers a positive pressure breath, followed in quick succession by a switch to negative pressure. It is used mainly with neuromuscular or fatigued patients with an ineffective cough (Draper & Ritson 2004). (It is recommended that you familiarise yourself with the cough assist device used in your local setting.)

Exercise/Mobilisation

If the patient is able to do exercises during the acute phase, mobilisation can be used to:

- **Increase lung volume** – Hough (2001) advocates that exercise is the optimum treatment for increasing lung volume and should always be considered in the first instance. However it is not always feasible in the acutely ill adult, and it should be graded to ensure that diaphragmatic breathing is achieved.

- **Improve gas exchange** – ventilation and perfusion become more even throughout the lung (Hough 2001).
- **Clear secretions** – as exercise increases lung volume, collateral ventilation is recruited, thus aiding the movement of secretions in distal airways. Hough (2001) found that active exercises were particularly beneficial and these can be incorporated into the patient's general rehabilitation. In addition, Hough (2001) found that mucus transport increased with exercise.

EZPAP® positive airway pressure system

This positive pressure, hand-held device, which amplifies an input of air or oxygen, is a common form of treatment. It provides a larger flow and volume, with less effort than unsupported breathing exercise (Elliott 2012, 2013).

Humidification

Any patient whose own respiratory system has been bypassed, or who has thick secretions, or who is using oxygen (via a face mask that is delivering over 5 litres/minute of oxygen), should receive humidification.

Hydration

Effective hydration, either by the oral or intravenous routes, will decrease sputum viscosity and allow effective mucociliary action (Hough 2001).

Incentive spirometry

This device gives visual feedback on the patient's performance of deep breathing exercises.

Intermittent positive pressure breathing (IPPB)

IPPB assists breathing through the use of a pressure-cycled ventilator. The device, once triggered by the patient's own inhalation, delivers positive pressure on inspiration and then allows passive expiration. The pressure, flow rate and trigger sensitivity can be altered according to the individual patient's needs.

Manual techniques (percussion)

Slow rhythmic clapping on patient's chest can moderately aid mucociliary transport (Hough 2001).

Positive expiratory pressure (PEP)

This involves active expiration through a one-way valve against a variable flow resistor. Common devices are the PEP mask and thera-PEP (Hristara- Papadopoulou *et al.* 2008). (It is recommended that you familiarise yourself with the device used in your local setting.)

Positioning

The patient can be repositioned in order to:

- **Increase lung volume** – functional residual capacity increases, which helps to facilitate maximal inspiration (Draper & Ritson 2004).
- **Increase gas exchange** – this is best applied to patients with unilateral lung pathology. In side lying, with the affected lung uppermost, the lower and better ventilated lung is then also better perfused, thus improving ventilation/perfusion (V/Q) matching (Hough 2001). For acute respiratory distress, with patients who are extremely hypoxic, the prone position aids the recruitment of lung tissue (Draper & Ritson 2004). This is usually only performed within the intensive care setting.
- **Decrease the work of breathing** – the aim is to support a patient's position so as to encourage relaxation of the upper chest and shoulders. This in turn eases the load on the patient's

inspiratory muscles. Positions may include: high side lying; sitting upright in a chair with the arms supported on pillows; relaxed standing; and forward-lean sitting. Hough (2001) explains that in this last position the diaphragm is domed and so works with greater efficiency.

- Clear secretions – gravity-assisted positions may be adopted to aid drainage of secretions from the affected areas (Hough 2001). However, in acute settings, head-down positions are best avoided, due to the number of contraindications, including hypertension, dyspnoea, recent surgery and cardiac failure (Draper & Ritson 2004).

Relaxation

Relaxation and stress reduction strategies are useful for reducing muscle tension and anxiety. Simple things, like positioning, reassuring the patient and offering them specific relaxation techniques, can all help.

Suction

Suction is a procedure that uses negative pressure to remove excessive or retained secretions from the main airway of patients who are not otherwise able to effectively clear those secretions. It may need to be preceded by other treatment techniques to ensure that secretions are accessible in the upper airway. Suctioning may be carried out via several devices, including a tracheostomy tube, a nasopharyngeal airway, an oropharyngeal airway or a minitracheostomy (see Chapter 8 on suctioning a tracheostomy tube).

Vibratory therapy (Acapella/Flutter)

Exhalation through these devices results in oscillations of expiratory pressure and airflow, which vibrate the airway walls (loosening mucus), decrease the collapsibility of the airways, and accelerate airflow, facilitating movement of mucus up the airways (Konstan *et al.* 1994)

The role of the physiotherapist after critical illness

Physiotherapy is an important intervention that prevents and mitigates the adverse effects of critical illness. The National Institute for Health and Care Excellence (NICE) and the European Respiratory Society and the European Society of Intensive Care Medicine recommend early assessment and management, including exercise prescription delivered by physiotherapists.

Early progressive rehabilitation delivered by physiotherapists is tailored to the patient's needs, depending on their level of consciousness, psychological status and physical strength, and is essential in order to keep functional decline to a minimum (Perme & Chandrashekar 2009). This early proactive approach by physiotherapists results in improved respiratory and cardiovascular function, better limb muscle strength and greater functional independence at hospital discharge, both in exercise capacity (Burtin *et al.* 2009) and the basic activities of daily living (ADLs) (Schweickert *et al.* 2009). It can also reduce the length of hospital stay and the subsequent financial costs (Burtin *et al.* 2009, Morris *et al.* 2008).

The physiotherapist develops an individualised rehabilitation plan that takes into account the specific and unique needs and interests of the patient and their family. The plan also includes input from other members of the multidisciplinary team and integrates rehabilitation into the patient's daily care needs. It is important that the whole team embrace a rehabilitation ethos that motivates the patient to be compliant and achieve their goals. Table 4.2 (below) explains the factors to be considered when formulating a rehabilitation programme.

Table 4.2 Considerations when prescribing exercise

Components of exercise prescription	Explanation	Examples
Type of exercise or activity	**Aerobic (endurance):** keeps the cardiovascular system healthy. May increase oxygen demand in critically ill patients during and after the exercise. Will improve overall fitness and stamina, ready for discharge home.	Mobilisation or exercise is a great example of endurance training for hospital-based patients, as it can be incorporated into their daily care and can be easily measured to demonstrate improvement.
	Strength: improves posture and balance and ability to do everyday tasks, such as walking up and down stairs, carrying shopping and other ADLs. Strengthening exercises are carried out in short bursts and it is best to rotate different muscle groups each day in order to avoid fatigue.	Physiotherapists may use the patient's own body to add resistance (as in squats or sit-to-stands from a low chair) or use small weights and resistance bands.
	Balance/Core stability: a strong foundation will improve the efficiency of all movements and prevent falls.	This may start with simple exercises (such as bridging and sitting on the side of the bed) and progress to the use of wobble boards and gym balls.
	Flexibility: by maintaining joint range and muscle length during critical illness, flexibility exercises will allow more freedom of movement on recovery, thus promoting independence with ADLs.	In the early stages, this may be a passive range of motion exercises, but can progress to active assisted and active exercises as the patient improves.
Exercise intensity	Every person responds differently to exercise. Finding the right intensity, and a balance between effort and rest, is essential.	Intensity can be measured objectively by monitoring HR and SaO_2 and the patient's ability to recover. In addition, a subjective measure (such as the Borg perceived exertion scale) can be utilised.
Exercise duration and frequency	Critically ill patients should gradually increase the duration of their exercise regarding endurance training, and should therefore follow the physiotherapist's advice. For strength training, where exercise intensity is	Rehabilitation can be divided into short bursts throughout the day, rather than one long session. A rehabilitation timetable is useful, to enable the patient and multidisciplinary team to work

Exercise duration and frequency (cont.)	higher, it should be in short sessions. Frequency will depend on the patient's previous exercise tolerance and their ability to recover from previous sessions. It is important to use different types of exercise in order to avoid fatigue or injury.	together and ensure that care needs and rehabilitation needs are all met, with adequate rest periods in between to allow for recovery and avoid fatigue. The physiotherapist may undertake gait re-education one day, followed by balance work the next day, and then strengthening exercises. This helps avoid fatigue and injury. Also, more varied exercise may encourage greater patient compliance. Activities can be functional activities (such as washing and dressing) that encourage independence and should therefore be utilised in a rehabilitation plan.
Precautions and contraindications	**Past medical history**: consider pre-existing conditions (such as osteoarthritis) that may be aggravated during rehabilitation. In addition, respiratory/cardiovascular conditions may affect endurance and exercise tolerance. Take the time to gain an understanding of the patient's previous ability, mobility aids and previous exercise tolerance.	Ensure that the patient has adequate pain relief for any musculoskeletal conditions. You should also ask about their ability to cope with their pre-existing conditions (such as how they pace ADLs if they have COPD) and try to help them recreate the real-life situation. If they have specific equipment, ask family members to bring it to the hospital so it can be utilised.
	Cardiovascular (CVS) status: review observations such as BP and HR and take into account inotropic demand. Review blood results such as haemoglobin and potassium. Discuss the patient's status with the multidisciplinary team.	In some instances, it may not be possible to mobilise a patient due to CVS instability, but consider other types of exercise that may be carried out in bed, while at all times monitoring CVS status. If unsure, discuss with a senior member of staff. On occasions it may not be possible to rehabilitate critically ill patients, but ensure that a respiratory review is undertaken.
	Oxygen demand: oxygen demand will be increased during and after exercise so the patient's oxygen requirement will need to be reviewed carefully before physiotherapy rehabilitation.	In some instances it may be necessary to increase oxygen delivery in order to meet the increased demand during exercise and for up to 2 hours after it. If the patient has a high oxygen

Precautions and contraindications (cont.)		demand, anaerobic (short bursts of strength) exercise might be more appropriate than aerobic (endurance) exercise.
	Apparatus: critically ill patients will often have many attachments (such as intravenous tubes, drains, oxygen tubes and catheters) but these should not restrict rehabilitation.	All equipment is portable, but requires careful planning. For instance, you may wish to request catheter leg bags. Consider the use of portable oxygen if required and mobile monitoring (such as a pulse oximeter).
	Surgical conditions: patients may have specific post-operative instructions following orthopaedic intervention (such as weight-bearing status or restricted range of movement). Or they may have restricted sitting following vascular or abdominal surgery, or their skin integrity may be compromised. Amputees will have an altered centre of gravity, affecting their balance, and may be grieving their lost limb.	Adjust treatments according to specific instructions and ensure that the patient has an appropriate follow-up appointment, which may include psychological support. Bear in mind that an altered weight-bearing status or amputation will increase the patient's exercise intensity during mobilisation.
	Altered neurology: following a cerebrovascular accident (stroke) or head injury, patients may have altered muscle tone, sensation and proprioception.	Ensure that all joints are protected and consider the use of splinting. Teach family members how to help the patient carry out passive stretches if required. Concentrate on quality (rather than quantity) of movement so as to ensure a good foundation for further recovery.
	Nutrition: ensure that the patient has adequate nutritional intake to enable them to participate in rehabilitation and manage any symptoms of nausea or vomiting.	Consider referral to a dietician if required and ask the multidisciplinary team to review the patient's medication. Discuss with patient if they have a preferred time of day for rehabilitation in order to avoid nausea and vomiting.

Conclusion

This chapter has outlined the role and interventions of a physiotherapist for patients with respiratory difficulties and those in post-intensive care. Simple interventions have been described and their benefits to the patient explained.

References and further reading

Agostini, P. & Knowles, N. (2007). Autogenic drainage: the technique, physiological basis and evidence. *Physiotherapy*. **93**, 157–63.

Borg, G.A. (1982). Psychophysical bases of perceived exertion. *Medicine and Science in Sports and Exercise*. **14**, 377–81.

Burtin, C., Clerckx, B., Robbeets, C., *et al.* (2009). Early exercise in critically ill patients enhances short-term functional recovery. *Critical Care Medicine*. **37** (9), 2499–505.

Draper, A. & Ritson, P. (2004). 'Respiratory Physiotherapy Treatments' in Harden, B. (ed.) *Emergency Physiotherapy*. Edinburgh: Churchill Livingstone.

Elliott, S. (2012). A study to investigate the clinical use and outcomes of EZPAP positive pressure device to determine its effectiveness as an adjunct to respiratory physiotherapy. *Association of Chartered Physiotherapists in Respiratory Care Journal*. **44**, 4–11

Elliott, S. (2013). A retrospective analysis of the use of EZPAP positive pressure device by respiratory physiotherapists. *Association of Chartered Physiotherapists in Respiratory Care Journal*. **45**, 4–14.

Hough, A. (2001). *Physiotherapy in Respiratory Care – An Evidenced-based Approach to Respiratory and Cardiac Management*. 3rd edn. Cheltenham, Nelson Thornes.

Hristara-Papadopoulou, A., Tsanakas, J. & Papadopoulou, O. (2008). Current devices of respiratory physiotherapy. *Hippokratia*. **12** (4), 211–28.

Konstan, M.W., Stern, R.C. & Doershuk, C.F. (1994). Efficacy of the flutter device for airway mucus clearance in patients with cystic fibrosis. *The Journal of Paediatrics*. **124** (5), 689–93.

Mazzeo, R.S. & Tanaka, H. (2001). Exercise prescription for the elderly. *Sports Medicine*. **31** (11), 809–18.

Morris, P.E., Goad, A.,Thompson, C., *et al.* (2008). Early intensive care unit mobility therapy in the treatment of acute respiratory failure. *Critical Care Medicine*. **36** (8), 2238–43.

National Institute for Health and Care Excellence (2009). *Rehabilitation after critical illness, CG83*. London: NICE. http://www.nice.org.uk/CG83 (accessed 8 June 2015).

Perme, C. & Chandrashekar, R. (2009). Early mobility and walking program for patients in intensive care units: creating a standard of care. *American Journal of Critical Care*. **18** (3), 212.

Pryor, J.A. & Prasad, S.A. (eds) (2002). *Physiotherapy for Respiratory and Cardiac Problems*. 3rd edn. Edinburgh: Churchill Livingstone.

Schweickert, W.D., Pohlman, M.C.,Pohlman, A.S., *et al.* (2009). Early physical and occupational therapy in mechanically ventilated, critically ill patients: a randomised controlled trial. *The Lancet*. **373** (9678), 1874–82.

5 Patient Safety

Jorge da Fonseca and Alistair Challiner

Patient safety should be everyone's responsibility and this chapter discusses how recent developments in the emerging discipline of patient safety can inform clinical practice and help mitigate some of the inherent risks to patients of caring for them. NHS England recently published a *Serious Incident Framework* (NHS England 2015), which summarises the lessons that have been learned.

Background

Doctors, nurses and medicine can be harmful to your health. Some 2500 years ago, Hippocrates gave healthcare practitioners the following advice: 'The physician must be able to tell the antecedents, know the present and foretell the future – must mediate these things, and have two special objects in view with regard to disease, namely, to do good, or to do no harm' (Hippocrates 400 BCE).

More recently, the landmark Institute of Medicine study 'To Err is Human' (Kohn *et al.* 2000) indicated the nature and extent of harm resulting from modern medical care by measuring adverse incidents (defined as incidents that result in patient harm resulting from medical care, rather than a disease process). The following year, in line with global trends, a study of two large London hospitals (Vincent 2001) described an adverse incident rate of 10.8%, with 5% of these incidents being preventable. These adverse incidents resulted in an additional 8.7 days in hospital per event and an extra cost of £290 per admission. When extrapolated to the entire NHS in 2001, this is estimated to have cost the health service an extra £2 billion and this does not include any litigation costs that may follow.

Delivering safe and effective healthcare, with compassion and respect for the patient, is the defining challenge facing modern practitioners in all healthcare professions. Individual technical competence is necessary, but arguably not sufficient, in the face of increasingly complex systems of healthcare delivery. The necessary patient safety knowledge, skills and attitudes have been defined by regulatory authorities (General Medical Council 2013, Nursing and Midwifery Council 2010), although these professional bodies do not provide details of how they might be acquired in day-to-day clinical practice. The World Health Organization has published its *Multi-professional Patient Safety Curriculum Guide* (WHO 2011), as well as its global initiatives such as 'Safe Surgery Saves Lives' and the 'Global Hand Hygiene Campaign'.

> ## Case scenario
>
> Some years ago, a 72-year-old man was seen in outpatients with arthritis of both hips. The right one was worse and a Right Total Hip Replacement (R THR) was planned and agreed to. However, when the patient was put on the waiting list the booking form was filled out saying 'Left THR' by mistake. The operating list was created using the booking form, stating 'L THR', and the junior doctor sent to consent the patient filled out the consent by copying the information from the operating list.
>
> When the patient arrived, he was anaesthetised and taken into theatre. He was placed on the operating table in the right lateral position and prepped and draped. The scrub nurse looked at the consent, which stated 'L THR'. The consultant surgeon arrived in theatre and stood on the side opposite the scrub nurse. He said 'Left is it' and asked for the knife. Meanwhile, a student nurse had been reading the notes while waiting for the surgeon and wondered why the entries stated he was coming for a 'Right THR', and yet they were prepped for the left. He didn't say anything, as he assumed they knew what they were doing and didn't feel it was his place to question seniors.
>
> The mistake was noted in recovery. The ward nurse was surprised at handover to find that her patient had undergone an 'L THR', when he had told her he had come in for an 'R THR'.
>
> After a brief investigation, the surgeon blamed the booking office for writing the wrong side on the operating list. The patient was told that he needed the left hip doing anyway, and that it was decided to do it once he was asleep, and the right one would be done in a few months' time.

Case analysis

This example raises a number of issues that are frequently associated with healthcare-associated harm, including communication and teamwork. How many other issues can you identify that led to the wrong side being done?

What should have happened?

- The consent form should have been completed by someone who was competent in completing the operation. That person should have asked the patient what operation they were having, and should have cross-referenced their answer with the notes. At the same time, the site of the operation should have been marked.

- Checks should have been made when the patient arrived for surgery, asking them what operation they were having and checking the site. This should have been repeated in the anaesthetic room, before the patient was anaesthetised.

The traditional approach to error analysis

Clearly, things went wrong in this case, and the traditional reaction is to find the culprit, punish them as an example to others, and enforce the rules more forcefully – in the hope that there won't be any more adverse incidents.

Who is to blame? More importantly, what *should* be done to prevent this happening again?

A superficial analysis of the situation might suggest an incompetent surgeon, hastily rushing to start a procedure (maybe so they can get away to the private hospital or the golf course), sloppy junior doctors not paying attention during the consent process, and somnolent anaesthetists and theatre staff breaking the known rules that require consent forms to be cross-checked with the patient and the clinical notes. The rules are clear and everyone knows what they should be doing. The system is complex, but safe, if everybody does their job competently, so what were they thinking?

According to this perspective, the 'bad' underperforming individuals are identified, punished and/ or retrained to improve their performance and help them try harder so that we can return to our perfect error-free system.

However, Reason (2000) provides evidence to challenge this traditional view, arguing that systems are inherently unsafe, with latent, error-producing faults at organisational levels. These errors are remote from the so-called 'sharp end' interface between the clinician and the patient, where the 'active' errors manifest. He argues that the 'sharp end' is not the source of the error – it is just where it manifests. Focusing on the individual therefore ensures that the latent errors inherent in the system remain 'trapped' and ready to harm the patient when they recur. To protect the patient from the inherent fallibility of humans working in a complex healthcare delivery system, the various layers of 'Swiss cheese with aligning holes', which permitted a patient to come to harm, need to be examined and understood. In this way, organisations can prevent the same harm occurring under similar circumstances (see Figure 5.1).

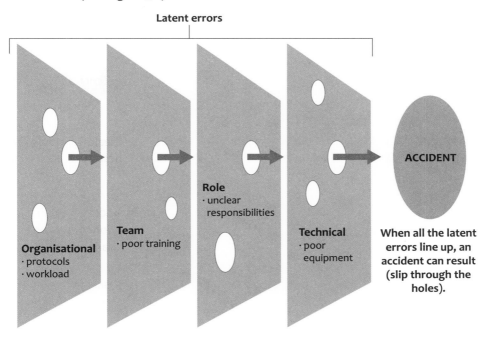

Figure 5.1 *'Swiss cheese model' of human error causation* (based on Reason 2000).

HOT TIP

The priority should be to prevent the error happening again in the future. Blaming an individual may therefore be counterproductive because it tends to encourage a culture of hiding mistakes.

The systems-based approach to error analysis

In the case outlined above, instead of searching for underperforming individuals, a systems-based analysis would consider a number of possible latent, error-producing conditions. Vincent's (1998) model for error analysis suggests looking at a number of areas:

1 Organisation and culture

- Management decisions
- Processes

    factors known as 'latent' conditions

2 Contributory factors

- Work setting
- Team factors
- Individual factors
- Task
- Patient factors

    error-producing conditions

3 Care delivery problems

- Unsafe acts
- Errors and violations

    factors known as active failures

4 Defences and barriers

- Other aspects in place to prevent errors

    incident.

Thinking about the case study:

- What national initiatives (such as A&E waiting time targets, bed pressure and accelerated discharge targets, time targets for various pathways, European working time directives and cost containment targets) could have contributed to pressures on the organisation?

- Did the doctors and nurses have overbooked clinics, or limited secretarial or trainee support? Was documentation absent or difficult to obtain? Or could poor IT have contributed to the initial mistake at the time of booking and subsequently?

- Was there pressure to proceed with the surgery at a time when the patient hadn't been seen and the list needed to start on time?

- Was the anaesthetist supervising more than one theatre or dealing with an emergency simultaneously?

- Did 'escalated' medical patients admitted to surgical wards influence how effectively staff were able to do their pre-operative preparation of this patient? Were they further distracted by pressure to discharge patients?

- Were any members of staff distracted by having to cover too many roles simultaneously? (For instance, were they carrying out multiple ward rounds, medicines rounds, talking to relatives and dealing with staff illness – all first thing in the morning?) How familiar were the individuals with the tasks required of them? (For instance, was there use of agency or locum staff versus permanent staff? And was there enough clinical leadership, training and support?)

- Were there language barriers? What was the rota? Was any member of staff working after a busy period on call, or with a fretful child overnight at home or expecting bailiffs in the morning? Did fatigue play a role?

All these factors are known to affect how clinical tasks are performed and could make complying with best practice difficult or impossible, with the best will and training in the world. For a robust analysis of the incident, all this needs to be considered in-depth to prevent repetition.

Hindsight bias

Another problem with the traditional analysis is 'hindsight bias'. When reflecting on an incident, it is easy to say what *we* would have done, as we know the outcome of the various decisions, and we are outside the situation. Dekker (2001) suggests that this retrospective reaction tends to focus on those closest to the event (proximal), rather than the system as a whole. It also emphasises the counterfactual aspects (i.e. lays out in detail what these people *could* have done to prevent the error), often in an extremely judgmental way. This leads to a poor understanding of the reasons underpinning what was done *at the time*, which may have seemed perfectly reasonable to the person who was actually involved. It needs to be remembered that, without the advantage of 'hindsight', others may well have done the same.

How does your organisation approach patient safety?

The systemic approach to patient safety is a much greater organisational challenge because key decision makers may find it difficult to prioritise patient safety against the demands of performance targets and operational production imperatives.

To find out if your organisation is ready for this systems-based approach, try answering these questions:

1. Is everyone, at all levels in the organisation, involved with and focused on safety?
2. On the occasions when safety and production goals collide, does safety always win?
3. Does the organisation not only welcome but actually reward staff for owning up to mistakes they make? (These mistakes point to important organisational issues that can be improved.)
4. When it comes to patient safety, are money, staff and time no object?

If you answered mainly 'no', then read on to find out how you can influence change in your organisation to improve patient safety and satisfy Care Quality Commission standards, among others.

Human factors

Often mistakenly thought to refer to the human causes of error, 'human factors' is in fact a field of engineering that studies the interaction between individuals (including pre-existing states such as fatigue, emotion and hunger) and the steps that precede a given task; the environment (such as noise, temperature, and perception and assessment of a situation) and the decision-making processes involved in that task; and finally the task and how it is performed (including equipment used and modes of communication).

Crew resource management (CRM), developed by the aviation industry, aims to optimise and structure the people, skills and resources required to manage an emergency.

The key principles of CRM are:

1. Know the environment
2. Anticipate and plan
3. Call for help early
4. Exercise leadership and followership
5. Distribute the workload
6. Mobilise all available resources
7. Communicate effectively
8. Use all available information
9. Prevent and manage fixation errors
10. Cross (double) check
11. Use cognitive aids
12. Re-evaluate repeatedly
13. Use good teamwork
14. Allocate attention wisely
15. Set priorities dynamically.

(Adapted from Rall & Gaba 2005.)

The *Team Strategies and Tools to Enhance Performance and Patient Safety* (STEPPS) programme, designed by the Agency for Healthcare Research and Quality and the US Department of Defense (AHRQ 2013), provides a practical online training programme that incorporates these principles in emergency and non-emergency situations. It emphasises the interplay between:

- Communication
- Leadership
- Situational awareness
- Mutual support.

These four skills are essential in order to deliver safe, efficient, adaptable and productive healthcare routinely and reliably. The STEPPS programme and supporting materials are available at no charge and are recommended as a valuable practical aid to safe practice. Simply visit: http://teamstepps.ahrq.gov/

Patient safety tools

Table 5.1: Examples of patient safety tools

SBAR – NHS Institute for Innovation and Improvement (2008)	I'M SAFE – Agency for Healthcare Research and Quality (2013)
This is a tool to frame critical conversations by detailing: - Situation - Background - Assessment - Recommendations	This tool was based on aviation but is now used in healthcare: **I** – Illness **M** – Medication **S** – Stress **A** – Alcohol/Drugs **F** – Fatigue **E** – Eating/Elimination

There are numerous tools available to assist with patient safety. Some of them will already be familiar in UK clinical practice – see Table 5.1 on previous page.

How can patient safety be improved?

In any organisation, the process of healthcare needs to be constantly evaluated, re-engineered and improved to mitigate for human factors.

The World Health Organisation's *Multi-professional Patient Safety Curriculum Guide* (WHO 2011) includes the following recommendations:

1. Avoid reliance on memory
2. Make things visible
3. Review and simplify processes
4. Standardise common processes and procedures
5. Routinely use checklists
6. Decrease the reliance on vigilance.

Medication errors

Human factors science can be applied to a common source of medical error – that of medication. Rather than simply exhorting doctors and nurses to be more careful, engineering the process may mitigate some of the inherent human fallibility. For instance, in some circumstances, automated prescription may be useful – to avoid typographical errors.

During the manufacturing process, much could be done to standardise drug labelling and packaging, and the collective purchasing power of a large healthcare organisation could be a catalyst to facilitate such changes. Figure 5.2 illustrates some confusing packaging labelling that could result in significant patient harm or death.

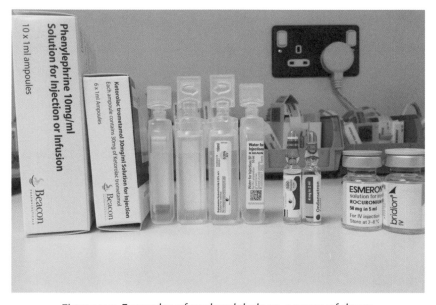

Figure 5.2 *Examples of unclear labels on a range of drugs.*

Re-engineering the drug cupboard, for instance by arranging drugs logically and complying with national guidelines, such as the National Essential Anaesthetic Drug List (Association of Anaesthetists of Great Britain and Ireland 2015), reduces the quantity of medication in the cupboard and, thus, the risk of error. It also enhances patient safety and offers a considerable cost saving.

Arranging drugs by class (rather than alphabetically) theoretically further reduces the risk of patient harm. Figure 5.3 shows an example of improved cupboard layout. However, the best arrangement will vary according to healthcare setting and situation, and this will need assessing in each case.

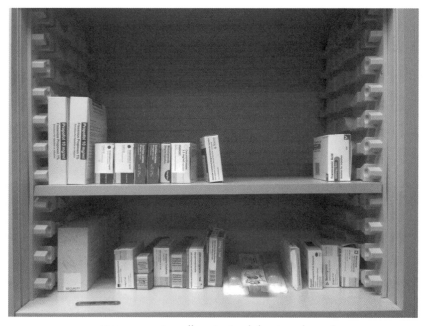

Figure 5.3 *A well-organised drug cupboard.*

Before administering drugs, remembering to use the World Health Organisation's 5Rs checklist (WHO 2011) also improves patient safety:

- Right patient
- Right drug
- Right dose
- Right route
- Right time.

Medical errors

Mistakes by healthcare professionals are the other major cause of adverse incidents, and two examples are briefly discussed below.

Spinal injection of Vincristine

In this case, at Queen's Medical Centre, Nottingham, a spinal injection of Vincristine (which is highly toxic if injected intrathecally) led to the patient's death (Toft 2001): http://www.who.int/patientsafety/news/Queens%20Medical%20Centre%20report%20%28Toft%29.pdf

Issues in this case include human factors, in that the prescription was *not* acted upon correctly and the junior doctor who gave the injection did not feel he could challenge the registrar who gave it to him. Vincristine should have been given intravenously and another drug given spinally.

However, there were also organisational issues regarding the training of doctors in giving chemotherapy, a lack of protocols or limited access to them, and communication failures.

Technical issues included the use of an identical labelling colour and font for the intravenous and spinal syringes and the fact that both could be attached to a spinal needle (Toft 2001).

These two drugs were not supposed to be given on the same day (to reduce the risk of error). However, staff had *changed* the dispensing protocol to avoid patients waiting, and this is why both drugs were in the same pack in the same fridge. The doctor assumed they were both to be given.

Elaine Bromiley

The case of Elaine Bromiley is described in 'Stories' in the Resources section of the Clinical Human Factors Group website: http://chfg.org/

Mrs Bromiley died following hypoxic brain injury, due to failed intubation for elective sinus surgery. The report on the incident suggests that corrective actions were undertaken but several mistakes were made: http://www.chfg.org/resources/07_qrt04/Anonymous_Report_Verdict_and_Corrected_Timeline_Oct_07.pdf

- The period of severe hypoxia lasted for over 20 minutes, during which the anaesthetists concentrated on trying to intubate (fixation error).
- Equipment was used incorrectly, suggesting that a training update was needed.
- Surrounding staff made suggestions without assertiveness, which were ignored or dismissed.
- An ENT surgeon was present who could have helped with a surgical airway.
- The difficult airway and 'can't intubate, can't ventilate' protocol could have been available as a poster on the wall in the operating theatre.

Adverse incident reporting

In his foreword to the World Health Organisation's Draft *Guidelines for Adverse Event Reporting and Learning Systems* (WHO 2005), Sir Liam Donaldson asserts that an effective incident reporting system is the cornerstone of safe clinical practice and is also an important tool to identify and prevent healthcare-associated patient harm. The WHO Guidelines list the four essential components in reporting as:

- Input
- Data
- Analysis
- Feedback.

This document provides a useful overview of the key issues in this important field, and also reiterates the point that the traditional punitive 'name, shame and blame' approach remains a significant barrier to effective reporting. Another helpful resource is Dekker's *Field Guide to Understanding Human Error* (Dekker 2006), a practical guide to conducting an investigation of an adverse incident using a more effective systems-based approach.

Finally, guidelines released by NHS England reflect current UK policy and best practice in this field (NHS Patient Safety Domain March 2015).

Duty of candour

Since the publication of the *Report of the Mid Staffordshire NHS Foundation Trust Public Inquiry* (Francis 2013), UK trusts have a legal obligation to disclose any occurrence of healthcare-associated patient harm to the patient and their family. This legal requirement to disclose is further supported by the General Medical Council, which considers disclosure to be an example of good professional practice.

Patients have a right to know about potential and actual harm from adverse incidents. They are also entitled to an explanation about what happened, discussion about any complications and an apology. This promotes public trust.

The Canadian Patient Safety Institute, in its *Canadian Disclosure Guidelines* (2008), emphasises that disclosure is *not* synonymous with admission of culpability or negligence and discourages the use of the term 'error'. This seems a good way of shifting the focus away from individual performance and towards consideration of the broader issues contributing to adverse incidents. Disclosure allows the legitimate expression of regret by the healthcare provider, in the context of a complete and factual account of events, and enables the provider to give an undertaking to ensure that the situation does not recur.

Rather than increasing the chances of litigation, evidence shows that an open disclosure process reduces the incidence of malpractice suits. It also restores trust in the therapeutic relationship (which has been undermined by an adverse incident) and helps the patient gain an understanding of what has happened to them (McDonald 2010). Further practical guidance can be found in publications describing such incidents. For instance, Harrison describes the personal and professional impact on doctors involved in adverse incidents and makes an eloquent and poignant case for supporting the secondary victims of medical error (Harrison 2014).

Conclusion

Avoidable mistakes cause significant mortality and morbidity. It is every healthcare practitioner's responsibility to help reduce risk by means of effective incident reporting and compliance with risk reduction strategies. Probably the most important organisational factors are: ensuring that everyone engages as a team member, allowing challenges to be accepted, and enabling learning from mistakes to be embedded in future practice.

References and further reading

Agency for Healthcare Research and Quality, in collaboration with the Defense Health Agency (2013). *Team Strategies and Tools to Enhance Performance and Patient Safety.* 2nd edn. Maryland: AHRQ.

Association of Anaesthetists of Great Britain and Ireland (2015). *The National Anaesthesia Drug List.* London: AAGBI.

Canadian Patient Safety Institute, Disclosure Working Group (2008). *Canadian Disclosure Guidelines: National Guidelines for Disclosure of Adverse Events.* Edmonton: CPSI.

Clinical Human Factors Group (2015). *Implementing Human Factors in Healthcare: 'How to' guide.* http://www.patientsafetyfirst.nhs.uk/Content.aspx?path=/interventions/humanfactors/ (accessed 11 June 2015).

Cook, R. (1998). *How Complex Systems Fail.* Chicago: Cognitive Technologies Laboratory, University of Chicago.

Dekker, S. (2006). *The Field Guide to Understanding Human Error.* Farnham: Ashgate Publishing.

Francis, R. (2013). *Report of the Mid Staffordshire NHS Foundation Trust Public Inquiry.* https://www.gov.uk/government/publications/report-of-the-mid-staffordshire-nhs-foundation-trust-public-inquiry (accessed 11 June 2015).

General Medical Council (2013). *Duties of a Doctor: Good Medical Practice.* London: GMC.

Harrison, R. (2014). Doctors' experiences of adverse events in secondary care: the professional and personal impact. *Clinical Medicine.* **14** (6), 585–90.

Hippocrates (400 BCE). *Of the Epidemics.* Book 1, Section 2. Part 5.

Kohn, L.T., Corrigan, J.M., & Donaldson, M.S. (eds) (2000). Committee on Quality and Healthcare in America, Institute of Medicine. *To Err is Human: Building a Safer Healthcare System.* Washington: National Academy Press.

McDonald, T. (2010). Responding to patient safety incidents: the seven pillars. *Quality and Safety in Health Care.* **19**.

NHS England Patient Safety Domain (March 2015). *Serious Incident Framework: Supporting learning to prevent recurrence.* London: NHS England.

Nursing and Midwifery Council (2010). *Standards for Competence for Registered Nurses.* London: NMC.

Rall, M. & Gaba, D. M. (2005). 'Human performance and patient safety' in R.D. Miller (ed.) *Miller's Anaesthesia.* Philadelphia: Elsevier Churchill Livingstone.

Reason, J. (2000). Human Error: models and management. *British Medical Journal.* **320**, 768–70.

Toft, B. (2001). *External Inquiry into the adverse incident that occurred at Queen's Medical Centre, Nottingham, 4th January 2001.* London: Department of Health.

Vincent, C. (2001). Adverse Events in British Hospitals: preliminary retrospective record review. *British Medical Journal.* **322**, 517–19.

Vincent, C. (1998). Framework for analysing risk and safety in clinical medicine. *British Medical Journal.* 316(7138), 1154-57.

World Health Organisation (2005). *Draft Guidelines for Adverse Event Reporting and Learning Systems.* Geneva: WHO.

World Health Organisation (2011). *Patient Safety Curriculum Guide: Multi-professional edition.* Geneva: WHO.

Useful websites

Agency for Healthcare Research and Quality. TeamSTEPPS.
http://teamstepps.ahrq.gov/

Clinical Human Factors Group (2007). The case of Elaine Bromiley.
http://www.chfg.org/resources/07_qrt04/Anonymous_Report_Verdict_and_Corrected_Timeline_Oct_07.pdf
(Accessed 11 June 2015)

Health Foundation (2011). Levels of harm.
http://www.health.org.uk/public/cms/75/76/313/2593/Levels%20of%20harm.pdf?realName=PYiXMz.pdf
(Accessed 11 June 2015)

The Joint Commission (2015). Hospital National Patient Safety Goals.
http://www.jointcommission.org/assets/1/6/2015_HAP_NPSG_ER.pdf (Accessed 11 June 2015)

NHS Direct (2009). World Health Organization Surgical Safety Checklist.
http://www.nrls.npsa.nhs.uk/resources/?EntryId45=59860 (Accessed 11 June 2015)

NHS Institute for Innovation and Improvement (2015). SBAR resources.
http://www.institute.nhs.uk/safer_care/safer_care/sbar_resources.html (Accessed 11 June 2015)

Nursing and Midwifery Council (2015). Duty of Candour.
http://www.nmc-uk.org/Get-involved/Consultations/duty-of-candour/ (Accessed 11 June 2015)

·A B C D E·

Airway

Assessing and managing the airway

Alistair Challiner and Sally A. Smith

This chapter will cover the assessment of a patient's airway and how to intervene using basic life support techniques. It will also describe how to use simple airway manoeuvres to maintain the airway, and how to use simple airway adjuncts.

Assessing the airway

It is imperative that patients are able to maintain their airway in order to breathe properly, and in order to protect themselves from aspirating secretions (potentially leading to aspiration pneumonia) or from blocking their airway with their tongue. The goal is to ensure a patent airway.

Assessing the airway is the first step in any assessment of an acutely unwell patient. Recognition of airway obstruction can be made using the 'look, listen, feel' technique.

Look

Look for the presence of cyanosis, a 'seesaw' breathing pattern, use of accessory muscles, tracheal tug (where, as the patient breathes in, you see the tracheal area move up and down as if being pulled), alteration of conscious level, any obvious obstruction (such as a foreign body or vomit), and whether the patient is in any form of distress (Resuscitation Council 2005, Tait 2012).

Listen

Listen for sounds such as gurgling, snoring, crowing, stridor or wheeze (see Table 6.1 below).

Feel

Feel for airflow on inspiration and expiration with the back of your hand or your cheek that has been moistened. If the airway is totally blocked, the patient will require emergency resuscitation. A totally blocked airway is signalled by a cyanosed patient, who is in deep distress and who may have no breath sounds.

In this situation, summon urgent help (put out a cardiac arrest call) and commence basic life support according to resuscitation guidelines.

Table 6.1 Partial airway obstruction sounds

Sound	Type of obstruction
Expiratory wheeze	Obstruction of lower airways, which tend to collapse and obstruct during expiration
Gurgling	Suggests presence of liquid or semi-solid material in upper airways
Snoring	Pharynx partially occluded by tongue or palate
Crowing	Laryngeal obstruction or spasm
Stridor	Obstruction above or at the level of the larynx

Simple manoeuvres

If a patient's airway is compromised, immediate measures must be taken to clear it. These include the head tilt, chin lift and jaw thrust (see Figures 6.1a, 6.1b and 6.1c 1b below).

Turn the patient onto their back and then open the airway using head tilt and chin lift:

- Place your hand on the forehead and gently tilt the head back.
- With your fingertips under the point of the chin, lift the chin to open the airway.

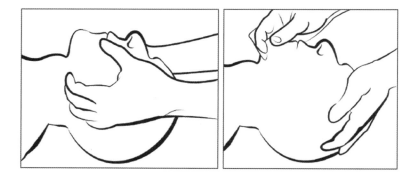

Figure 6.1 *Techniques for opening an airway: (a) jaw thrust; (b) head tilt and chin lift.*

If the airway is compromised in any way, high-flow oxygen (15LPM) will need to be administered and saturations via pulse oximetry (SpO2) will have to be monitored. It is also imperative to get help quickly from someone who is skilled in advanced airway techniques (such as the on-call anaesthetist).

Using airway adjuncts to maintain the airway

Sometimes patients require their airway to be maintained using an airway adjunct. This enables easy suctioning of secretions, and administration of oxygen.

Inserting an oropharyngeal airway

Oropharyngeal airways, such as the Guedel (see Figure 6.2), are used for patients who have an obstructed airway due to reduced consciousness, usually because the tongue falls back in the mouth.

An oropharyngeal airway ensures that the tongue is moved forward and reduces obstruction, thus enabling the patient to breathe.

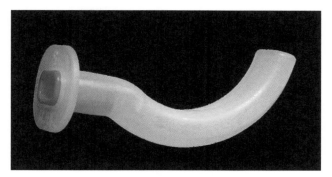

Figure 6.2 **An oropharyngeal airway**

The size of the adjunct to be used is assessed by lining up the airway against the side of the patient's cheek and ensuring the flange is level with the front teeth and the end is at the angle of the jaw line. Insert the airway upside down (in other words, curling upwards) so its concavity is directly upward, until the soft palate is reached. Then rotate the airway 180° degrees, so that the concavity is directed inferiorly and the airway is slipped into place over the tongue. This ensures that the tongue doesn't block the airway as the device is being inserted.

Oropharyngeal airways are coughed out by patients when they begin to be able to manage their own airway. If the patient tolerates the oropharyngeal airway, it means they have no protective gag reflex. They are therefore at risk of aspiration of their gastric contents. Skilled help is required, as the patient may need intubation. If the patient is breathing, they would be safer lying on their side so that any secretion or regurgitation drains from the mouth.

Inserting a nasopharyngeal airway

Nasopharyngeal airways are useful for patients who are not necessarily unconscious, but do have a compromised airway, or have difficulty in expectorating secretions, as occurs in patients with myasthenia gravis, or Guillain-Barré syndrome, or someone with a decreased conscious level.

The choice of airway is generally a size 3 for a female and 4 for a male. Lubricate the tube and then pass it into the right nostril, as if aiming in a straight line from the front to the back of the head, directing it posteriorly and towards the ear (not up and over, as you may feel inclined to do, parallel to the palate). Gently pass the nasopharyngeal airway through the nostril into the oropharynx, rotating slightly, until the flange rests against the nostril.

This procedure can cause some trauma to the nasal passages, so a gentle smooth movement is required. If you have difficulty, you can try the other nostril.

Suctioning the airway using a Yankauer sucker

This technique is useful for removing oral secretions from the mouth. The sucker is bent in the middle so that, as you pass it into the oral cavity, your hand does not occlude your view.

Attach the sucker to the suction tubing and pass the catheter into the mouth, removing secretions gently. Always make sure you can see the tip of the catheter; never pass it beyond direct vision. If the patient needs ventilating, remember to limit suctioning to the minimum required to clear secretions, as the patient is not receiving oxygen while suctioning is being carried out.

Giving oxygen via a bag-valve mask

Administering oxygen via a bag-valve mask is an advanced technique, which is usually taught on advanced life support courses and requires two people to undertake. Ward staff members may be able to assist by either holding the mask securely onto the patient's face with both hands, or squeezing the bag gently. For training and competence in this manoeuvre, please refer to your own resuscitation training teams.

Indications for the insertion of a supraglottic airway or an endotracheal tube

Supraglottic airways (SGAs) include laryngeal masks (LMAs) and I-gels®. An LMA needs air to be injected into a 'cuff' to secure a seal, whereas an I-gel® requires no inflation as it is sealed by means of a silicone gel-filled cuff. SGAs are more frequently used to maintain an airway in an unconscious patient (as in anaesthesia or a cardiac arrest situation). They are useful in an emergency situation in the ward because they can be inserted by practitioners who have received training, but who are not necessarily anaesthetists.

An SGA acts as a mask over the larynx and is therefore easier to maintain than holding a face mask. The airway is inserted into the mouth and, in the case of an LMA, the cuff is inflated to the correct volume. SGAs can only be used in patients with no airway reflexes (as in a cardiac arrest) and they are used to administer ventilation via a bag-valve device. Aspiration is still a risk but no more than with a face mask (Mort 2011).

Endotracheal tubes are the preferred device for maintaining the airway in a patient who may go on to require mechanical ventilation in an intensive care environment. The technique requires hands-on training and should be performed by a skilled practitioner.

Placing a patient in the recovery position

There are several ways of undertaking this maneouvre, each with its own advantages. No single position is perfect for all patients. The position should be stable, near a true lateral position with the head dependent (lower), and with no pressure on the chest to impair breathing (Resuscitation Council (UK) 2015).

Training is required, usually from the resuscitation team, in order to undertake this maneouvre competently. Briefly, it involves positioning the person on their side, protecting their airway and ensuring their limbs are safely positioned. One person can undertake this, although in a hospital setting two or more people can position the patient more effectively.

Conclusion

Assessing the airway is the first step in assessing an acutely unwell patient. The goal is to ensure a patent airway at all times, and several airway adjuncts and manoeuvres can be used to achieve this.

Practitioners can learn these skills through basic and advanced resuscitation training in their own hospitals. However, with any patient whose airway is compromised, it is essential to call for expert help immediately.

References and further reading

Mort, T.C. (2011). The Supraglottic Airway Device in the Emergent Setting: its changing role outside the operating room. *Anesthesiology News Guide to Airway Management.* 59–71
http://www.anesthesiologynews.com/download/sga_angam11.pdf (accessed 13 April 2015).

Resuscitation Council (UK) (2005). *A systematic approach to the acutely ill patient.*
https://www.resus.org.uk/pages/alsABCDE.htm#airw (accessed 13 April 2015).

Resuscitation Council (UK) (2015). *Adult Basic Life Support.* https://www.resus.org.uk (accessed 29 November 2015).

Sun Kyung Park (2015). Comparison of the I-Gel and the Laryngeal Mask Airway Proseal during General Anesthesia: A Systematic Review and Meta-Analysis. *PLOS One.* **10** (3): e0119469.
http://www.ncbi.nlm.nih.gov/pmc/articles/PMC4374933/ (accessed 8 April 2015).

Tait, D. (2012). 'Assessing, recognising and responding to acute and critical illness' in D. Tait, D. Barton, J. James and C. Williams

Useful websites

iGel information sheet
http://www.chinookmed.com/i-gel-information-sheet.pdf (Accessed 13 June 2015)

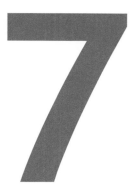

7 Temporary tracheostomies

Philip Woodrow

Tracheostomies are a medical intervention to solve a medical problem. This chapter discusses care for adult patients with existing temporary tracheostomies (see Figure 7.1 below). Authoritative guidelines are available from the National Confidential Enquiry into Patient Outcome and Death (2014), the Intensive Care Society (2014) and St George's Healthcare NHS Trust (2007).

After finishing this chapter, you should be able to describe what tracheostomies are, why they are used, and how to care for a patient with a tracheostomy. Although not specifically described, paediatric tracheostomies are generally similar, with smaller equipment.

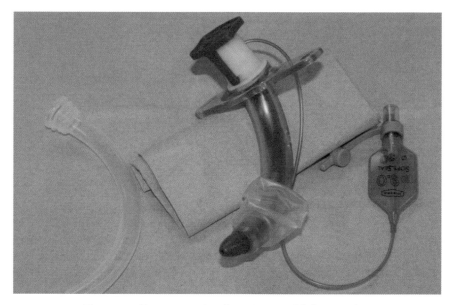

Figure 7.1 *Temporary tracheostomy, with inner tube.*

Types of tracheostomy

A tracheostomy is a stoma in the trachea, created to facilitate breathing or artificial ventilation. The procedure that creates the tracheostomy is called a tracheotomy.

There are three types of tracheostomy:

- Permanent
- Temporary
- Mini-tracheostomy.

Temporary tracheostomies are the type most frequently encountered in acute hospitals. Permanent tracheostomies are created when part of the upper airway has been removed, usually because of cancer. Well-formed permanent stomas do not always need tubes, but if tubes are present they will not have cuffs. Mini-tracheostomies are not an airway, but a means of access for tracheal suction. They are rarely used, and will not be discussed here.

Because no gas exchange occurs until air reaches the alveoli, the space between where air enters the body (normally the nose and/or mouth) and the alveoli is called 'dead space'. Normal adult dead space is about 150ml. During expiration, this space is filled with the oxygen-poor and carbon-dioxide-rich air from the lungs. Therefore during inspiration, the first approximately 150ml of air to reach the alveoli is this same oxygen-poor and carbon-dioxide-rich air. Normal (healthy) resting adult tidal volumes (breath sizes) of 300–500ml leave sufficient good-quality (21% oxygen, 0.04% carbon dioxide) air for the volume of dead space not to cause problems. But shallow breathing (which commonly occurs with respiratory failure) increases the proportion of poor-quality air reaching the lungs, resulting in hypoxia, and often hypercapnia. Creating a tracheostomy approximately halves dead space volume and so, with severe respiratory failure, significantly increases the quality of air (and quantity of oxygen) reaching the alveoli. It also reduces the quantity of re-breathed carbon dioxide, thus improving carbon dioxide clearance.

Case scenario

A man with a seven-year history of COPD was admitted three weeks ago, with an acute exacerbation. This necessitated admission to intensive care, where he was ventilated for 18 days. On the fifth day, he had a percutaneous tracheostomy formed and is now making a slow but steady recovery. He is transferred to a medical ward, where you admit him. His tracheostomy is size 7.5mm and its cuff remains inflated.

After reading this chapter, plan this patient's nursing care for the next few days.

Percutaneous tracheostomies

Historically, tracheostomies were created surgically – a surgical incision was used to create the stoma. Permanent tracheostomies are almost invariably surgical, but most temporary tracheostomies are now created using a 'percutaneous dilational tracheostomy' (Nolan & Kelley 2011). Percutaneous tracheostomies are typically created by anaesthetists. A specially designed needle makes a hole into the trachea, which is then stretched with a guidewire and dilators, until the tracheostomy tube can be inserted. Difficult airways and other problems may necessitate surgical, rather than percutaneous, creation (Regan 2009).

Tube size

To maintain patency, a tube is inserted into a temporary stoma. Most adult tubes are internal diameter (ID) size 7.0, 7.5, 8.0 or 8.5mm, although smaller and larger sizes are available. The size is moulded into the plastic on the flange at the side of the tube, and printed on the bladder.

Problems associated with tracheostomy care

Tracheostomies expose patients to various problems, some of which can be life threatening. Care should therefore be taken to reduce risks and problems to patients. According to the National Confidential Enquiry Into Patient Outcome and Death (NCEPOD 2014), staff caring for patients with tracheostomies must be trained in:

- Humidification
- Cuff pressure
- Monitoring and cleaning of the inner cannula
- Resuscitation.

Other aspects of care discussed here are:

- Communication
- Nutrition
- Deep suction
- Wound care.

NCEPOD (2014) also recommend using bedhead signs to guide safe tracheostomy care.

Humidification

The upper airway warms, moistens and filters inhaled air. Much of the warming and moistening occurs in the nasal cavity, which is bypassed by tracheostomies. Colder and dryer air entering the lower airways can cause damage to cilia and encrustation of lower airways (Wilkes 2011). Humidification is therefore essential. The Intensive Care Society (2014) provides a ' humidification ladder' (see Table 7.1 below).

Table 7.1 The humidification ladder

HME
(Buchanan bib, 'Swedish nose' – heat moisture exchanging filter placed over a tracheostomy tube)
Self-ventilating patient (no oxygen)
Cold water bath
Self-ventilating patient (on oxygen)
HME for breathing circuit
Ventilated patient with minimal secretions
Monitor effectiveness (less likely to be effective if required for more than five days).
Heated water bath (active humidification)
Ventilated patient with thick secretions
Self-ventilating patient (on oxygen) with thick secretions
If secretions are still difficult to clear, add saline nebulisers or mucolytics and ensure adequate hydration.

(Adapted from Intensive Care Society (ICS) 2014, p. 22.)

Cuff pressure

Temporary tracheostomies have a cuff around the outside, which can be inflated with air to protect the patient's airway. However, if cough and gag reflexes are present (as they are in most ward patients), the cuff does not usually need to be inflated. If you are unsure whether a cuff needs to be inflated or deflated for a particular patient, you should seek medical advice.

If inflated, most cuffs usually hold about 5ml, varying mainly with tracheostomy size. If the cuff pressure exceeds capillary pressure, ulcers (pressure sores) may develop in the trachea. Tracheal ulcers can cause permanent tracheal stenosis. Pressure inside inflated cuffs should therefore be checked at least every 8 hours (ICS 2014) with a cuff pressure manometer (see Figure 7.2). Cuff pressure should not exceed 25cmH$_2$O (ICS 2014), and should be documented at least once each shift (NCEPOD 2014).

Many cuff pressure manometers display a 'safe' range, typically in green. However, the range displayed on manometers sometimes exceeds guidelines. If pressure above 25cmH$_2$O is needed to prevent a leak, the tube may be too small (ICS 2014). In this case, further advice should be sought from an anaesthetist or the critical care outreach team.

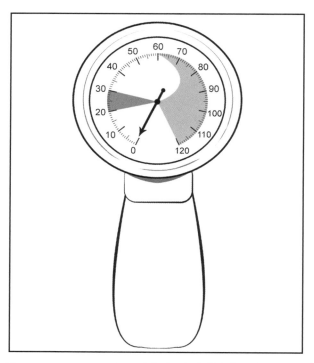

Figure 7.2 Cuff pressure manometer with shaded dial showing normal (dark grey) and high-pressure ranges in cmH$_2$O.

Cuffs do not create a perfect seal. Saliva and other fluids often accumulate above the cuff, usually trickling past into the lungs. Some tubes have subglottic drainage ports. If these are present and the cuff is inflated, the drainage ports should either be connected to continuous drainage devices or initially aspirated every 1–2 hours (reducing the frequency according to the volume aspirated). Otherwise, excessive secretions usually have to be removed using oral or nasopharyngeal suction.

Inner cannulae

Most, though not all, temporary tracheostomies are manufactured to accommodate inner cannulae. These inner cannulae can be easily removed, to enable cleaning. They should be changed at least every 4 hours if patients have productive chests, and at least 8-hourly with all other patients (ICS 2014). Most inner cannulae are designed to allow them to be cleaned (with sterile water), but some are single-use items. Readers should always check the manufacturer's instructions.

If the tube does not have an inner cannula, it is likely to become partly or fully occluded with encrusted secretions. In this case, it should normally be changed every 7–14 days (ICS 2014).

If the tracheostomy is obstructed, removing the inner cannula usually restores airway patency (ICS 2014).

Resuscitation

An occluded tracheostomy equals respiratory arrest, so an airway *must* be established. As in any arrest situation, help should be summoned urgently. Occlusion is usually caused by encrusted secretions, so removal of the inner tube often resolves the problem (ICS 2014). However, if this fails, the whole tube should be removed (ICS 2014). Unless the stoma is less than a week old, it will usually remain patent. If necessary, suction can be performed through the open stoma (ICS 2014). The ICS (2014) suggests keeping a tube the same size and one size smaller for use in an emergency situation.

If the tracheostomy cuff is inflated, or the patient has had a laryngectomy, face-mask oxygen should not be used, as the upper airway is *not* patent (NCEPOD 2014, ICS 2014).

Following resuscitation, ideally a tube of the same size should be re-inserted. If a similar size tube cannot be inserted, either the stoma may be dilated with tracheal dilators, or a tube that is a half-size or one size smaller should be attempted.

Wards should have a 'difficult airway trolley', with the same contents and organisation as in the local operating theatres (NCEPOD 2014). In addition, endoscopy equipment should be immediately available (NCEPOD 2014).

HOT TIP

Emergency resuscitation equipment should be kept near the bed space of any patient with a temporary tracheostomy (ICS 2014). This equipment includes:

- Operational suction unit with tubing and Yankauer sucker
- Appropriately sized suction catheters
- Gloves, aprons and eye protection
- Spare tracheostomy tubes: one same size and one a size smaller

- Tracheal dilators
- Rebreathing bag and tubing with connection
- Tracheostomy disconnection wedge
- Tracheostomy tube holder and dressing
- 10ml syringe (if tube cuffed)
- Suture cutters (if tube stitched into place).

You will need to consider the safety issues within your locality for keeping syringes and suture cutters by the bedside; if there are concerns, you should follow local policy to ensure that these are easily accessible in an emergency.

Staff caring for patients with a temporary tracheostomy should check this equipment at each shift, ensuring that the suction equipment works. They should also check the size of tube used for the patient – internal diameter size is usually printed on the 'bladder'.

General problems associated with tracheostomies
Communication

Tracheostomy tubes are sited below the vocal cords. If cuffs are inflated, no air passes through the cords, causing loss of voice. Loss of speech is frightening and isolating. Staff should explain to patients, and their families, that loss of voice is caused by the tube, and that when the tube is removed, or the cuff deflated, the patient's speech should return.

While patients are unable to speak, staff should optimise other means of communication. The means used will vary according to individual patients, staff and the aids available, but may include:

- Lip-reading
- Sign language
- Writing
- Picture/letter/word boards
- Laptop-style computer aids.

When acute disease subsides, the voice may be restored by utilising:

- One-way speaking valves
- Fenestrated tubes.

Speaking valves allow air to enter the tracheostomy, retaining benefits from reduced airway dead space but preventing exhalation through the tube. It is therefore essential that cuffs are fully deflated *before* placing speaking valves on the tubes. With the tracheostomy blocked, exhalation is forced around the tube, and so through the vocal cords. Alternatively, ' fenestrated' tubes, with small holes on the curve of the tube, allow sufficient air to escape through the vocal cords. Fenestrated tubes are seldom used in acute care.

Discourage patients from placing a finger over the tracheostomy to speak. Each square centimetre of skin may harbour three million organisms (Mercuri 2012), so this can place three million bacteria 75ml away from the alveoli that are recovering from pneumonia.

Various artificial 'voice boxes' are available for people with permanent tracheostomies, but these are only likely to be seen in acute (non-ENT) wards if patients already have them when admitted.

Nutrition

Because the oesophagus is adjacent to the trachea, tracheostomy tubes make swallowing difficult, especially if the cuff is inflated (Amathieu *et al.* 2012). Traditionally, inflated cuffs were considered a contraindication to feeding. However, the Intensive Care Society (2014) now recommends individual assessment of patients, and attempting feeding with sips. If that fails, they recommend referral to speech and language therapists. Even with cuffs deflated, dysphagia often persists (Romero *et al.* 2010). Nutrition is fundamental to health, and malnourishment delays recovery. Until the patient is able to eat orally, an alternative means of nutrition should therefore be supplied (such as nasogastric feeding). Dieticians should be actively involved, and the patient's diet should be closely monitored, especially when oral intake is resumed.

Weak cough

Although cough and gag reflexes may be present, many patients with tracheostomies have weak coughs. While some patients are able to clear their own sputum, others may require help to prevent sputum retention. Some patients may be able to cough secretions to the end of the tracheostomy, only requiring staff to remove secretions from the tip of the tube – often a clean Yankauer catheter is best for this. But if coughs are too weak to achieve this, a (sterile) soft suction catheter should be used to remove secretions from just above the carina.

Safe suction requires skill, so it should only be performed by someone competent to carry out the procedure. Trusts may provide training on suction technique. Staff, such as respiratory physiotherapists or members of the critical care outreach team, are usually able to demonstrate and assess technique.

Suction pressures should be low; many practitioners limit pressure to 20kPa. Most Trusts have a clean glove policy for suction (readers should check the policy in their local healthcare setting). Normal adult suction catheter sizes are FG 10, 12 and (sometimes) 14, usually colour-coded black (FG10), white (FG 12) and green (FG 14). Formulae have been devised for calculating which size to use, but it is safer to use the smallest size that will be effective. FG 10 is effective with watery secretions (such as saliva), but FG 12 is often needed for mucus. If FG 12 fails to remove secretions, FG 14 should be tried. With children, or very small adults, FG 8 or smaller may be needed, due to the smaller size of the airway. With mini-tracheostomies, only FG 10 or smaller will pass through the lumen.

The suction catheter should be advanced into the trachea, quickly but gently, and reach below the tube but above the carina, ideally about 1cm above the carina. The xiphisternum is a useful marker, and life-size anatomical models of the trachea may be useful for staff to familiarise themselves with the location. Most patients will cough once the catheter is in the trachea, and cough more violently should the catheter touch the carina.

Once in place, suction should be applied (usually by occluding the side port on the catheter). The suction catheter should then be withdrawn smoothly, maintaining suction. During suction, the patient will be unable to breathe, so the process should be completed within 5–10 seconds (but watch the patient, not a clock; holding your own breath during suction is a useful guide). After suction, reassess the patient, and determine whether further suction is needed. If it is, allow the patient to take some breaths and stabilise before further suction passes. A new sterile catheter should be used for each pass.

The National Confidential Enquiry into Patient Outcome and Death (NCEPOD 2014) cites the UK National Tracheostomy Safety Project's suggestion of suctioning at least every 8 hours. However, the Intensive Care Society recommends assessing the individual patient's suction needs (ICS 2014). As suction can cause trauma, routine suctioning is *not advisable.*

Wound care

Before routine re-dressing of tracheostomy sites, staff should check for:

- Specific medical instructions (e.g. a new tracheostomy may need to remain undisturbed for a period of time)
- Specific wound care product instructions (e.g. many dressings are designed for daily replacement but some may remain in place longer if they are not soiled).

Re-dressing can only be safely undertaken with two people. The assistant is simply required to hold the tube in place once the tube-holder has been removed, so the assistant may be anyone who is competent to undertake the task. Once the assistant is holding the tube, the tube holder and old dressing are discarded.

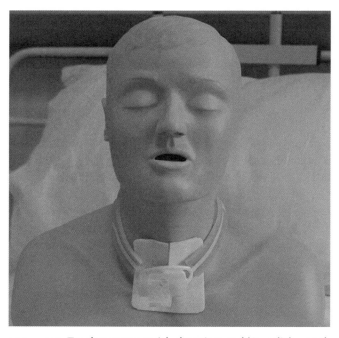

Figure 7.3 Tracheostomy with dressing and 'Swedish nose'.

Some holders can be cleaned and reused but this is rarely practised in acute care where new holders are usually applied daily. Excessive secretions around the stoma may be removed with a sterile suction catheter (soft catheters are easiest). The wound should then be cleaned with saline (ICS 2014), using aseptic technique. This should include cleaning underneath the plastic flange, which should also be dried before applying the new dressing. Tracheostomy tubes are now seldom stitched to skin, but if there are stitches, sterile cotton buds are often easiest for cleaning.

Most tracheostomy wound dressing pads have two distinct sides. Check which side should be placed against the skin – some dressings can be visually deceptive. Tube holders are often custom-made, with two different lengths. Both lengths usually have Velcro® fastenings, which are placed through the holes in the flange. The longer length is then passed behind the patient's neck, and attached to the shorter length with a further Velcro® fastening (see Figure 7.3).

The tube-holder should be just tight enough to place two fingers between it and the patient's neck (Docherty & Bench 2002). If it is any slacker, it may fail to hold the tube in place; if tighter, it may cause discomfort.

Changing and removing tubes

Tubes should be changed at least every 30 days, or sooner if required by the manufacturer (ICS 2014). Tubes should only be changed or removed by someone who is competent to undertake this task (see Chapter 9 – Changing a tracheostomy tube). Most Trusts will have policies stating who should change tracheostomy tubes. Generally, this will include:

- Anaesthetists
- Critical care outreach team members
- Specialist/experienced respiratory staff.

Decannulation increases the 'work of breathing' (the muscular effort and energy 'cost', especially of oxygen) by 30% (Chadda *et al.* 2002). Respiratory function should therefore be closely monitored after decannulation. Following removal of the tube, the stoma site should be covered with an occlusive dressing, such as hydrocolloid. Initially, there are usually secretions that require sterile swabs beneath the dressing. If the dressing becomes displaced, looks soiled, or otherwise causes concern, it should be replaced. Otherwise, intact dressings should remain in place as long as they are needed and comply with the manufacturer's instructions.

Conclusion

Caring for patients with tracheostomies requires skill and knowledge. Where tracheostomies are rarely seen, staff have few opportunities to develop these skills and are likely to forget knowledge that is not frequently needed.

The tracheostomy *is* the patient's airway, so maintaining patency is vital. Staff should seek advice about any aspect of care that they are unsure about, and take opportunities to develop their skills under competent supervision. Unless other ward staff are experienced in tracheostomy care, the critical care outreach team should be included within the multidisciplinary team. Tracheostomies are increasingly being used in various clinical areas, many Trusts therefore provide or purchase study days about tracheostomy care, which staff should attend.

References and further reading

Amathieu, R., Sauvat, S., Reynaud, P., Slavov, V., Luis, D., Dinca, A., Tual, L., Bloc, S. & Dhonneur, G. (2012). Influence of the cuff pressure on the swallowing reflex in tracheostomized intensive care unit patients. *British Journal of Anaesthesia.* **108** (4), 578–83.

Chadda, K., Louis, B., Benaïssa, L., Annane, D., Gajdos, P., Raphaël, J.C. & Lofaso, F. (2002). Physiological effects of decannulation in tracheostomized patients. *Intensive Care Medicine.* **28** (12), 1761–67.

Docherty, B. & Bench, S. (2002). Tracheostomy management for patients in general ward settings. *Professional Nurse.* **18** (2), 100–104.

Intensive Care Society (2014). *Standards for the care of adult patients with a temporary tracheostomy.* London: ICS.

Mercuri, L.G. (2012). Avoiding and managing temporomandibular joint total joint replacement surgical site infections. *Journal of Oral and Maxillofacial Surgery.* **70** (10), 2280–89.

National Confidential Enquiry into Patient Outcome and Death (2014). *On the Right Trach?* London: NCEPOD.

NHS Quality Improvement Scotland (2007). *Best Practice Statement: Caring for the Patient with a Tracheostomy.* Edinburgh: NHS Quality Improvement Scotland.

Nolan, J.P. & Kelley, F.E. (2011). Airway challenges in critical care. *Anaesthesia.* **66** (2), 81–92.

Regan, E.N. (2009). How to care for a patient with a tracheostomy. *Nursing.* **39** (8), 34–39.

Romero, C.M., Marambio, A., Larrondo, J., Walker, K., Lira, M.-T., Tobar, E., Cornejo, R. & Ruiz, M. (2010). Swallowing dysfunction in nonneurologic critically ill patients who require percutaneous dilational tracheostomy. *Chest.* **137** (6), 1278–82.

St George's Healthcare NHS Trust (2007). *Guidelines for the Care of Patients with Tracheostomy Tubes.* London: St George's Healthcare NHS Trust.
https://www.stgeorges.nhs.uk/gps-and-clinicians/clinical-resources/tracheostomy-guidelines/ (accessed 14 June 2015).

Wilkes, A.R. (2011). Heat and moisture exchangers and breathing system filters: their use in anaesthesia and intensive care. *Anaesthesia.* **66** (1), 31–39.

Useful websites

UK National Tracheostomy Safety Project
http://www.tracheostomy.org.uk/ (Accessed 14 June 2015)

Intensive Care Society (2014). Standards for the Care of Adult Patients with a Temporary Tracheostomy.
http://www.ics.ac.uk/ics-homepage/guidelines-and-standards/ (Accessed 14 June 2015)

St George's Healthcare (2015). Tracheostomy guidelines.
https://www.stgeorges.nhs.uk/gps-and-clinicians/clinical-resources/tracheostomy-guidelines/ (Accessed 14 June 2015)

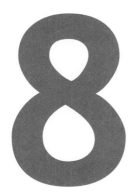

Suctioning a tracheostomy tube

Sally A. Smith

This chapter will describe how to suction a patient's tracheostomy tube safely and effectively. The purpose of suctioning a tracheostomy is to remove any secretions and to maintain patency of the airway. If the tube is not suctioned regularly, there is a danger that it may occlude and block the airway, which could lead to a respiratory or cardiac arrest (Intensive Care Society 2014).

Frequency of suctioning

Patients who have a tracheostomy require regular tracheal suction in order to:

- Maintain airway patency
- Prevent collapse of the lung, due to the small airways becoming blocked by secretions
- Reduce the risk of infection
- Maintain patient comfort.

The frequency of suction required will depend on the patient's needs and should be assessed and charted accordingly. Factors that should be assessed are:

- The patient's ability to cough and clear their own secretions
- The amount and consistency of secretions
- The patient's oxygen saturation and arterial blood gases
- The presence of any infection
- The size of suction catheter required.

Essential bedside equipment

The following safety equipment should be kept beside any patient who has a tracheostomy. Some of the items can be kept in a small plastic box within easy reach, in case a problem occurs. Such boxes for tracheostomy care are easily ordered from NHS supplies departments.

The bedside equipment should include:

- Oxygen supply (tested and functioning) with appropriate adapters
- Suction (tested and functioning) with pressure range 13.5–20kPa (120–150mmHg)
- Correct size suction catheters (see calculation method below)
- Yankauer suction catheter
- Bottled sterile water (labelled and dated)
- Gloves (non-sterile and disposable) and aprons
- Eye protection or full-face protection (if available)
- Humidification equipment (e.g. tracheostomy mask, T-piece, 'Swedish nose' – whichever is in use; all patients must have some form of humidification)
- Anaesthetic face mask, disposable bag-valve device, catheter mount, swivel connector
- Oxygen saturation monitor
- Tracheal dilators or Cottell's nasal speculums (sterile)
- Spare tracheostomy tubes (one the same size and one a size smaller)
- Spare inner tubes
- Sterile bowl and sterile water (labelled 'for cleaning inner tubes')
- 10ml syringe, water-based lubricant, tapes and dressing (keeping syringes by the bedside is controversial – please refer to your local policy)
- Patient call bell, communication devices, notepad and pen.

Calculating the required suction catheter size

It is important to select the correct size suction catheter. If the catheter is too large, it will occlude the tracheal tube, which may cause hypoxia. It is recommended that the catheter should be no more than half the internal diameter of the tracheal tube (St George's Healthcare NHS Trust 2015).

To calculate the appropriate suction catheter size, you need to deduct 2 from the tracheostomy tube size and then multiply the result by 2.

For example, if the tracheostomy tube size is 8:

$8 - 2 = 6$

$6 \times 2 = 12$

Therefore, for a size 8 tube, the correct suction catheter size would be French gauge (FG) 12. NB: For mini-tracheostomies, you should use a maximum size 10 FG suction catheter.

Essential suctioning equipment

The equipment required for suctioning a tracheostomy is:

- Functional suction unit with suction set at 13.5–20kPa (120–150mmHg)
- Sterile suction catheters (size determined as above)
- Gloves and aprons
- Bottled sterile water (labelled 'for cleaning suction tubing'; include date when opened and change water every 24 hours)
- Sterile 0.9% saline and syringe (in case they are needed)
- Oxygen therapy, wall flowmeter, tracheal mask

- Yankauer suction catheter
- Protective eyewear (goggles or visor)
- Sputum trap if required
- Correct coloured bag for disposal of waste.

The suctioning procedure

Step 1

First prepare the patient for the procedure, explaining what you are going to do and why. Ensure that the patient has privacy, and check that you have all the required equipment ready. This enables the patient to give verbal or non-verbal consent to the procedure and allows them to feel reassured. It is important to maintain the patient's dignity.

Step 2

Wash your hands. Put on a disposable apron, gloves and protective eyewear.

Step 3

It is advisable to monitor the patient's oxygen saturations during the procedure to check for hypoxia or any changes. You may need to increase the amount of oxygen they are receiving if they desaturate when receiving suction.

Step 4

If the patient has a fenestrated tube in situ, it is advisable to change the fenestrated inner tube to a non-fenestrated tube before suctioning. Suctioning with a fenestrated inner tube in situ may cause mucosal damage. The outside of the tracheostomy tube should be held firmly while the inner cannula is removed and the replacement inner cannula inserted. Holding the outside stabilises the tracheostomy tube, to reduce the risk of displacement, and maintains patient comfort.

Step 5

Turn on the suction apparatus and attach a sterile suction catheter. Ensure that the pressure is checked before use. It should be 13.5–20kPa (120–150mmHg). High pressures may cause mucosal damage. Put a glove on the dominant hand and *only* touch the sterile suction catheter with this hand. Introduce the suction catheter into the tracheostomy tube. Do not apply suction at this point. Gently but quickly insert it to 0.5–1.0cm beyond the tip of the tracheostomy tube or until the patient coughs. Then withdraw the catheter approximately 0.5 cm and apply suction. Withdraw the catheter slowly, applying suction continuously. This should take no longer than 15 seconds.

Step 6

Gentleness is essential. Damage to the mucosal area can cause trauma and infection. The catheter should go no further than the carina. Continuous suction is most effective in clearing secretions, but the catheter must be kept moving. Prolonged suction will result in hypoxia.

Step 7

Release the suction, remove the catheter and glove and discard, and re-apply the patient's oxygen supply immediately.

Step 8

Observe the patient throughout the procedure for any signs of distress or discomfort. This will also enable you to assess their response to suction therapy and how well they tolerate it.

Step 9
Rinse the suction tubing through with water. It is prudent to change the bottle of water for this use daily, and you should also change the suction tubing every day. This reduces the risk of bacterial growth. Ensure that the suction reservoir is not full, and change when required.

Step 10
Using a fresh clean glove and a sterile catheter, repeat the procedure until the secretions are cleared and the patient is breathing comfortably. Allow the patient sufficient time to recover between suction passes, especially if the oxygen saturation is low (ensure pre-oxygenation) or if the patient coughs several times.

Step 11
If you feel that the secretions are very tenacious, it may be worth considering saline nebulisers, but most definitely humidification for the patient. Do not forget to refer the patient to the physiotherapist for further care.

Step 12
Report your findings in the patient's notes.

Hold your own breath as you carry out the suctioning. If you begin to feel you need to take a breath, then you know the patient also needs to!

References and further reading

Burton, M.A. & Ludwig, L.J.M. (2014). *Fundamentals of Nursing Care: Concepts, Connections and Skills*. Philadelphia: FA Davis.

Nance-Floyd, B. (2011). Tracheostomy Care: An Evidence-Based Guide to Suctioning and Dressing Changes. *American Nurse Today*. **6** (7), 14–16.

Intensive Care Society (2014). *Standards for the Care of Adult Patients with a Temporary Tracheostomy*. http://www.ics.ac.uk/ics-homepage/guidelines-and-standards/ (accessed 14 June 2015).

St George's Healthcare (2015). *Tracheostomy Guidelines*. https://www.stgeorges.nhs.uk/gps-and-clinicians/clinical-resources/tracheostomy-guidelines/ (accessed 14 June 2015).

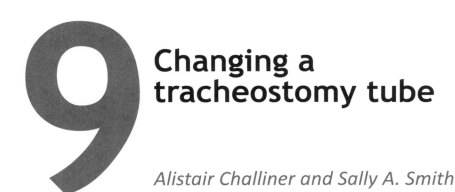

9 Changing a tracheostomy tube

Alistair Challiner and Sally A. Smith

Tracheostomy tubes with an inner cannula should be changed every 28 days or according to the manufacturer's recommendations. The decision to change a tracheostomy tube should be made by the attending physician in conjunction with experienced personnel and the physiotherapy team. A physician or anaesthetist should perform the tracheostomy tube changes, unless individual departments have expanded nurse role procedures in place. The person carrying out the procedure must be suitably skilled and competent.

The following equipment is required to change a tracheostomy tube:

- Dressing pack
- Correctly sized tracheostomy tube (a spare tracheostomy tube one size smaller should be within easy reach)
- Tube holder
- 10ml syringe (for cuffed tubes)
- Sachet or clean tube of water-soluble lubricant
- Sachet of normal saline 0.9%
- Tracheostomy dressing
- Sterile gloves
- Protective eye wear
- Tracheal dilators.

The tube changing procedure

Step 1

Explain the procedure to the patient and give the rationale for the tracheostomy tube change. The patient should give consent for the procedure (unless they are sedated, unconscious or the tracheostomy change is an emergency). It is safer to perform the procedure when an anaesthetist is available to deal with any difficulties that may arise. Planned tracheostomy changes (not urgent ones) should therefore take place during 'normal' working hours.

Step 2
It is recommended that patients are 'nil by mouth' for 3–4 hours before the tracheostomy change and nasogastric feeding should also be stopped. If a nasogastric tube is in place, this should be aspirated prior to the procedure. As the airway is unprotected when the tracheostomy tube is removed, starving the patient (or aspirating the nasogastric tube) will reduce the risk of aspiration during the procedure.

Step 3
Position the patient in bed in a semi-recumbent position, ensuring that the neck is extended and the patient is comfortable. Extending the neck allows for easier removal and insertion of the tracheostomy tube. The patient should feel as relaxed and comfortable as possible when preparing for the procedure.

Step 4
Wash your hands and prepare the dressing trolley.

Step 5
Pre-oxygenate the patient (if they are receiving oxygen) with 100% concentration for at least 2 minutes. Take care with patients with chronic obstructive pulmonary disorder; it may be more appropriate to increase their inspired oxygen by 20%, rather than delivering 100%. During the tracheostomy change, the patient will not receive oxygen and may be at risk of hypoxia.

Step 6
Two skilled practitioners should perform the procedure – one to remove the old tracheostomy tube and one to insert the new tube. This will ensure that the procedure is performed as cleanly and swiftly as possible. Both practitioners should wear eye protection. The first person should open the new tracheostomy tube onto the opened dressing pack and put on sterile gloves.

Step 7
If the tracheostomy is cuffed, check for air leaks in the cuff of the new tube by inflating it and deflating it, using the 10ml syringe.

Step 8
Lubricate the tracheostomy tube sparingly with water-soluble lubricant.

Step 9
Remove the old dressing and clean around the tracheostomy site.

Step 10
The second person (if necessary) suctions to remove secretions. When the patient stops coughing, release the tracheostomy ties. The tube may be more difficult to remove when the patient is coughing because the neck muscles may tense.

Step 11
There are two ways of changing the tube. One is to use the obturator (introducer) provided with the new tube. The other is to use an airway exchange device that acts as a guide to 'rail road' the new tube over, preventing insertion into tissue instead of the trachea.

- **If using the obturator**, check that it can be removed ready for the insertion of the new tube. Remove the old tube in an 'out, then down' movement on expiration. Then insert the new tube into the stoma, using the introducer in the tracheostomy tube lumen. Make sure that the first movement is at 90° to the cervical axis, then gently rotate down to allow the tube to pass into the trachea. This reduces the risk of creating a false anterior passage in the pretracheal space (Johnson *et al.* 2013). Remove the obturator immediately.

  • **If using an airway exchange device** (such as a sterile suction catheter with the suction controller cut off), it should be threaded down the old tracheostomy tube as a guide, just beyond the tip of the tracheostomy tube. The old tube can then be removed, and the new tube threaded over the guide catheter (or bougie), using an 'up and over' action, preferably on exhalation.

Step 12

Immediately remove the guide catheter (bougie) and observe the patient for signs of respiratory distress. Inflate the cuff and re-administer oxygen. Feel for respiration via the tracheostomy tube and observe the chest movements. Auscultate for equal air entry. The flow of air will be felt via the tracheostomy tube if it is in the correct position. Ensure that both lungs are inflating equally.

Step 13

If the tube insertion fails or the patient appears distressed and cyanosed, insert the tracheal dilators, remove the tube and insert a smaller-sized tube.

Step 14

If the new tube fails, administer oxygen via the stoma or maintain the patient's airway via the oral route and give oxygen via a mask. If airflow is not felt, the tracheostomy tube should be removed and a smaller one inserted (ensuring that it is well lubricated). The track may not have formed or the tracheostomy tube may have been advertently blocked during insertion. An arrest call should be put out in this case.

Step 15

Ensure that the patient is comfortable and breathing without difficulty.

Step 16

Observe the site for bleeding and, if applicable, ensure that the cuff is inflated. Excessive bleeding should be reported to the attending physician. A small amount of bleeding is common due to trauma at the stoma site. An inflated cuff will prevent aspiration of blood. Excessive bleeding may require further treatment.

Step 17

Record the tube change in the patient's notes, with the time, date, size and type of tube, including any complications that occurred during the procedure. You will need to insert the sticker that comes with the new tube in the patient's notes.

References and further reading

Intensive Care Society (2014). *Standards for Care of Adult Patients with Temporary Tracheostomies.* Standards and Guidelines. London: ICS.

Johnson, W.A., Pinto, J.M., Paz, M. & Baroody, F.M. (2013). *Tracheostomy Tube Change.* http://emedicine.medscape.com/article/1580576-overview (accessed 15 June 2015).

Lindman, J.P., Morgan, C.E., Peralta, R. et al. (2015). *Tracheostomy.* http://emedicine.medscape.com/article/865068-overview (accessed 15 June 2015).

NHS Greater Glasgow and Clyde (2014). *Changing a Tracheostomy Tube.* http://www.nhsggc.org.uk/about-us/professional-support-sites/shock-team/guidelines-for-care-of-patients-with-a-tracheostomy-tube/changing-a-tracheostomy-tube/ (accessed 15 June 2015).

St George's Healthcare (2015). *Tracheostomy guidelines.* https://www.stgeorges.nhs.uk/gps-and-clinicians/clinical-resources/tracheostomy-guidelines/ (accessed 14 June 2015).

▪ A B C D E ▪

Breathing

10 Obtaining and interpreting arterial blood gases

Ann M. Price and Sally A. Smith

Breathing is vital to maintain life and essential in order to transport oxygen and carbon dioxide between the external environment and the internal body systems. This chapter will focus on the practicalities of obtaining arterial blood samples in the ward setting and will give you a basic understanding of arterial blood gas (ABG) interpretation.

Assessment of signs and symptoms of breathing/respiration difficulties have been comprehensively addressed in Chapters 2 and 3. It is vital to assess the patient fully *before* undertaking arterial blood gases. Arterial blood gases assist in directing treatment and observing effect but they do not replace physical examination of the patient, which is essential in order to make a diagnosis.

Throughout this book, the authors refer to situations when you should consider obtaining arterial blood gases. Please read the chapters that are relevant to your own healthcare setting, to understand when ABGs may be indicated. Please also remember that specialist staff (who are trained in obtaining samples, processing them and interpreting the results) are vital for the patient's safety. They ensure that accurate information is provided and treatment is managed effectively. Experienced members of the team (such as critical care outreach and the medical emergency team) should therefore be utilised to assist with arterial blood gas sampling and interpretation as required.

Radial arterial puncture

This section outlines the technique for obtaining an arterial blood sample from the radial artery. Radial artery samples are often required in ward areas when caring for acutely ill patients, and blood gases are like a window to a patient's body, informing the practitioner of key physiological changes. A common reason for taking an arterial sample is to assess oxygenation, ventilation and the acid–base status during acute illness – for example, in a patient who becomes acutely breathless, or who is receiving non-invasive ventilation, or who is a diabetic in crisis.

Radial arteries are small but close to the skin's surface and can often be located quite easily. Before a sample is taken, collateral circulation must be checked using Allen's test (see Table 10.1).

Table 10.1 Allen's test

1	Ask the patient to clench their hand tightly for several seconds.
2	Compress both the radial and ulnar arteries, occluding them.
3	Ask the patient to open their hand, which should appear blanched.
4	Remove the pressure from the ulnar artery, whilst maintaining pressure over the radial; colour should return quickly to the palm from the ulnar artery.
5	If colour does not return quickly, do not take arterial gases from this arm, as circulation to the limb may be compromised.

It is also important to ensure there are no contraindications to sampling, such as poor collateral circulation, or cellulitis around the site. Other considerations include: impaired coagulation, liver disease or low platelets.

Equipment needed for taking the blood sample

The essential items are:

- Cleaning agent
- Gauze
- Blood gas syringe
- Dressing.

Local anaesthetic (EMLA cream or lidocaine) is optional – please follow your own hospital's procedures. Subcutaneous infiltration of the skin with lidocaine via a 23 G needle (and allowing time for it to work) will make the procedure more comfortable for patients. This is particularly so when repeated samples are required and finding the artery is difficult.

Blood sampling procedure

This procedure is that given by Bucher (2001). Other examples can be found online (Geeky Medics Medicine 2014) or sourced in other texts (Foxall 2008, Mallett *et al.* 2013).

Step 1
Explain to the patient what you are about to do.

Step 2
Clean the site.

Step 3
Palpate the artery.

Step 4
With the bevel of the needle facing upward, insert the heparinised syringe (ideally a designated blood gas syringe) into the artery at an angle of 30–45°.

Step 5
A pulsatile backflow of blood into the syringe indicates that the artery has been punctured.

Step 6
Stabilise the syringe and withdraw the sample.

Step 7

Remove, then apply pressure with sterile gauze to the puncture site for 5 minutes, or until the puncture has stopped bleeding.

Ongoing care

Ensure that the site is checked for haematoma formation every 15 minutes for the first half hour, then every 30 minutes for the next 2 hours.

Arterial blood sample analysis

Arterial blood samples should be capped, gently agitated (not shaken, as the sample will haemolyse) and processed through a blood gas analysis machine as quickly as possible. Each blood gas analysis machine has recommended procedures for processing samples, and staff must follow these instructions to ensure that accurate information is obtained. In cases where processing may be delayed, the sample can be transported in ice to reduce sample decay.

Staff processing gas samples should ensure that they are familiar with local policy. They should also be aware of signs indicating that the sample may have degraded and the results may be inaccurate.

Interpreting arterial blood gases

The most important aspect of arterial blood gas interpretation is to be able to recognise normal ones and therefore to know when something is abnormal – identification of the specific abnormalities comes with practice.

This brief guide aims to give you a logical method of identifying abnormal arterial blood gases, based on Mays' (1995) tic-tac-toe method. When two of these three components (pH, CO_2 or HCO_3) fall into the same category, you should be able to identify which type of condition the patient has.

The values considered normal for arterial blood gases vary slightly, depending which book you read. However, a fairly standard 'normal' has been stated by Jevons & Ewens (2012) and these values are shown in Table 10.2 (below):

Table 10.2 What is normal?

Measurement	Range
PH	7.35–7.45
PCO_2 (carbon dioxide)	4.5–6.0kPa
PO_2 (oxygen)	10.0-12kPa on air
HCO_3 (bicarbonate)	22–26mmol/litre
Base excess (BE)	-2 to +2
Saturation	>95%

PO_2 and PCO_2 indicate the 'partial pressure' of oxygen and carbon dioxide gases within the artery – thus it is always presented in this way.

pH

The pH indicates the acidity or alkalinity of the blood. Blood is normally very slightly alkaline. Because the blood pH is usually in such a narrow range (just 0.10), slight changes towards acid or alkaline have significant effects on the body. Most of the effects on blood gases are an attempt to bring the pH back to a normal range (Figure 10.1).

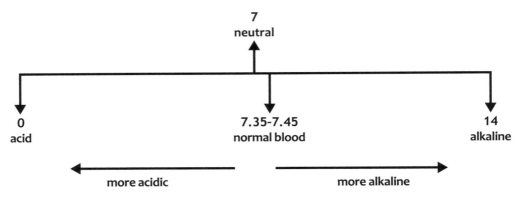

Figure 10.1 *Acid and alkaline ranges.*

The pH reflects hydrogen ions (H+) in the blood. High H+ concentration leads to acidosis (pH >7.35), and low H+ leads to alkalosis (pH.7.45).

The role of carbon dioxide

Hydrogen ions are formed when carbon dioxide (CO_2), a waste product of respiration, combines with water – thus CO_2 is considered to be an acid. In respiratory failure, CO_2 will increase and so lead to acid build-up. In hyperventilation, CO_2 will drop and so lead to alkalosis.

Table 10.3 Carbon dioxide values

Acidic	Normal	Alkaline
pH <7.35	pH 7.35–7.45	pH >7.45
PCO_2 >6.0kPa	PCO_2 4.5–6kPa	PCO_2 <4.5kPa
Respiratory acidosis		Respiratory alkalosis

Respiratory acidosis will often be accompanied by poor saturations and low oxygenation (PO_2 <10.5kPa). However, there is no need to remove oxygen masks from patients with suspected respiratory failure in order to take an arterial blood gas, because their pH and CO_2 alone will indicate this.

The role of bicarbonate

Bicarbonate (HCO_3) is the main alkaline substance in body fluids. HCO_3 binds with excess hydrogen ions to reduce the concentration and maintain pH within normal limits. When HCO_3 rises (as in prolonged vomiting and Cushing's syndrome), a metabolic alkalosis will develop. In diarrhoea and renal failure, HCO_3 falls and a metabolic acidosis results.

Table 10.4 Bicarbonate values

Acidic	Normal	Alkaline
pH <7.35	pH 7.35–7.45	pH >7.45
HCO3 <22mmol/litre	HCO3 22–26mmol/litre	HCO3 >26mmol/litre
Metabolic acidosis		Metabolic alkalosis

Compensation

The body quickly compensates pH for an acidosis and alkalosis to provide the best environment for cell function. Compensation is easy to recognise – if you have a normal pH (7.35–7.45) but CO_2 and HCO3 are abnormal, you have a compensated arterial blood gas. The nature of the compensation will depend on the original problem – for example, respiratory acidosis will be compensated by a rise in HCO3. A quick method to work out compensation is shown in Examples 1 and 2 below.

Example 1

Acidic	Normal	Alkaline
	pH 7.36	
CO2 7.0kPa		HCO3 34mmol/litre

When analysing compensation in an arterial blood gas, you take the pH from the mid-point of the normal range – thus, below 7.40 is acid and above 7.40 is alkaline. The above example for a compensated respiratory acidosis (shown in the 'Acidic' column) therefore becomes:

Acidic	Normal	Alkaline
pH <7.40	pH 7.36	
CO2 7.0 kPa		HCO3 34mmol/litre
Respiratory acidosis		Metabolic compensation

Example 2

Acidic	Normal	Alkaline
	pH 7.42	
CO2 7.0 kPa		HCO3 34mmol/l

The CO_2 and HCO3 are unchanged but the pH is above 7.40. This therefore becomes:

Acidic	Normal	Alkaline
	pH 7.42	pH >7.40
PCO2 7.0 kPa		HCO3 34mmol/litre
Respiratory compensation		Metabolic alkalosis

Example 3

You can have *partial compensation*, where the pH has not returned to normal but the PCO_2 and HCO_3 are abnormal. The two factors will be in one column and the compensation on its own in the opposing column. For example:

Acidic	Normal	Alkaline
		pH 7.47
PCO_2 7.0kPa		HCO_3 34mmol/litre
Partial respiratory compensation		Metabolic alkalosis

Combined metabolic and respiratory problems

Occasionally you will see a combination of metabolic and respiratory components – acidosis is most common, often in a cardiac arrest situation. The patient has multiple problems to get a combination effect.

Example 4

Acidic	Normal	Alkaline
pH <7.35		pH >7.45
CO_2 >6.0kPa		PCO_2 <4.5kPA
HCO_3 <22mmol/l		HCO_3 >26mmol/litre
Combined respiratory and metabolic acidosis		Combined respiratory and metabolic alkalosis

Oxygen and saturation

If arterial oxygen levels (PO_2) are below 10.0kPa, the patient is described as 'hypoxic'. Thus, a patient with a low pH, a high PCO_2 and a low PO_2 would be described as having 'a respiratory acidosis with hypoxia'.

Saturations should be greater than 95% in normal adults. A saturation of 92–95% indicates that the patient's respiratory state may worsen, even though they may have a normal PO_2 level at that point. Saturations below 92% can indicate severe problems in transporting oxygen around the body. In such cases, urgent treatment is needed.

Base excess

Base excess (BE) is displayed on arterial blood gas results and indicates the amount of compensation the body is having to make to maintain a normal pH. Thus, a base excess of -12 is a severe level of compensation, whereas results nearer to -2 to +2 (normal values) will be less acute. For the purpose of working out acidosis and alkalosis, base excess is not needed.

Try working out the following examples (answers are given at the end of this chapter). For each one, you may find it helpful to copy the following table and fill in the columns:

Acidic	Normal	Alkaline

Scenario 1
The patient is in respiratory distress. Blood gases are pH 7.30, PCO2 6.9kPa, HCO3 24mmol/litre and PO2 9.8kPa.

Scenario 2
A patient is suspected of having renal failure. Blood gases are pH 7.30, PCO2 5.2kPa, HCO3 18mmol/litre and PO2 11.8kPa.

Scenario 3
A patient is admitted with a four-day history of diarrhoea. Blood gases are pH 7.46, PCO2 6.3kPa, HCO3 34mmol/litre and PO2 11.6kPa.

Scenario 4
A male patient has just been put on a ventilator and his blood gases are pH 7.48, PCO2 3.8kPa and HCO3 24mmol/litre and PO2 is 11.6kPa.

Scenario 5
A woman has been admitted with chronic renal failure – her blood gases are pH 7.37, PCO2 4.2kPa, HCO3 19mmol/litre and PO2 is 11.6kPa.

Scenario 6
A man who has had COPD for several years is admitted with acute-on-chronic respiratory failure due to pneumonia. His blood gases are pH 7.32, PCO2 7.2kPa, HCO3 33mmol/litre and PO2 is 9.5kPa.

Scenario 7
A patient is having a cardiac arrest. Blood gases are pH 7.29, PCO2 7.1kPa, HCO3 16mmol/litre and PO2 22kPa.

Conclusion

This chapter has offered a practically based overview of arterial blood sampling and interpretation. The key to accurate blood gas analysis is practice. If that is not feasible, it is vital to call on the advice of experienced practitioners. Above all, remember that blood gas analysis can never replace careful physical examination. The most important aspect is to 'look', 'listen' and 'feel', as this gives a more useful and immediate indication of the patient's clinical condition.

References and further reading

Bucher, L. (2001). 'Arterial puncture' in D.J. Lynn-McHale & K.K. Carlson (eds). *AACN Procedure Manual for Critical Care*. Philadelphia: WB Saunders.

Foxall, F. (2008). *Arterial Blood Gas Analysis: An Easy Learning Guide*. Keswick: M&K Publishing.

Geeky Medics Medicine (2014). *How to Take an Arterial Blood Gas (ABG) – OSCE Guide*. http://www.geekymedics.com (Accessed 16 June 2015).

Jevons, P. & Ewens, B. (2012). *Monitoring the Critically Ill Patient.* 3rd edn. Oxford: Wiley-Blackwell.

Mallett, J., Albarran, J. & Richardson, A. (2013). *Critical Care Manual of Clinical Procedures and Competencies.* Chichester: John Wiley & Sons Ltd.

Mays, D. (January 1995). Turn ABGs into child's play. *RN Journal.* 36–39.

Answers (Scenarios 1-7)

Scenario 1: Respiratory acidosis with hypoxia.

Scenario 2: Metabolic acidosis.

Scenario 3: Metabolic alkalosis with some compensation because PCO_2 is slightly high.

Scenario 4: Respiratory alkalosis.

Scenario 5: Compensated metabolic acidosis.

Scenario 6: Respiratory acidosis with some compensation.

Scenario 7: Combined metabolic and respiratory acidosis with too much oxygen being given.

11 Oxygen therapy

Debbie King

O xygen therapy can be defined as 'the administration of oxygen at concentrations greater than those found in ambient air'. It is used as a quick and simple way to avoid hypoxic tissue damage (Driscoll *et al.* 2008). However, oxygen therapy is not risk free. Indeed, in some cases, poor oxygen management has led to or contributed to patient death (National Patient Safety Agency 2009).

This chapter discusses the physiology of oxygen therapy, and describes indications for oxygen therapy in the acute ward. It then discusses the administration of supplemental oxygen, including prescription, the devices used (including high flow oxygen and humidification), monitoring, documentation and discontinuation of oxygen therapy. Lastly, there is a brief discussion of cautions that need to be observed when using oxygen therapy.

The role of oxygen in the body

All the body's cells rely on oxygen to meet their metabolic needs. Maintaining an adequate supply of oxygen is therefore essential in order to maintain cellular homeostasis.

Oxygen delivery to the cells occurs in three stages:

1. Oxygen first moves from the alveolus to the pulmonary capillaries, down a concentration gradient.

2. Oxygen is then carried, in the blood, to the cells. Around 2% of the oxygen is dissolved in plasma and the remaining 98% is bound to the haemoglobin in the red blood cells. The haemoglobin molecule contains four haem units and is said to be 100% saturated when all four haem units have oxygen attached to them. Thus, it can be seen that the body's capacity to carry oxygen depends on both the ability of the lungs to oxygenate the haemoglobin and the amount of haemoglobin in the blood.

3. Finally, the oxygen moves from the haemoglobin to the cells, down a concentration gradient (Porth 2010).

Oxygen therapy increases the pressure of oxygen in the blood by raising the concentration gradient at the alveolar pulmonary capillary level. This increases the concentration of oxygen diffusing into the arterial blood.

Indications for oxygen therapy

Oxygen therapy is used to treat hypoxaemia and should be given to all breathless hypoxaemic and critically ill patients (Driscoll *et al.* 2008). Hypoxaemia refers to low oxygen tension (or partial pressure) of oxygen in the blood. This is commonly measured non-invasively by oxygen saturation readings, or invasively by arterial blood gas readings.

Hypoxaemia can result from (Grossman & Porth 2014):

- Inadequate oxygen in inspired air
- Disease of the respiratory system
- Dysfunction of the neurological system
- Alterations of circulatory function.

If left untreated, hypoxaemia results in tissue hypoxia (Grossman & Porth 2014). In severe cases, it may lead to loss of consciousness, rapid organ failure and death (Driscoll *et al.* 2008).

Prescription and administration of oxygen therapy

Oxygen should be administered by staff who are trained in oxygen administration and they should follow local and national protocols. Oxygen is a drug and should therefore be prescribed on a designated document. However, in an emergency situation, oxygen should always be given first and documented later (Driscoll *et al.* 2008).

A prescription should include:

- The target saturations to be achieved – this will normally be 94–98% in acutely ill patients and 88–92% for patients at risk of hypercapnic respiratory failure (hypercapnia being defined as carbon dioxide levels above 4.6–6.1kPa)
- The starting dose of oxygen
- The initial mode of delivery
- Whether the oxygen should be administered continuously or PRN.

Staff should select the most appropriate device and flow rate and be empowered to titrate the oxygen to achieve the prescribed oxygen saturation (Driscoll *et al.* 2008).

Oxygen delivery devices

Oxygen delivery devices may be classified as variable or non-variable delivery devices. Variable flow devices deliver an oxygen concentration that depends on the flow of oxygen and the patient's breathing pattern. Non-variable devices deliver a fixed concentration, regardless of the patient's breathing pattern.

Nasal speculum

A nasal speculum is a variable flow device that can deliver low- and medium-dose concentrations of oxygen. Oxygen can be delivered at up to 6 litres per minute (LPM), although patients may experience discomfort with flow rates greater than 4LPM. Nasal cannulae allow the patient to eat, drink and speak, and are less likely to be affected by movement of the patient's face. In addition they are not associated with the claustrophobia sometimes experienced by patients when wearing an oxygen mask.

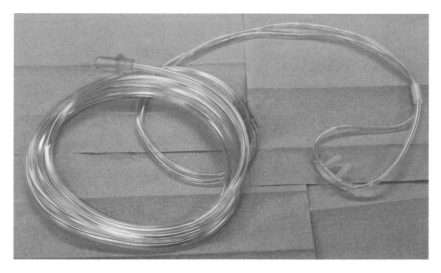

Figure 11.1 *A nasal speculum.*

Simple mask

A simple face mask is a variable flow device that will deliver oxygen concentrations of 40–60%, at an oxygen flow rate of 5–10LPM. As this device may deliver oxygen in concentrations above 50%, it is not recommended for patients who need low-dose oxygen therapy.

These masks cannot be used with an oxygen flow rate below 5LPM, as there is the risk of an increased resistance to breathing, and a risk of re-breathing carbon dioxide (BTS 2008). Although the device may be used with patients who have hypoxaemic respiratory failure, it should not be used with patients who are at risk of hypercapnic respiratory failure.

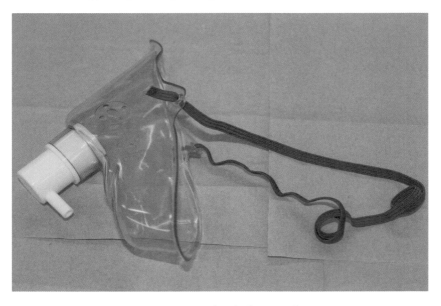

Figure 11.2 *A simple face mask.*

Venturi mask system

The Venturi mask system is a fixed flow device that will deliver a constant percentage of oxygen. It can deliver oxygen at 24%, 28%, 35%, 40% or 60%, depending on the valve fitted (the valves are usually different colours). Each valve has the flow of oxygen needed to deliver that percentage printed on it.

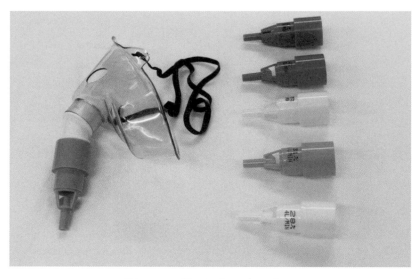

Figure 11.3 Venturi mask system.

Non-rebreathing system

This is a variable flow system that will deliver high-flow oxygen, and is suitable for use in emergency and trauma cases. A flow rate of 10–15LPM will deliver concentrations of 60–90% oxygen.

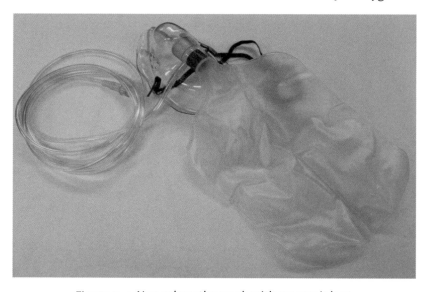

Figure 11.4 Non-rebreathe mask with reservoir bag.

Table 11.1 Overview of oxygen delivery devices

(based on Driscoll *et al.* 2008)

Device	Type of flow	Use	Cautions
Nasal cannula	Variable flow device	Low- to medium-dose oxygen therapy; 1–6LPM flow rates give approximately 24%–50% oxygen.	Uncomfortable with flow rates above 4LPM
Simple face mask	Variable flow device Should not be used with flow rates <5LPM.	Medium-dose oxygen therapy. Not suitable for patients at risk of hypercapnic respiratory failure, or those requiring low-dose oxygen therapy.	Flow rates of 5–10LPM give approximately 40–60% oxygen.
Venturi mask system	Fixed flow device	Delivers a constant, accurate concentration of oxygen. Suitable for all patients, including those at risk of carbon dioxide retention.	Need to ensure that the flow rate set is correct for the oxygen percentage required.
Non-rebreathing system	Variable flow device	High-dose oxygen therapy. Flow rates of 10–15LPM give approximately 60–90% oxygen. Can be used in emergency and trauma cases.	This is for short-term use, as the high oxygen flow dries the respiratory system.

Monitoring of oxygen therapy

Oxygen saturation — the fifth vital sign

A total of 98% of the oxygen passing over the alveolar membrane is carried in the bloodstream, attached to haemoglobin. The term 'oxygen saturation' refers to the extent to which the haemoglobin is saturated with oxygen. This is one of the methods used to determine the level of hypoxaemia.

Oxygen saturation levels are measured using a pulse oximeter. Pulse oximetry must therefore be available wherever emergency oxygen is used (Driscoll *et al.* 2008). Patients should have their oxygen saturation levels measured for at least 5 minutes after starting oxygen therapy. Oxygen saturations should be measured again an hour after starting oxygen therapy, and then after 4 hours (Driscoll *et al.* 2008).

Subsequently, stable patients may then have their oxygen saturation measured four times a day, along with their vital signs and early warning score. Should the concentration of inspired oxygen need increasing to maintain target saturations, then oxygen saturations should be monitored for a further 5 minutes after the increase (Driscoll *et al.* 2008). However, staff should use their clinical judgement, and refer to local policies, for monitoring saturation levels more frequently or continuously in unstable or at-risk patients.

It is important to remember that using pulse oximetry to estimate levels of oxygen in the blood has a number of limitations (see Table 11.2 below).

Table 11.2 Limitations of oxygen saturation monitoring

(based on Driscoll *et al.* 2008).

Limitation	Consequence and recommendation
Poor peripheral perfusion	The accuracy of the measurement is reduced. Ensure that there is a good pulse pressure, to ensure accuracy of the readings. Using the probe on different fingers or toes or on the ear lobes may result in an improved pulse pressure.
Anaemia	Normal pulse oximetry measurements may be obtained in the presence of 'anaemic hypoxia'. As oxygen saturation readings do not measure haemoglobin, it is recommended that full blood count measurements should also be undertaken.
The presence of carbon monoxide levels (e.g. in smokers after having smoked a cigarette)	It is suggested that heavy smokers may benefit from a slightly higher target saturation range.
Skin pigmentation	This may result in over- or under-estimation of pulse oximetry readings.
Nail varnish and false nails	These can result in artefacts in readings. Ensure that nail varnish and false nails are removed before measuring oxygen saturation.
It does not give measurements for pH or carbon dioxide levels.	It is recommended that an arterial blood gas sample should be taken where clinically indicated.

Documentation

The oxygen saturation result should be documented on the observation chart, along with the oxygen delivery system, the patient's respiratory rate, pulse, blood pressure, temperature and early warning score (Driscoll *et al.* 2008).

Humidification

Patients receiving oxygen therapy may develop dehydrated airways due to inhaling a dry gas. This may result in viscous sputum that is difficult to expectorate (Woodrow 2007).

Humidification is the addition of water to a volume of gas (Smith & Ball 2012). It is not routinely needed for patients receiving low-flow oxygen or short-term high-flow oxygen (Driscoll *et al.* 2008). However, it may be required for patients who need high-flow oxygen therapy for more than 24 hours, those who have discomfort caused by upper airway dryness, or those who have viscous secretions and who are having difficulty expectorating (Driscoll *et al.* 2008). Humidification may be achieved by the use of a variety of devices (Smith & Ball 2012) or by the use of nebulised normal saline (Driscoll *et al.* 2008)

Apart from externally humidifying oxygen, the patient needs to be well hydrated – either by encouraging oral fluids, if possible, or by the use of intravenous or subcutaneous fluids (Woodrow 2007).

High-flow oxygen devices

Simple oxygen delivery devices often fail to meet the needs of patients with high oxygen requirements. Although non-invasive ventilation (NIV) has been associated with improved outcomes in this group of patients, it can be poorly tolerated, which may lead to the need for invasive ventilation (Kernick & Margary 2010).

High-flow oxygen devices offer an alternative for patients with type one respiratory failure. These devices may also be used for patients with chronic obstructive airway disease or asthma (Price *et al.* 2008). High flow (greater than 15LPM) humidified oxygen is delivered to spontaneously breathing patients via a nasal cannula, attached to a heat-humidified high-flow blended oxygen circuit (Kernick & Margary 2010). This high-flow oxygen meets the patient's needs, and the addition of warmth and humidification ensures their comfort and reduces the problems associated with inhaling a dry gas at high flow.

Discontinuing oxygen therapy

With treatment, most conditions that require the administration of supplemental oxygen will improve. The patient's improvement will be confirmed by a reduction in their early warning score. The amount of supplemental oxygen given can then be reduced – in line with the prescribed target oxygen saturations. Generally oxygen can be discontinued when the patient can maintain target saturations of 94–98% on air. After discontinuing oxygen, oxygen saturations should be monitored for 5 minutes, then re-checked after an hour (Driscoll *et al.* 2008).

Cautions

To reduce the risk of oxygen being connected to the wrong outlet device, outlets that deliver other gases should be removed from the wall or covered with a specially designed outlet cover when not in use (Driscoll *et al.* 2008).

Oxygen supports combustion and therefore patients should never smoke, and inflammable materials should never be used, during oxygen therapy (Ashurst 1995).

Conclusion

This chapter has discussed some factors that contribute to the safe administration of oxygen therapy. However, it should be read in conjunction with local policies and guidelines. Also, please note that the British Thoracic Society is due to publish updated guidelines in 2015.

References and further reading

Ashurst, S. (1995). Oxygen therapy. *British Journal of Nursing.* **4** (9), 508515.

British Thoracic Society (BTS) (2008). *Emergency Oxygen Use in Adult Patients.* https://www.brit-thoracic.org.uk/guidelines-and-quality-standards/emergency-oxygen-use-in-adult-patients-guideline/ accessed 20 July 2015).

Driscoll, B., Howard, L. & Davison, A. (2008). BTS guideline for emergency oxygen use in adult patients. *Thorax.* **63** (V1) https://www.brit-thoracic.org.uk/document-library/clinical-information/oxygen/emergency-oxygen-use-in-adult-patients-guideline/emergency-oxygen-use-in-adult-patients-guideline/ (accessed 26 November 2014).

Grossman, S. & Porth, C. (2014). *Porth's Pathophysiology, Concepts of Altered Health States.* 9th edn. London: Lippincott Williams & Wilkins.

Kernick, J. & Margary, J. (2010). What is the evidence for the use of high flow nasal cannula oxygen in adult patients admitted to critical care units? A systematic review. *Australian Critical Care.* **23**, 53–70.

National Patient Safety Agency (2009). *Rapid Response Report. Oxygen Safety in Hospitals*. London: NPSA. http://www.nrls.npsa.nhs.uk/resources/?entryid45=62811 (accessed 26 November 2014).

Porth, C. (2010). *Essentials of Pathophysiology: concepts of altered health states*. 3rd edn. Philadelphia: Lippincott, Wilkins & Williams.

Price, A., Plowright, C., Makowski, A. & Misztal, B. (2008). Using a high-flow respiratory system (Vapotherm) within a high dependency setting. *Nursing in Critical Care*. **13** (6), 298–304.

Smith, S. & Ball, D. (2012). Humidification devices. *Anaesthesia and Intensive Care Medicine*. **13** (9), 413–16.

Woodrow, P. (2007). Caring for patients receiving oxygen therapy. *Nursing Older People*. **19** (1), 31–35.

12 Pleural chest drains

Philip Woodrow

This chapter discusses drains used in the lungs, rather than cardiac chest drains. After finishing this chapter, you should be able to describe what pleural chest drains are, why they are used, and how to care for patients with pleural chest drains.

Background

There are two main body systems in the chest – the heart and lungs. Abnormal collections in either might require drainage. Chest drains inserted between the pleura of the lungs may drain air (pneumothorax), blood (haemothorax), pus (pyothorax) or fluid exudate/transudate (pleural effusion).

Case scenario

A 30-year-old man, with no past medical history, was playing football when he became suddenly breathless. Despite receiving 15 litres of oxygen via a reservoir bag face mask ('100% oxygen'), he remained distressed and unable to breathe adequately, with very low oxygen saturations.

Following a chest x-ray in the accident and emergency department, a spontaneous pneumothorax was diagnosed and a chest drain inserted. He rapidly became less breathless, and his oxygen saturations improved. He has now been transferred to the respiratory ward for chest drain management.

Pathophysiology

Each lung is surrounded by two layers, called pleura. Between the inner (visceral or pulmonary) and outer (parietal) pleura is a space containing a very small film of fluid – usually about 10ml. This thin film of fluid enables the two pleura to slide over each other, preventing friction when breathing.

Negative intrathoracic pressure normally ensures that the pleura remain adjacent to each other. This negative pressure is lost if the pleural wall ruptures, causing collapse (inwards) of the lung wall. Most pneumothoraces are spontaneous, caused by breakdown of a bleb, or blister (MacDuff *et al.* 2010) but a minority are caused by trauma, including thoracic surgery and other procedures.

Spontaneous pneumothoraces

Spontaneous pneumothoraces typically occur in two groups of people (Roskelly & Smith 2011):

- Otherwise healthy adults, usually tall men
- Older people with emphysema or other chronic/severe lung diseases.

Pneumothoraces can be classified as either simple or tension.

- A **simple pneumothorax** is one in which part of the lung has simply collapsed, causing loss of space for ventilation.
- A **tension pneumothorax** is one in which the leak persists, creating a 'one-way valve' that draws more air into the pleura with every inward breath. As this air cannot escape, tension pneumothoraces cause progressive lung collapse with each breath, often mediastinal shift, and potentially cardiac tamponade with pulseless electrical activity (PEA) cardiac arrest. A tension pneumothorax is therefore an emergency (Roskelly & Smith 2011).

Pleural effusions

Pleural effusions, abnormal fluid collections in the pleural space, are often smaller than a pneumothorax, so they may resolve spontaneously. Larger collections need drainage. They are usually caused by exudate, but can be caused by transudate.

- **Exudate** may occur with infection, cancer, trauma, surgery or other diseases causing tissue damage to the pleura.
- **Transudate** occurs when fluid is pulled abnormally into the pleural space, which may happen with heart failure, hypoproteinaemia (e.g. liver disease or nephrotic syndrome) or occasionally other conditions creating abnormal osmotic pull (e.g. peritoneal dialysis).

Testing pleural fluid for protein can identify whether fluid is transudate (<30 grams per litre of protein) or exudate (>30 grams per litre of protein).

Malignant pleural effusions, caused by lung cancer, necessitate repeated chest drain insertion, often for prolonged periods. Drainage occlusion and pleural infections are relatively common with malignant pleural effusions (Medford & Maskell 2005).

Treatment

A pneumothorax, or pleural effusion, is usually diagnosed by chest x-ray, although breathlessness, (new) asymmetrical breathing, absence of lung sounds and (often) clinical history may indicate diagnosis. Underlying causes (such as infection) should be treated, and system support (such as oxygen) is usually needed. However, the main treatment for abnormal collections of air, blood, pus or other fluid in the lungs is to remove it.

A small (<20%) pneumothorax may be treated by percutaneous needle aspiration (PCNA), but larger collections are removed with chest drains. Air is usually best removed by inserting drains higher in the lungs (air rises), while fluid is usually removed by placing drains lower (fluid falls).

Chest drains

A chest drain is the tube inserted into the patient for drainage. If a drain is left in place, it will be attached to a collection chamber. Being below the patient, the collection chamber creates a siphon, which drains by means of gravity. In everyday practice, the collection system is often erroneously referred to as a 'chest drain', as the drain actually sits between the lung pleura.

In the past, wide-bore (24–28 FG) chest drains were often used. Although these are still available, and might be used in an emergency or for a haemothorax (Light 2011), larger tubes are more painful and create many complications. For these reasons, smaller drains (10–14 FG), which are equally effective, are usually now used (Fysh *et al.* 2010, Davies *et al.* 2010, Cafarotti *et al.* 2011, Galbois *et al.* 2012).

Placement of chest drains

The optimal site for insertion of a chest drain is the fifth intercostal space, anterior to the mid-axillary line. This is more comfortable than posterior placement, and leaves a less obvious scar.

The larger drains are inserted using a surgical technique under local anaesthesia, placing the tube through the intercostal muscle, with subsequent suturing to close the incision. Larger drains are usually used in major trauma or during surgery, when there is a need to drain blood and clots.

To drain non-blood fluid, the Seldinger technique is commonly used. This method involves passing a wire through a needle and subsequent dilation of the track and insertion of the drain. It is carried out most safely when guided by ultrasound.

When inserting a chest drain based on chest x-ray findings, it is essential to check which side the drain is to be placed, to avoid the risk of injuring the wrong side of the thorax.

A tension pneumothorax is an emergency, necessitating urgent treatment from an experienced practitioner. In this case, a cannula is placed in the mid-clavicular line (in the second intercostal space, just above the third rib), to decompress it.

Protection from infection

A seal or valve is needed to prevent infection entering the pleura. Historically, the seal was created by placing the drainage tube in sterile water. This is called an 'under water seal drain' or UWSD (see Figure 12.1). Although UWSDs are still used, they are increasingly being replaced by 'dry' collection systems (see Figure 12.2), which use a mechanical ('Heimlich') valve to prevent back-flow.

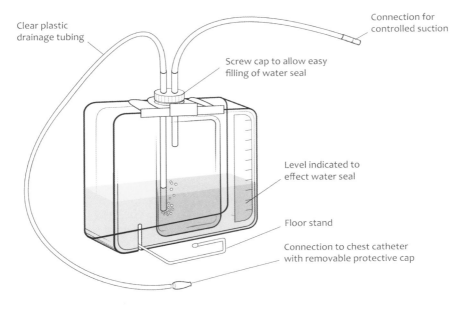

Figure 12.1 *Under water seal drainage system.*

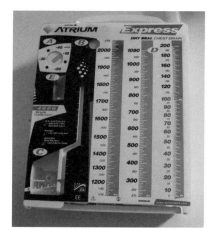

Figure 12.2 A 'dry' drainage system.

With under water seal systems, an exit tube above the water line allows air to escape, so the drained fluid can fill the chamber. Dry chambers use an exit valve for the same purpose. In the past, exit tubing was often connected to external suction, in the belief that this increased drainage. Although this seems logical, there is little evidence that additional suction increases drainage, and using it is more likely to cause pulmonary oedema (MacDuff et al. 2010). National guidelines therefore discourage adding vacuum suction. If suction is used, -10 to -20cmH$_2$O is recommended (Havelock et al. 2010).

HOT TIP

Unless suction is used, drainage relies on gravity, which will only work if the collection chamber is below the patient's chest. If the chamber is above the patient's chest, backflow can increase the size of the pneumothorax. Make sure that patients and visitors are aware of the reasons why the chest drain must never be lifted to or above the level of the chest.

Monitoring and management of pleural drainage

The wound dressing should be inspected at least once each shift, and the site should be securely covered with a non-adhesive dressing. Jones (2011) recommends using a transparent adhesive dressing, but 'keyhole' cannula or tracheostomy dressings will often create a more effective seal. Dressings used should be recorded in the care plan. If visibly soiled or infected, dressings should be changed. Otherwise, they should be left intact as long as needed and as recommended by the manufacturer.

Connections between the drain and the collection chamber should be checked to ensure that they are secure and airtight (disconnection would increase the pneumothorax). If suction is used (see below), the pressure should be checked at least once each shift. Collection chambers should only be changed when they are full, to minimise the risk of infection from changes (Allibone 2003, Durai et al. 2010).

Chest drains should be monitored for:

- Swinging (if suction is not used)
- Bubbling
- Draining.

Air draining causes bubbling in the water (dry systems usually include a small chamber of water for observing this). Fluid drained will not bubble, but will accumulate in the collection chamber. If external suction is used, drains will not swing. Swinging may cease because the drain is blocked, or because the patient's chest has re-expanded (Gallon 1998).

With under water seal systems, the initial fluid level should be marked. Almost invariably, manufacturers use plastic that can be written on. The drainage level should therefore be marked frequently (at least each shift) and measured (at least each day). Volume, colour and type of drainage should be recorded; if infection is suspected, a sample may be required for microscopy.

Rapid initial drainage may cause pulmonary oedema, so if more than 1500ml drains in the first hour, the drain should be clamped (Havelock *et al.* 2010). Respiratory observations (rate, depth, saturation, supplementary oxygen – see Chapter 2) should be monitored regularly (normally at least every 4 hours) while the chest drain is in place.

Flushing catheters

Narrow chest drains may get blocked by clots. National guidelines recommend flushing regularly with 20–30ml saline via a three-way tap (Davies *et al.* 2010). However, as the drain (rather than the collection chamber tubing) is likely to be the site of blockage, flushing is unlikely to be effective unless flushed into the pleura. This procedure should only be undertaken by experienced specialists. Thrombolytics, which used to be recommended for preventing blockage, are not beneficial (Davies *et al.* 2010).

Clamping

Clamping tubing can convert a simple pneumothorax into a tension pneumothorax. Tubing should therefore only be clamped when it is unavoidable, for as little time as possible, and with a member of staff in constant attendance. The only indications for clamping are:

- Disconnection
- Rapid drainage (see above)
- Changing collection chambers
- Moving collection chambers above the patient (avoid if possible)
- Briefly (1 hour), following sclerosant instillation (Roberts *et al.* 2010).

Pain management

Unnecessary pain was the second-largest cause (after fatalities) for chest drain-related claims against the NHS Litigation Authority between 1995 and 2006 (National Patient Safety Agency 2008). Pain on inspiration will discourage deep breathing, and this will predispose the patient to chest infections. To reduce this risk, sufficient analgesia should be prescribed, and patients should be assessed for pain.

Position

Sitting semi-upright helps people breathe more effectively, and assists drainage (Allibone 2003). Early mobilisation reduces mortality (Martinson *et al.* 2001) and should therefore be encouraged. Most collection chambers used today are relatively small and durable, and often provide easy ways to be carried. However, patients (and carers) should be reminded that chest drain collection chambers must always be kept below chest level, otherwise pneumothoraces may recur.

Removing chest drains

Removal of chest drains is a medical decision. In the past, drains were often clamped for 24 hours before removal, but there is no evidence that this is beneficial (Havelock *et al.* 2010). If this is requested, the request should be documented. Expert advice is divided between advising the holding of breath in and out during removal (Bell *et al.* 2001). Physiologically, neutral intrathoracic pressure (from holding breath out), rather than negative intrathoracic pressure (from holding breath in), would seem more advisable.

Fine-bore tubes (FG 10–14) are not usually sutured. If sutures are used, they should be 'mattress' sutures, which require two people for removal (Havelock *et al.* 2010). Following removal, an occlusive dressing (such as a hydrocolloid) should be placed over the drain site. Lung re-expansion should then be checked with a chest x-ray, and the patient's respiratory function should be closely monitored for 24 hours, as pneumothoraces can recur.

Conclusion

Chest drains are a medical solution to a medical problem. If left in place, the drain and collection system exposes patients to various risks, which can be kept to a minimum with skilled care. Chest drains should therefore be managed on wards that are familiar with their use (Havelock *et al.* 2010), and care should follow national and local guidelines.

References and further reading

Allibone, L. (2003). Nursing management of chest drains. *Nursing Standard.* **17** (22), 45–54.

Bell, R.L., Ovadia, P., Abdullah, F., Spector, S. & Rabinovici, R. (2001). Chest tube removal; end-inspiration or end-expiration? *Journal of Trauma.* **50** (4), 674–77.

Cafarotti, S., Dall'Armi, V., Cusumano, G., Margaritora, S., Meacci, E., Lococo, F., Vita, M.L., Porziella, V., Bonassi, S., Cesario, A. & Granone, P. (2011). Small-bore wire-guided chest drains: Safety, tolerability, and effectiveness in pneumothorax, malignant effusions, and pleural empyema. *The Journal of Thoracic and Cardiovascular Surgery.* **141** (3), 683–87.

Davies, H.E., Davies, R.J.O. & Davies, C.W.H. (2010). BTS Pleural Disease Guideline Group. 2010. Management of pleural infection in adults: British Thoracic Society pleural disease guideline 2010. *Thorax.* **65** (2), ii41–ii53.

Durai, R., Hoque, H. & Davies, T.W. (2010). Managing a chest tube and drainage system. *AORN Journal.* **91** (2), 275–80.

Fysh, E.T.H., Smith, N.A. & Lee, Y.C.G. (2010). Optimal chest drain size: the rise of the small-bore pleural catheter. *Seminars in Respiratory Critical Care Medicine.* **31** (6), 760–68.

Galbois, A., Meurisse, Z.S., Kernéis, S., Margetis, D., Alves, M., Ait-Oufella, M., Baudel, J.-L., Offenstadt, G., Maury, E. & Guidet, B. (2012). Outcome of spontaneous and iatrogenic pneumothoraces managed with small-bore chest tubes. *Acta Anaesthesiologica Scandinavica.* **56** (4), 507–12.

Gallon, A. (1998). Pneumothorax. *Nursing Standard.* **13** (10), 35–39.

Havelock, T., Teoh, R., Laws, D. & Gleeson, F. (2010). Pleural procedures and thoracic ultrasound. *Thorax.* **65** (2), ii61–76.

Jones, S.K.B. (2011). *Chest Tube Dressings: A Comparison of Different Methods.* PhD Thesis. Ann Arbor, Michigan: University of Oklahoma/Proquest.

Light, R.W. (2011). Pleural controversy: optimal chest tube size for drainage. *Respirology.* **16** (2), 244–48.

Macduff, A., Arnold, A. & Harvey, J. (2010). Management of spontaneous pneumothorax. *Thorax.* **65** (2), pp. ii18-31.

Martinson, B.C., O'Connor, P.J. & Pronk, N.P. (2001). Physical inactivity and short-term all-cause mortality in adults with chronic disease. *Archives of Internal Medicine.* **161** (9), 1173–80.

Medford, A. & Maskell, N. (2005). Pleural effusion. *Postgraduate Medical Journal.* **81** (961), 702–710.

National Patient Safety Agency (2008). *Rapid Response Report: Risks of chest drain insertion.* NPSA/2008/RRR03.

O'Hanlon-Nichols, T. (1996). Commonly asked questions about chest drains. *American Journal of Nursing.* **96** (5), 60–64.

Roberts, M.E., Neville, E., Berrisford, R.G., Antunes, G. & Ali, N.J. BTS Pleural Disease Guideline Group (2010). Management of a malignant pleural effusion: British Thoracic Society pleural disease guideline 2010. *Thorax.* **65** (2), ii32–ii40.

Roskelly, L. & Smith, A.P. (2011). 'Respiratory Care' in L. Dougherty & S. Lister (eds). *The Royal Marsden Hospital Manual of Clinical Nursing Procedures.* 8th edn. Oxford: Wiley-Blackwell. 534–614.

13

Pulmonary oedema in acute heart failure

Julie Macinnes and Simon Merritt

Acute heart failure is a common cause of admission to hospital and is the leading cause of admission in people 65 years and older in the UK. It is characterised by respiratory distress, oedema and haemodynamic instability. It is potentially life-threatening so rapid treatment is essential.

After finishing this chapter, you should be able to define acute heart failure, understand its causes, rapidly assess a patient with acute heart failure, and understand how to manage acute heart failure.

Background

Acute heart failure occurs when there is a sudden reduction in the heart's ability to pump enough blood to meet all the body's needs. The body reacts by retaining fluid and constricting blood vessels in an attempt to increase blood volume and maintain pressure.

Acute heart failure has a poor prognosis, with 11% of patients likely to die in hospital and 30% dying within a year (National Institute for Cardiology Outcomes Research (NICOR), cited in NICE 2014). Improved outcomes are reported in cases where patients have early and continuing input from a dedicated, specialist heart failure team (NICE 2014). Immediate treatment goals are: to treat symptoms, restore oxygenation, improve haemodynamics and organ perfusion, and limit cardiac and renal damage.

Case scenario

A 65-year-old woman on the medical ward has been transferred from the coronary care unit after a recent myocardial infarction. You are concerned because she has suddenly become short of breath, pale and sweaty. Her observations are: respiratory rate 30 breaths per minute, oxygen saturations 89% on 35% oxygen, pulse 130 beats per minute, and blood pressure 120/90mmHg.

What would you do to stabilise and treat her? What investigations might she require?

The pathophysiology of acute heart failure

Acute heart failure occurs when neurohormonal mechanisms (involving the nervous system and hormones) are activated within the body (see Figure 13.1).

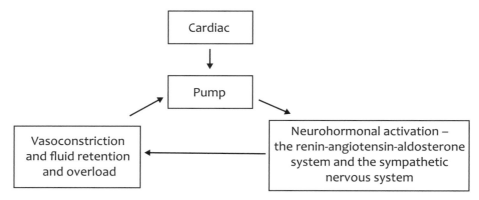

Figure 13.1 The vicious cycle of acute heart failure

Neurohormonal activation

A heart that is failing to pump blood effectively cannot generate enough pressure to drive the circulation. The drop in blood pressure stimulates the kidneys to produce a hormone called renin. This hormone triggers a cascade of chemical reactions, called the renin-angiotensin-aldosterone system (RAAS), which results in the kidneys retaining salt and water.

The increased fluid causes an increase in the pulmonary capillary pressure and an accumulation of fluid in the alveoli, which impairs gas exchange, resulting in hypoxia. This extra fluid is directly responsible for the symptoms of heart failure, including breathlessness and peripheral oedema (fluid accumulation in the tissues, commonly the feet and ankles).

In addition, the release of adrenalin and noradrenalin from the adrenal glands, together with stimulation of the sympathetic nervous system, causes the blood vessels to constrict – to try and increase the blood pressure. This also results in an increase in heart rate (tachycardia), which can trigger arrhythmias, most commonly atrial fibrillation. Pale, clammy skin is also a feature of sympathetic activity. Vasoconstriction and fluid overload put further strain on an already damaged heart and worsen the failure – hence, the vicious cycle.

Hypoxia

Hypoxia is a lack of sufficient oxygen in both the blood and tissues. The lower level of normal, in terms of partial pressure of oxygen in the bloodstream, is 11kPa; anything below this is termed hypoxia. If the pO_2 is <8kPa, then the patient is said to be in respiratory failure.

The causes of acute heart failure

Coronary artery disease is the most common cause of cardiac dysfunction. Acute heart failure can occur secondary to myocardial infarction, in which the death of part of the myocardium (heart muscle) reduces the heart's ability to pump effectively. Other, less common, cardiac causes include valvular disease (aortic or mitral), acute myocarditis (infection of the heart muscle), or an arrhythmia. Other non-cardiac causes include fluid overload (such as through over-enthusiastic post-operative fluid replacement), severe hypertension, or secondary to drug effects (for example, beta-blockers or tricyclic antidepressants). All these put strain on the heart and can precipitate acute heart failure.

In a ward environment, many cases of acute heart failure will result from a sudden deterioration in cardiac function in people with existing, chronic heart failure. This is termed 'decompensated' chronic heart failure, and characterises heart failure as a long-term condition punctuated by episodes of acute heart failure.

Assessing a patient with acute heart failure

Assessment, as well as management, of a patient with acute heart failure should be performed using the **ABCDE** method (see Chapter 2 for an overview of assessing and monitoring the acutely ill patient).

A-Airway

On assessment, the patient from the case scenario is short of breath and unable to talk in full sentences. You notice that she is agitated, but not confused. The fact that she is talking to you, and is alert, indicates that her airway is fine for now and not the major problem.

B-Breathing

The patient is sitting upright, with her legs hanging over the side of the bed. While assessing her breathing, you observe both sides of her chest are moving equally. Her respiratory rate is now 40 breaths per minute and her trachea is central. Percussion of her chest is equal and resonant throughout both lung fields. Auscultation reveals crackles that are audible during expiration, when listening posteriorly.

Her oxygen saturation has been measured at 89% (on 35% oxygen via a Venturi mask). An arterial blood gas should be performed (see Table 13.1 below). In acute heart failure, the PaO_2 would be lower than expected, considering the concentration of inspired oxygen being administered. Depending on its severity, there may also be a metabolic or respiratory acidosis.

Table 13.1 Arterial blood gas results on 35% oxygen

Arterial blood gas	Result
Oxygen	40%
PaO_2	7.5kPa
$PaCO_2$	4.2kPa
pH	7.44
Saturation	85%
Base excess	-1
Bicarbonate	21mmol/litre

A chest x-ray can be useful to determine the degree of pulmonary oedema (NICE 2014). This x-ray would classically show 'white, fluffy clouds' in the lung fields and the presence of bilateral perihilar alveolar oedema, giving a 'butterfly' appearance. It will also reveal the size of the heart and the presence of any pleural effusions that can occur in heart failure. Pulmonary congestion was evident on the case scenario patient's chest x-ray.

It is helpful, but not imperative, to perform your examination by first inspecting the patient and their surroundings, then palpating, percussing and finally auscultating. The patient from the case scenario is detailed here. However, it is important to note that in an emergency situation, assessment and treatment occur simultaneously (rather than one after the other, as described here).

C-Circulation

Assessment of this patient's circulation starts with the general observation that she is pale, which suggests she may be anaemic or has reduced peripheral perfusion. Her pulse is 130 beats per minute (regular) and feels weak. Her blood pressure was measured at 120/90mmHg several minutes ago.

Measuring jugular venous pressure

The jugular venous pressure (JVP) is 4.5cm. A raised JVP indicates fluid overload in the venous system.

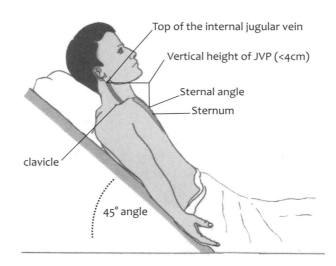

Figure 13.2 Measuring jugular venous pressure
(Diagram used with permission, adapted from Scott & Macinnes 2006, p. 506)

1. Ensure the patient is positioned on their back at an angle of 45° with their head resting on a pillow and their neck relaxed. (Note that patients who are breathless may find it difficult to lie in this position.)

2. Ask the patient to flex their neck slightly and look straight ahead.

3. Identify the pulsation of the internal jugular vein (it is normally visible just above the level of the clavicle). You will see the internal jugular vein pulsate twice for every one heartbeat (except if there is atrial fibrillation). Note the top of the pulsation.

4. Estimate the vertical height from the sternal angle to the top of the pulsation – it should be less than 4cm.

5. To locate the sternal angle, run your fingers along the clavicle to the midline – this point is the sternal notch. By running your fingers down the sternum at this point for a few centimetres, the sternal angle can be felt as a palpable 'lump'.

Monitoring heart rate and rhythm

Auscultation of the patient's heart reveals three separate heart sounds: the first two are close together and the third follows after a short gap. Together they sound like a horse galloping. This is a third heart sound, producing a so-called 'gallop' rhythm, which can be characteristic of heart failure. A laterally displaced apex beat is also characteristic.

The patient should be attached to a cardiac monitor to monitor her heart rate and rhythm. It is important to view a 12-lead ECG because she may be suffering from another myocardial infarction or may have an arrhythmia that has precipitated her failure, or more commonly this can occur as a consequence of heart failure. Table 13.2 outlines the 12-lead ECG findings commonly associated with heart failure. In this case, the ECG reveals a sinus tachycardia with resolving ST segment elevation and Q waves in the anterior leads (V1–V4).

Table 13.2
Common 12-lead ECG findings associated with heart failure

ECG finding	Characteristics and significance
Changes indicating acute myocardial infarction	ST segment elevation, deep Q waves and T wave inversion
Sinus tachycardia or tachyarrhythmias	Commonly atrial fibrillation
Broad QRS complexes (>2.5 small squares)	Indicates asynchrony between the left and right ventricles
Hypertrophy	Tall R waves and deep S waves in the anterior leads
M-shaped P waves; 'p mitrale'	Indicates mitral valve disease

The 'gold standard' for diagnosing acute heart failure is the echocardiograph (NICE 2014). This is essentially an ultrasound of the heart, which shows how well the heart is pumping. The measurement of an ejection fraction is an important diagnostic and prognostic indicator and should be performed within 48 hours of suspected acute heart failure. It quantifies the amount of blood pumped from the heart, compared to what is left. Normally, the ejection fraction in heart failure is <40%.

Another important diagnostic tool is the blood test B-type natriuretic peptide (BNP). A BNP of less than 100ng/litre helps to rule out a diagnosis of heart failure (NICE 2014). In this case scenario, an ejection fraction of 35% was reported and the BNP level was 400ng/litre.

D-Disability

Next, you need to assess the patient's level of alertness. This can be done using the 15-point Glasgow Coma Scale (see Chapter 34) or, more simply, the AVPU scale (see Chapter 2). This patient is agitated but alert and orientated, with a GCS of 15 and 'A' on the AVPU scale. In very severe heart failure, patients may become confused and drowsy, with reduced conscious level.

E-Exposure, environment and other aspects

Exposure involves a whole body assessment to observe for peripheral oedema. The case scenario patient has mild ankle oedema. Her skin is intact and she does not report any pain. Her body temperature should be measured, as this might indicate a chest infection, which may have precipitated her current deterioration. The temperature in this case scenario is 36.1°C, measured using a tympanic thermometer. In addition to ABGs and BNP, blood should be taken for full blood count (FBC), C-reactive protein (CRP), urea and electrolytes (U&Es), liver function tests (LFTs), thyroid function tests (TFTs), and the cardiac marker Troponin (TnT or TnI) in order to detect a further myocardial infarction (NICE 2014).

It is also important to measure the effects of under-perfusion of the vital organs, by means of renal function tests such as GFR (glomerular filtration rate). In heart failure, GFR will frequently be reduced from the normal range of 100–130ml/min. In this scenario, blood test results were all within normal limits – with the exception of Troponin I, which was raised as a result of the patient's recent infarct.

Assessment is an ongoing process and it is vital to continually reassess the patient, especially if their condition changes or following any treatment. Track and trigger systems (early warning scores) should be used to highlight any deterioration in the patient's condition to enable prompt intervention. Chapter 1 discusses early warning systems in greater detail.

Management of acute heart failure

Restoring oxygenation is an urgent priority. In the case scenario, increasing the patient's oxygen concentration (using a mask and non-rebreathe bag with 15 litres oxygen) to achieve oxygen saturations of >95% will help her breathing, as will placing her in an upright sitting position. Continuous positive airway pressure (CPAP) may be considered in severe dyspnoea if accompanied by acidaemia (NICE 2014). This provides a higher oxygen concentration and will also 'force' some of the pulmonary fluid out of the alveoli and back into the circulation. The application of CPAP is discussed in more detail in Chapter 16 on non-invasive ventilation.

Since treatment involves the administration of intravenous drugs, one or preferably two venous cannulae need to be inserted. Initial management of acute heart failure consists of pharmacological treatment. The aim is to relieve the symptoms of fluid overload using diuretic therapy (NICE 2014). An intravenous bolus of a loop diuretic, such as furosemide, usually at a dose of 40–80 mg, may be given. This may be followed by an IV infusion to achieve optimal diuresis. Furosemide is also an effective venodilator which reduces the work of the heart. The patient should start to improve relatively quickly, within 30–60 minutes. If they do not, then it is imperative to reassess, and seek assistance.

Spironolactone may be added. This is an aldosterone antagonist and so helps prevent further build-up of fluid. In this case scenario, 80mg furosemide was given. Ultrafiltration is an invasive treatment, which removes sodium from the blood. It is usually only considered when there is confirmed diuretic resistance in acute heart failure. Patients undergoing ultrafiltration will only do so within a critical care environment so a discussion of this intervention is beyond the scope of this chapter.

Venodilators, such as nitrates, should not be given routinely (NICE 2014) but might be considered if, for example, the patient has severe hypertension or valve disease. A glyceryl trinitrate (GTN) infusion relieves pulmonary congestion, dilates the renal arteries and so increases perfusion and diuresis. The usual concentration is 50mg of GTN in 50ml of 0.9% saline, prescribed at 0–10mg per hour, titrated according to blood pressure.

NICE (2014) does not recommend the routine use of opiates. However, opiates may be considered for some patients, as they reduce the heart's workload (due to venodilation) and reduce anxiety.

Diamorphine (2.5–5mg) and morphine sulphate (5–10mg) are often effective. Opiates reduce the sympathetic drive and relax the patient. In this scenario, 2.5mg IV diamorphine was given.

Diuretics, nitrate and opiates will all cause a drop in blood pressure. It is therefore essential that blood pressure is monitored frequently – half-hourly or hourly, depending on the patient's condition. A significant drop in systolic blood pressure (to <100mmHg or a mean arterial pressure of <70mmHg) should be reported immediately.

Inotropes, such as dobutamine and dopamine, should not be routinely administered (NICE 2014) but can be considered in acute heart failure where there is potentially reversible cardiogenic shock. In this situation, the patient should be transferred to a coronary care unit or high dependency unit where level 2 care can be provided. Cardiogenic shock is beyond the scope of this chapter but is discussed in Chapter 23.

The patient described in the case scenario received 15 litres oxygen via a non-rebreathe mask, which increased her oxygen saturation to 95% and reduced her respiratory rate. Administering 80mg IV furosemide and 2.5mg diamorphine resulted in effective diuresis and reduced anxiety. Her blood pressure was reduced to 100/60mmHg.

In acute heart failure, the use of a loop diuretic, such as furosemide, is the first-line treatment. Opiates, venodilators (such as GTN) and inotropes can be useful in specific circumstances.

The importance of monitoring acute heart failure

Regular monitoring of vital signs, including blood pressure, heart rate, rhythm, respiratory rate and SpO$_2$, are indicated in this patient. These would normally be performed half-hourly or hourly, depending on how stable the patient is. Vital signs should also include a 'patient at risk' or early warning score. A fluid chart should be commenced and completed accurately, with hourly fluid input and output recorded, particularly if the patient has been catheterised. Initially, it is helpful to calculate the ongoing fluid balance on an hourly basis, but once the patient has improved this can be reduced to four-hourly. Once the patient is more stable, daily weights give a good indication of fluid status.

Blood tests are required daily, particularly to detect a deterioration in renal function. Any deterioration in the patient's condition should be promptly reported to the clinical team caring for the patient and the specialist heart failure team if available, and re-assessment should be undertaken (see Chapters 2 and 3 on monitoring of acutely ill ward patients).

Once the patient is stabilised, it is important to commence medication that will preserve cardiac function in the longer term, improve the prognosis and prevent further hospital admissions due to acute exacerbation of heart failure. Beta-blockers, such as bisoprolol, reduce the work of the heart and should be started whilst in hospital, ensuring that the patient's condition remains stable for 48 hours before discharge. An angiotensin-converting-enzyme inhibitor (ACEI) such as ramipril, and an aldosterone blocker, such as spironolactone should also be considered.

Patients should be assessed by the medical team for their suitability for device therapy. For example, cardiac resynchronisation therapy (CRT) is usually combined with an implantable cardioverter defibrillator (ICD). Alternatively, the patient may be suitable for surgical intervention such as a valve replacement or repair or a heart transplant. In this case scenario, patient education and referral to specialist community heart failure nurses, where available, would also be beneficial.

HOT TIP

Remember, the echocardiograph is the 'gold standard' for the diagnosis of acute heart failure. The blood test B-type natriuretic peptide (BNP) helps to rule out a diagnosis of acute heart failure.

References and further reading

National Institute for Health and Care Excellence (NICE) (2014). *Acute Heart Failure: Diagnosing and managing acute heart failure in adults. Clinical Guideline 187* https://www.nice.org.uk/guidance/cg187 (accessed 3 April 2015).

Riley, J. (2014). Practical issues in acute heart failure management. *British Journal of Cardiac Nursing.* **9** (1), 18–23.

Spiers, C. (2011). Cardiac auscultation. *British Journal of Cardiac Nursing.* **6** (10), 482–86.

Scott, C. & MacInnes, J. (2006). Cardiac assessment: putting the patient first. *British Journal of Nursing.* **15** (9) 502–508.

14 Chronic obstructive pulmonary disease

Ann M. Price and Simon Merritt

In the UK, around 1 million people have currently been diagnosed with chronic obstructive pulmonary disease (COPD). However, there is thought to be gross under-diagnosis and the true number may be closer to 3 million (NICE 2011) (see Box 14.1). The annual cost to the National Health Service is around £800 million, and COPD is responsible for approximately 30,000 deaths per year (NICE 2011). As COPD is a preventable disease, there has been an emphasis on tackling it through health promotion (such as anti-smoking campaigns) and legislation.

Box 14.1 Why is COPD under-diagnosed?

There are a number of reasons why COPD is grossly under-diagnosed, not least the feeling among smokers that their symptoms are self-induced and 'par for the course', so why bother a doctor about them? Other reasons include a relatively large reserve in lung capacity (meaning that considerable lung destruction must occur before the development of significant symptoms) and the fact that COPD is often misdiagnosed as asthma or bronchitis.

By the end of this chapter, you will be able to define COPD, and understand its aetiology and pathology. You will also know how to assess, monitor and manage a patient with an acute exacerbation of COPD in a ward environment.

Background

COPD is characterised by airflow obstruction that is not fully reversible. The symptoms get progressively worse, and exacerbations may occur with sudden worsening of symptoms (NICE 2010). The main cause of COPD is cigarette smoking, although some people have symptoms due to occupational hazards; COPD is therefore considered a preventable disease.

COPD is diagnosed based on the patient's age (>35 years), the presence of a risk factor (usually smoking), shortness of breath, a cough (often productive) and wheezing (NICE 2011). Also, the clinician will perform a respiratory examination and spirometry measurements (demonstrating airflow obstruction), assess the degree of breathlessness using the Medical Research Council (MRC) dyspnoea scale and consider other investigations, such as blood tests and a chest x-ray (NICE 2011).

An exacerbation of COPD is 'characterized by a change in baseline dyspnea, cough, and/or sputum, that is beyond normal day-to-day variations, is acute in onset, and may warrant additional treatment in a patient with underlying COPD' (Lodewijckx et al. 2011, p. 1446). An exacerbation of COPD is an additional burden, leading to increased mortality rates, increased readmission rates and higher cost (Lodewijckx et al. 2011).

Case scenario

A 65-year-old man was admitted to the medical assessment unit (MAU) with a six-day history of progressive shortness of breath and a cough productive of thick green sputum. Although his Ventolin inhaler had initially helped with his breathing, it no longer seemed to be making any difference. Normally he was able to walk to his local newsagent's without stopping (500 metres), but on the day he came to the MAU he could manage no more than 5 metres.

His GP had diagnosed him with COPD two years earlier and he had been commenced on a salbutamol (Ventolin) and eformoterol (Oxis) inhaler. His last spirometry, eight months previously, revealed a forced expiratory volume (FEV_1) of 1.1 and a forced vital capacity (FVC) of 2.0 (see Box 14.2). He suffered from at least three chest infections per year, though none as bad as this one. He continued to smoke 10 cigarettes per day and had done so for the last 45 years.

Although he had already received treatment from the admitting medical doctor prior to coming to the ward, his shortness of breath had worsened and he had become a little confused. The staff nurse caring for him was concerned and asked you to review him.

If you were the doctor or nurse asked to review this patient, what assessment and observations would you perform, and how would you stabilise him?

Pathophysiology and aetiology

The damage in COPD is secondary to a smoking-induced chronic lung inflammation which causes airway narrowing and diffuse damage to the lung parenchyma (substance of the lung). In the larger airways, there is an increase in the size and number of the mucous glands, leading to increased production of thick mucus. Examination of the medium-sized airways reveals thickened and excessively contracted smooth muscle, while the smaller airway walls are oedematous and infiltrated with inflammatory cells. The alveoli have been variably damaged or destroyed (Braun & Anderson 2011). The extent of these changes differs in every patient.

Tests used to assess the severity of COPD are forced expiratory volume (FEV_1) and forced vital capacity (FVC). A ratio of FEV_1/FVC of <0.7 post bronchodilator is considered indicative of COPD (NICE 2010).

Box 14.2 FEV₁ and FVC

FEV₁ is the amount of air the patient can exhale in 1 second. It is reduced in COPD because of the narrowed airways.

FVC is the total amount of air the patient can exhale after a maximal inspiration. It is usually maintained in early COPD but decreases as the disease progresses, due to air trapping and lung destruction.

Age, sex, height and ethnicity all affect FEV₁ and FVC. Tables of normal values have been produced and are readily available. For example: http://patient.info/doctor/spirometry-calculator

Exacerbations

COPD exacerbations are commonly due to viral and bacterial infections of the tracheobronchial tree and to air pollution (NICE 2010). Typically the patient produces more mucus than usual, which is usually thicker and discoloured (green suggests a bacterial infection). Commonly implicated viral organisms are *rhinovirus* (common cold), *influenza*, *parainfluenza* and *coronavirus*, while bacterial pathogens include *Haemophilus influenza, Chlamydia pneumoniae, Streptococcus pneumoniae* and *Moraxella catarrhalis.* The cause of the exacerbation may be unidentifiable in up to 30% of cases (NICE 2004).

The pathophysiology of a COPD exacerbation comprises a catabolic state, airway narrowing, an increase in ventilation/perfusion (V/Q) mismatch (see Box 14.3) and an increase in both the volume and purulence of sputum. It is diagnosed predominantly from the patient's history. However, a chest x-ray (CXR), arterial blood gas (ABG) and lung function tests can also be useful.

Box 14.3 Ventilation perfusion (V/Q)

V = ventilation of lung

Q = perfusion (by blood) of the lung

In normal lungs, most of the alveoli are both ventilated and perfused, giving normal V/Q matching, which is essential for efficient gas exchange. In COPD there is variable destruction of both alveoli and pulmonary blood vessels. This results in areas of lung that are either ventilated but not perfused (dead space) or perfused but not ventilated (shunt), causing V/Q mismatch. This leads to inefficient gas exchange and, when advanced, severe hypoxia. An extreme example of dead space is a pulmonary embolus, and shunt in severe consolidation of the lung in pneumonia.

The full NICE clinical guidelines CG101 for COPD are available online at: https://www.nice.org.uk/guidance/cg101

Assessment

The assessment, as well as management, of a patient with an exacerbation of COPD should be performed using the **ABCDE** method.

On arrival in the MAU, the staff nurse should attach a cardiac and blood pressure monitor and an oxygen saturation probe and undertake a full set of vital sign recordings (for more on monitoring, see Chapter 2). It is helpful to perform the examination by first inspecting the patient and their surroundings, then palpating, percussing and finally auscultating.

The assessment of the patient from the above case scenario will be described here. However, it is important to note that, in an emergency situation, assessment and treatment would occur simultaneously (rather than one after the other, as described below).

A-Airway

On arrival at the patient's bedside, you find him lying down (which is clearly making it harder for him to breathe). He is very agitated and refuses to wear his oxygen mask. His lips and tongue and the tips of his fingers have turned a blue/grey colour. However, he is talking in full sentences, albeit nonsensical ones, and you can hear his expiratory wheeze from the end of the bed. Since he is alert and talking, you assess his airway as intact, but you are a little concerned about his confusion and so you decide to keep a very close eye on his level of consciousness. Any change in this may impact on his airway.

B-Breathing

His respiratory rate is 25 breaths per minute and his oxygen saturation is 94% on 40% oxygen, via a Venturi mask (when he keeps it on). Inspection of his chest reveals a decrease in chest expansion when he takes an inward breath; palpation of his trachea reveals it to be central. Percussion produces a rather hyper-resonant note, like tapping on a hollow wall. When auscultating his chest, you notice that his breath sounds are quieter than you would expect and that he has long polyphonic expiratory wheezes (see Table 14.1).

Table 14.1 Added breath sounds (based on Murray & White 1999 and Douglas *et al.* 2005)

Crackles (crepitations)	Non-musical or popping sounds mainly heard during inspiration caused by: • Reopening of occluded small airways, as in pulmonary fibrosis and pulmonary oedema • Air bubbling through secretions, as in bronchiectasis and consolidation. Crackles can either be fine or coarse. *Fine crackles* sound like very fine Velcro® being undone and suggest the presence of pulmonary oedema or fibrosis. *Coarse crackles* sound like a supermarket plastic bag being crunched and suggest bronchiectasis or consolidation. In the acute situation, it can sometimes be difficult to determine whether crackles are fine or coarse so the above is useful only if combined with the other examination findings. Asking the patient to cough is essential when crackles are auscultated, because they are not deemed significant if they disappear on coughing.
Wheezes	Musical or whistling sounds produced by air passing through narrowed airways, as in asthma and COPD. They mainly occur on expiration.
Pleural rub	Creaking sounds produced by movement of inflamed pleural surfaces – for example, in pleurisy. This is usually associated with pleuritic pain.

C-Circulation

Assessment of this patient's circulation begins with the observation that the blue/grey discolouration of his fingertips and lips has diminished, and his hands are now warm to touch and appear well perfused. His palms are erythematous (red). His pulse is 96 beats per minute and feels very strong; the character of this pulse is 'bounding'. A bounding pulse and erythematous palms can be an indication of carbon dioxide (CO_2) retention. His blood pressure is elevated, at 150/90mmHg, and jugular venous pressure (JVP) (see Chapter 13) is normal at 3cm. His heart sounds, although quiet, are also normal. Mild peripheral oedema is noted.

Assessment must be ongoing. It is important to continually reassess, especially if the condition of the patient changes or if you have given any treatment. Remember ABCDE.

D-Disability

It has already been noted that this patient is confused. It is therefore unsurprising that formal assessment of his alertness and mental disability reveals his Glasgow Coma Score to be 14/15 (see Chapter 34) and 'A' on the AVPU scale (see Box 2.1 on AVPU assessment, p. 12).

E-Exposure

Finally, the patient is systematically exposed to ensure that there are no other physical signs. There are none. However, his temperature is 38.2°C.

Investigations

A departmental chest x-ray had already been done and it revealed flattened diaphragm and hyper-expanded lung fields. There was no indication of any other pathology. The arterial blood gas was performed on 40% oxygen (delivered via Venturi mask) and the results are reproduced in Table 14.2.

Table 14.2 Arterial blood gas results at 40% oxygen

PaO_2	16.2kPa
$PaCO_2$	6.9kPa
pH	7.32
Saturations	98%
Base excess	+2
Bicarbonate	26mmol/litre

The results reveal a mild acute respiratory acidosis, with a high PaO_2. This may be partly due to over-enthusiastic oxygen therapy, and the oxygen concentration should therefore be reduced.

Respiratory failure type 1:

PaO_2 of less than 8kPa

In type 1 respiratory failure, the $PaCO_2$ is either normal or low. If left untreated, it has the potential to progress to type 2.

Respiratory failure type 2:

PaO_2 of less than 8kPa

Elevated $PaCO_2$ (i.e. over 6.0kPa).

If the $PaCO_2$ is sufficiently elevated, a respiratory acidosis can develop (pH drops <7.35). This has adverse prognostic implications.

Severity

Worrying features, specific to this case, include confusion, which may lead to poor compliance with treatment, and the presence of a bounding pulse and red palms, indicating possible CO_2 retention. Paradoxically, a normal (>95%) oxygen saturation is almost as concerning as a low one in this situation. Many patients with moderate to severe COPD have chronically low levels of oxygen and their bodies have, to some extent, adapted to this. Therefore, an individualised saturation target should be agreed (88–92% may be appropriate).

Elevating saturation in susceptible patients increases the risk of CO_2 retention and respiratory acidosis (NICE 2010). This occurs through a combination of a decrease in the central drive to breathe (a tendency to hypoventilate, causing a reduction in respiratory rate) and a worsening of the ventilation/perfusion mismatch in the lungs. High concentrations of oxygen may result in areas of the lung that are ventilated but not perfused by blood (i.e. increasing V/Q mismatch). See Box 14.3 (p. 111) for an explanation of V/Q mismatch.

It is important that medical staff administer oxygen to a hypoxic patient with COPD. However, this needs to be done in a controlled manner, with frequent monitoring of arterial blood gases and frequent clinical assessment.

Management

A-Airway

It has already been established that this patient's airway is intact. With any patient who is having breathing difficulties, it is helpful to sit them upright because this considerably improves the mechanics of breathing.

Although high-flow oxygen can potentially cause harm in COPD by sometimes leading to a high carbon dioxide level, its use is occasionally necessary. In the short term, a profound hypoxia is more likely to result in serious harm to the patient than a high carbon dioxide level. Therefore *in an emergency situation* (i.e. while waiting for senior assistance to arrive), sufficient oxygen should be administered to increase the saturation to 90% (but not higher), without thought for the carbon dioxide level.

B-Breathing

We already know that the patient in this case scenario is suffering from a mild respiratory acidosis, thought to be secondary to excess oxygen. It would therefore be wise to reduce the concentration until his saturations drop to 90–92%. In this case, the oxygen was reduced to 28% via a Venturi mask. It is important to repeat the arterial blood gas 20–30 minutes after altering the oxygen concentration, to ensure that the PaO_2 remains over 8kPa and that the pH is improving (becoming less acidotic).

If these variables are not improving, the use of non-invasive ventilation (NIV) should be considered (see Chapter 16). However, with the use of standard therapy (as discussed below), which includes controlled oxygen therapy, 20% of acidotic COPD patients will normalise their pH without the need for NIV (NICE 2010). See Figure 14.1 (algorithm for acute respiratory failure).

ABGs need to be monitored on a regular basis until the patient's condition has stabilised.

Bronchodilator drugs including short-acting beta-2 agonists (SABA), such as salbutamol, and short-acting muscarinic antagonists (SAMA), such as ipratropium, via nebuliser, would be the next treatment to start (see Box 14.4). These drugs are useful in treating bronchoconstriction, which is one of the many problems in COPD. Bronchodilators can also help to reduce air trapping, and therefore hyper-expansion. This reduces the sensation of breathlessness and improves the patient's tidal volume and minute ventilation.

Salbutamol has relatively short-lived effects and can be repeated on an almost continuous basis in the acute phase if required. The effects of ipratropium last for 4–6 hours. It should therefore be administered four to six times daily.

Box 14.4 Bronchodilators

Salbutamol: This short-acting beta-2 agonist is usually administered via a handheld inhaler or a nebuliser. In selected cases it is used intravenously. However, there is very rarely an indication to do this in COPD. It works via stimulation of beta-2 adrenoreceptors in the airway, and results in relaxation of bronchial smooth muscle. Common side effects include tremor, tachycardia and hypokalaemia.

Ipratropium bromide: This short-acting muscarinic antagonist can be taken via a handheld inhaler or nebulised. It works by competitively inhibiting muscarinic receptors on the airway smooth muscle, leading to bronchodilation by reducing vagal tone. Possible side effects consist of dry mouth, dilated pupils, urinary retention and constipation, but they are rarely troublesome.

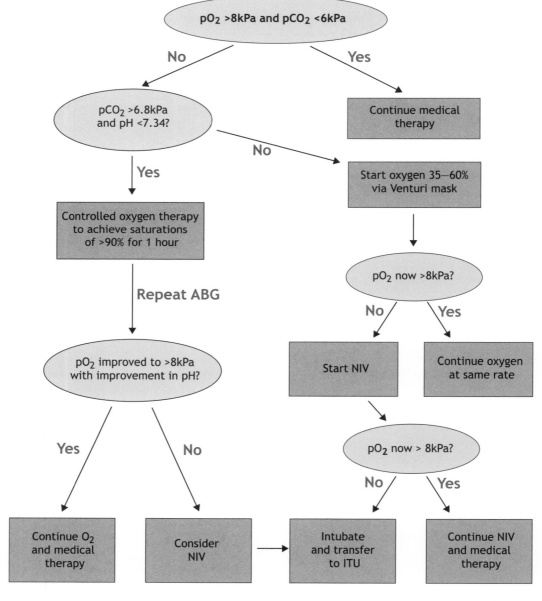

Figure 14.1 *Algorithm for acute respiratory failure (adapted from ATS/ERS COPD guidelines 2004).*

For the patient in the scenario, you should commence a nebuliser containing 2.5mg salbutamol and 500mcg ipratropium bromide. Once this nebuliser has finished, you reassess the patient and find that his respiratory rate has decreased a little and his oxygen saturations have improved. However, he remains quite wheezy so you decide to give him another 2.5mg of salbutamol immediately. He is prescribed both drugs to be nebulised four-hourly on the drug chart, with extra doses of salbutamol as required. Chest physiotherapy (see Chapter 4) is another useful adjunct to treatment of the COPD exacerbation, especially to aid expectoration and teach more efficient and comfortable ways of breathing.

It is essential that this nebuliser is driven on air, and not oxygen, to avoid the problems with carbon dioxide retention described earlier. Supplemental oxygen can be given simultaneously using nasal prongs — usually at a rate of 1—4 litres.

If the patient's breathlessness continues despite SABA and SAMA inhalers in an acute exacerbation, NICE (2010) recommends the use of theophyllines such as aminophylline (see Box 14.5) or, if the hypercapnic state continues, non-invasive ventilation (NIV). Other therapies that may be considered are long-acting beta-2 agonists (LABAs), long-acting muscarinic antagonists (LAMAs) and the use of inhaled corticosteroids (ICS). See NICE 2010 for full algorithms.

Box 14.5 Aminophylline

Aminophylline belongs to a class of drugs know as theophyllines, which work by inhibiting an enzyme called phosphodiesterase. In COPD their use may not be beneficial in mild to moderate cases, and there is a risk of side effects. However, they should be considered in severe cases where inhaled bronchodilators are insufficient.

Theophyllines cause relaxation of bronchial smooth muscle and therefore bronchodilation. They may also have positive effects on diaphragmatic contractility, and cardiac output. Sanders *et al.* (1980) suggested that, in addition to bronchodilating, aminophylline also appears to increase the respiratory drive. However, it seems that this is of relatively little importance.

Aminophylline is only a weak bronchodilator. It has many drug interactions and a narrow therapeutic ratio so side effects are common and include tachycardia, nausea, cardiac arrhythmias and convulsions. Aminophylline may be started as an infusion and may need a loading dose unless the patient is already on oral theophylline; drug levels should be measured.

Circulation

Circulation is not usually a major problem in the patient with an exacerbation of COPD except for the tachycardia commonly associated with nebulised salbutamol. However, it is good practice to establish intravenous access and take routine bloods for full blood count, urea and electrolytes, CRP and blood cultures in all acutely unwell patients. In this confused and drowsy patient, in whom compliance may be an issue, it would be wise to give the first dose of antibiotics intravenously.

Antibiotics are not always needed in a COPD exacerbation. Their prescription should depend on the presence of at least one of the following: a history of a change in colour of the sputum to green, an increase in its volume or purulence, consolidation on the chest x-ray, a temperature >37.5°C or a significant elevation in white blood cell count +/- CRP. Unless the patient is very unwell, oral dosing of amoxicillin, clarithromycin or doxycycline would normally be reasonable.

The poor baseline level of lung function means that patients with an exacerbation of COPD can take a considerable time to get better. However, the treatment described above will usually serve to stabilise most patients. The unwell COPD patient requires close monitoring and continual reassessment by the medical team; any further deterioration must be spotted early and treated appropriately.

NIV in a COPD exacerbation

This topic is thoroughly covered in Chapter 16. For this reason, only a few pertinent points are covered here. Non-invasive ventilation (NIV) is an effective and often life-saving treatment option and should be available in all hospitals admitting acutely unwell patients with COPD. It should be used in the presence of a persistent respiratory acidosis that has proved unresponsive to controlled oxygen therapy and nebulised bronchodilators (NICE 2010).

Ideally, before instituting NIV a decision should be made as to whether the patient is suitable for admission to the intensive care unit for intubation and ventilation. This decision should be taken by the senior doctor present, after consultation with the patient (if possible) and with their family. This decision is usually based on the patient's level of pre-morbid functioning and the presence or absence of co-morbidities. If there is any doubt as to the patient's wishes, the patient would ideally be intubated and ventilated for a limited period, with treatment withdrawn at a later date if it becomes futile.

There are usually concerns about admission to the intensive care unit and the difficulties of weaning this group of patients from mechanical ventilation. However, there is evidence to the contrary. For example, Esteban et al. (2002) found that patients receiving mechanical ventilation due to decompensated COPD had a significantly lower mortality than patients receiving mechanical ventilation because of acute respiratory failure of other aetiologies. The same authors also found a reduced length of mechanical ventilation for COPD, compared to patients with acute respiratory distress syndrome (ARDS).

Pulmonary rehabilitation

Patients with COPD are prone to repeated exacerbations and readmission to hospital. The British Thoracic Society (BTS 2013) recommends that COPD patients should be assessed for a pulmonary rehabilitation programme, with the aim of reducing dyspnoea, increasing muscle strength and aiding their psychological wellbeing. NICE (2010) suggests that when patients are discharged from hospital they should be referred for a pulmonary rehabilitation programme. Currently, the availability of these programmes varies but they may be important in order to reduce readmission rates.

Conclusion

The patient in this case scenario was treated by reducing his oxygen concentration to 28% via a Venturi mask, and with nebulised salbutamol (2.5mg) and ipratropium (500mcg). Routine bloods, including blood cultures, were taken and initial doses of antibiotics (amoxycillin and clarithromycin) were given intravenously. Despite an initial improvement in his clinical condition, after 1 hour his arterial blood gases had deteriorated (pH 7.25). It was also noticed that he had become drowsier. After consultation with the outreach team and the medical registrar on call, he is commenced on NIV (see Chapter 16). COPD is clearly a complicated disease and patients are prone to exacerbations and readmissions. Patients should be reminded that stopping smoking, even after many years, may help to reduce symptoms.

References and further reading

Braun, C.A. & Anderson, A.M. (2011). *Pathophysiology: A Clinical Approach.* 2nd edn. Philadelphia: Lippincott, Williams & Wilkins.

British Thoracic Society (BTS) (2013). BTS Guideline on Pulmonary Rehabilitation in Adults. *Thorax: An International Journal of Respiratory Medicine.* **68** (2). https://www.brit-thoracic.org.uk/document-library/clinical-information/pulmonary-rehabilitation/bts-guideline-for-pulmonary-rehabilitation/ (accessed 17 March 2015).

Douglas, G., Nicol, F. & Robertson, C. (eds) (2005). *Macleod's Clinical Examination.* 11th edn. Edinburgh: Churchill Livingstone.

Esteban, A., Anzueto, A., Frutos, F., Alia, I., Brochard, L., Stewart, T.E. *et al.* (2002). Characteristics and outcomes in adult patients receiving mechanical ventilation: a 28 day international study. *Journal of the American Medical Association.* **287**, 345–55.

Lodewijckx, C., Sermeus, W., Panella, M., Deneckere, S., Leigheb, F., Decramer, M. & Vanhaecht, K. (2011). Impact of care pathways for in-hospital management of COPD exacerbation: A systematic review. *International Journal of Nursing Studies.* **48**, 1445–56.

Murray, S.E. & White, B.S. (1999). *Critical Care Assessment Handbook.* Philadelphia: WB Saunders.

National Institute for Health and Care Excellence (NICE) (2010). *Chronic Obstructive Pulmonary Disease: clinical guidance 101.* http://www.nice.org.uk/guidance/cg101 (accessed 17 March 2015).

National Institute of Health and Care Excellence (NICE) (2011). *Chronic Obstructive Pulmonary Disease: costing report.* http://www.nice.org.uk/guidance/cg101/resources/cg101-chronic-obstructive-pulmonary-disease-update-costing-report2 (accessed 17 March 2015).

Sanders, J.S., Berman, T.M., Bartlett, M.M. & Kronenberg, R.S. (1980). Increased hypoxic ventilatory drive due to administration of aminophylline in normal men. *Chest.* **78**, 279–82.

Useful websites

British Thoracic Society
http://www.brit-thoracic.org.uk/ (Accessed 23 June 2015).

15 Asthma

Ann M. Price and Simon Merritt

Asthma is the most common chronic respiratory disease in the UK, so all health professionals working in an acute medical environment should have a good working knowledge of its signs, symptoms and treatment. The World Health Organisation (2011) estimates that 235 million people suffer from asthma. Asthma UK estimates that 5.4 million people in the UK are suffer from asthma and that three people die per day as a result of asthma. Many of these deaths are preventable.

After reading this chapter, you will understand the pathophysiology of asthma, how to judge the severity of an attack and how to start urgent treatment.

Background

According to Braun & Anderson (2011, p.347): 'Asthma is a chronic inflammatory disorder of the airways that results in intermittent or persistent airway obstruction because of bronchial hyperresponsiveness, inflammation, bronchoconstriction and excess mucous production.'

Diagnosing asthma is not always straightforward, since wheezing can be associated with a number of different medical conditions (see below). Some patients have therefore been informed that they have asthma when they actually have a different condition. However, whatever the cause, the principles of assessing an acutely unwell wheezing patient follow the same ABCDE format.

The main causes of wheeze are:

- Viral or bacterial respiratory tract infection
- COPD
- Congestive cardiac failure
- Bronchiectasis
- Localised airway obstruction (such as a tumour or foreign body)
- Vocal cord dysfunction
- Cystic fibrosis.

Pathophysiology

The exact cause of asthma is unclear but it is usually triggered by an allergen, such as dust, smoke or mould. However, there are numerous potential triggers, including exercise, temperature changes and illness (Braun & Anderson 2011).

Exposure to a trigger produces a hypersensitive reaction, which leads to chemical mediators being released. This causes oedema and narrowing of the airways through inflammation and bronchoconstriction (Braun & Anderson 2011). The wheezing is due to concurrent bronchospasm and can be exacerbated by excess mucous production, which limits air flow further.

Airway inflammation

Asthma is a chronic inflammatory disease of the airways, characterised by airway epithelial damage, increased numbers of mucus-secreting cells and an inflammatory reaction. The allergen initiates the inflammation, which activates Mast cells, releasing various mediators including histamine, leukotrienes and prostaglandins (Braun & Anderson 2011). This exacerbates the bronchospasm, swelling and mucous production, leading to mucous plugs.

Chronic inflammation of the airways causes eosinophil infiltration and cytokines (see Box 15.1), resulting in epithelial injury and structural changes in the airway structure. This change in airway structure is termed 'airways remodelling'. Over a long period of time, in a subgroup of asthmatics, this can lead to fixed (i.e. irreversible) airways obstruction.

Box 15.1 Cytokines

Cytokines are proteins, which are released by cells of the immune system, after exposure to an antigen. They act as intercellular signals in generating an immune response. They can have either pro-inflammatory or anti-inflammatory effects.

Diagnosis

The diagnosis of asthma depends upon the presence of suggestive symptoms such as (BTS 2014):

- Wheeze
- Shortness of breath
- Cough
- Chest tightness.

Characteristically, the shortness of breath may be worse during the night and first thing in the morning. These symptoms may be triggered by exercise, pollens, dust and cold or after taking aspirin/beta blockers (BTS 2014).

Several objective tests are used to assist in the diagnosis of asthma. The British Thoracic Society (2014) recommends the use of forced expiratory volume (FEV_1), the amount of air the patient can exhale in 1 second, and peak expiratory flow (PEF). Spirometry is most commonly used, and a reduction in expected values (with the signs and symptoms) is suggestive of asthma. Repeated readings may be needed to assess the patient and get a better clinical picture of the presenting condition (see Box 15.2).

Box 15.2 Peak expiratory flow (PEF)

The normal PEF (sometimes referred to as PEFR peak expiratory flow rate) values for a particular individual depend upon their height, age, sex and, to a lesser extent, their ethnicity. Tables of normal values are available from a number of sources. There are also simple programs that can be downloaded to a desktop computer or mobile device, which will calculate the values. One such program can be found at http://www.peakflow.com/top_nav/normal_values/index.html

Non-steroidal anti-inflammatory drugs (NSAIDs), especially aspirin, will precipitate an asthma attack in about 5% of asthmatic patients so their use should be avoided in this group of patients. Exactly why these patients are particularly susceptible is not completely understood. However, this phenomenon occurs almost exclusively in patients who have both nasal polyps and asthma.

It is known that NSAIDs interfere with the cyclo-oxygenase (COX) pathway, eventually leading to the metabolism of a substance called arachidonic acid to produce leukotrienes. These are known to induce bronchospasm in susceptible patients.

Asthma severity

It is crucial to judge the severity of an asthma attack, the PEF, pulse (bpm), blood pressure (BP), oxygen saturations and the patient's ability to complete a sentence in one breath. All give very important prognostic information, and will guide both treatment and the need for critical care, as illustrated in the case scenario below.

Case scenario

A 19-year-old asthma patient was admitted two days ago with a severe asthma attack. She has recovered quickly and is due to go home the next day. However, she has become increasingly wheezy throughout the morning and has used three nebulisers in the last 4 hours. You are concerned that this happened within 10 minutes of taking her morning medication and you think maybe one of the tablets is at fault. You study the drug chart and at once spot that she has been given a 400mg dose of ibuprofen (a non-steroidal anti-inflammatory drug), which you remember can cause asthma attacks in some asthmatics.

You go at once to see the patient. She appears very short of breath and you can hear her wheezing from the end of the bed. Oxygen therapy has been commenced. Her observations are as follows:

- Respiratory rate – 40 breaths per minute
- Oxygen saturation (Spo2) – 91% on 40% oxygen via mask
- Pulse – 115 beats per minute
- BP – 150/96mmHg.

What would you do to stabilise and treat the patient? What investigations would you perform?

Table 15.1 Levels of severity of acute asthma attacks in adults

Moderate asthma exacerbation	<ul><li>Increasing symptoms</li><li>PEF >50–75% best or predicted</li><li>No features of acute severe asthma</li></ul>	
Acute severe asthma	Any one of:<ul><li>PEF 33–50% best or predicted</li><li>Respiratory rate >25/min</li><li>Heart rate >110/min</li><li>Inability to complete sentences in one breath</li></ul>	
Life-threatening asthma	Any one of the following in a patient with severe asthma:	
	Measurements:<ul><li>PEF <33% best or predicted</li><li>SpO_2 <92%</li><li>PaO_2 <8kPa</li><li>'Normal' $PaCO_2$ (4.6–6.0kPa)</li></ul>	Clinical signs:<ul><li>Silent chest</li><li>Cyanosis</li><li>Poor respiratory effort</li><li>Arrhythmia</li><li>Exhaustion</li><li>Altered conscious level</li><li>Hypotension</li></ul>
Near-fatal asthma	Raised $PaCO_2$ and/or requiring mechanical ventilation with raised inflation pressures	

Reproduced from British Thoracic Society Scottish Intercollegiate Guidelines Network (2014). British Guideline on the Management of Asthma. Thorax. 69 (1), 84. Copyright year 2015, with permission from BMJ Publishing Group Ltd.

Refer to the BTS/SIGN guidelines for a thorough review of asthma and its evidence-based acute and chronic management:

https://www.brit-thoracic.org.uk/guidelines-and-quality-standards/asthma-guideline/

Assessment (ABCDE)

Assessment, as well as management, of a patient with an asthma attack should be performed using the ABCDE method. The assessment of the patient from the case scenario will be detailed below. You should also pay particular attention to the indicators of asthma severity listed in Table 15.1 (above).

It is helpful to perform your examination by first inspecting the patient and their surroundings, then palpating, percussing and finally auscultating. However, please note that in an emergency situation assessment and treatment would occur simultaneously (rather than one after the other, as described below).

On arriving at the patient's bedside, a full set of vital signs recordings needs to be obtained if this has not already been carried out (see Chapters 2 and 3). A cardiac and blood pressure monitor should be attached to the patient as well as an oxygen saturation probe to measure pulse oximetry (SpO2). You can immediately hear the patient wheezing. She is sitting bolt upright and gripping on to the sides of the beds with her hands, thus enabling the use of her accessory muscles of respiration. She is able to talk, but can only manage a few words at a time before taking another breath. She tells you that she is frightened and asks you to help her. You also establish that she has been ventilated on the intensive care unit in the past. This immediately worries you and indicates the severity of her asthma.

A-Airway

Since she is alert and talking to you, her airway is fine at present. However, you appreciate that the principal problem in asthma is broncho-constriction (narrowing of the airways) and realise that this must be addressed as soon as possible.

B-Breathing

Her respiratory rate is 40 breaths per minute and oxygen saturation is 91% on 40% oxygen via a Venturi mask. Inspection of her chest shows equal but mildly reduced chest expansion and the use of accessory muscles already described. Palpation of her trachea reveals it to be central. Percussion of her chest is normal. Auscultation reveals a diffuse polyphonic wheeze (see Box 15.3) throughout the chest anteriorly and posteriorly. Breath sounds are normal in volume. At this stage you measure her peak expiratory flow (PEF). She has great difficulty performing the manoeuvre. But, after three attempts, she manages 200l/min, which you calculate to be about 40% of her best peak flow.

Box 15.3 Wheeze

A wheeze is a musical sound that results from the passage of air through narrowed airways. It principally occurs on expiration. It is a prominent feature of both asthma and chronic obstructive pulmonary disease (COPD).

C-Circulation

Assessment of this patient's circulation reveals a tachycardia of 115 beats per minute and an elevated blood pressure of 150/96mmHg. Her jugular venous pressure (JVP) is difficult to see, due to the contraction of the sternocleidomastoid muscle (one of the accessory muscles) but it doesn't appear unduly elevated. Her heart sounds are also difficult to elicit, due to the loud wheezes.

D-Disability

Since she is alert and orientated, formal assessment of her alertness and mental disability gives a Glasgow Coma Score (GCS) of 15/15 or 'A' on the **AVPU** (**A**lert, **V**erbal, **P**ain, **U**nconscious) score.

E-Exposure

The last part of your assessment comprises full exposure of the patient to ensure that there are no other physical signs that have been missed thus far. You find a red band around her right ankle, revealing an allergy to ibuprofen. You later learn that it was getting in the way when it was around her wrist and so it was moved yesterday. You move it back to her wrist. The patient's temperature is 36.8°C.

Investigations

Having recently read the British Thoracic Society (BTS 2014) guidelines on asthma, you appreciate that a chest x-ray is not routinely recommended in acute asthma, unless the patient has life-threatening asthma with atypical symptoms, is not responding to treatment or is suspected to have pneumonia or a pneumothorax. A chest x-ray is therefore not required at present.

Arterial blood gases (ABGs) are recommended in acute asthma if the patient's saturations are less than 92% (BTS 2014), which they are in this case. This is because there is an increased risk of hypercapnia (see Chapter 10 on obtaining and interpreting arterial blood gases). The results of the ABG are reproduced in Table 15.2.

Table 15.2 Case scenario arterial blood gas results

Oxygen	40%
PaO_2	8.9kPa
$PaCO_2$	4.0kPa
pH	7.45
Saturations	91%
Base excess	+2

HOT TIP

Remember that assessment is an ongoing process and it is important to continually reassess, especially if the patient's condition changes (whether it improves or gets worse). You also need to assess the patient's response to any treatment given.

The ABG reveals hypoxia and hypocapnia (a low $PaCO_2$) – see Table 15.2 above. (Refer to Chapter 10 for more detail about interpreting ABGs.) If the $PaCO_2$ was normal, this would be extremely worrying and would mean the attack would be classified as life threatening (see Table 15.1, p. 124). A high $PaCO_2$ would also be a worrying sign of near-fatal asthma so checking ABGs for deterioration is also important, depending on the patient's response to treatment.

Severity of attack

Worrying features, specifically relevant to this case, would include any of the signs of life-threatening or near-fatal asthma. It is worth noting that this patient has been ventilated on the intensive care unit before, which usually indicates severe long-standing asthma. She has a peak flow of 40% predicted, a respiratory rate of 40 breaths per minute, a heart rate of 115 beats per minute, and is unable to complete sentences in one breath, which indicates that she has acute severe asthma.

Management
A-Airway

It has already been established that this patient's airway is intact. However, any patient who is short of breath will derive considerable improvement if they are sat up at a 90° angle. This upright position helps them use their accessory muscles of respiration.

B-Breathing

'Breathing' will be the principal therapeutic target in the treatment of any acute asthma attack. The use of high-flow oxygen is encouraged in asthma, and the aim should be to keep the oxygen saturations above 92%. It is important to remember that, although oxygen can help to correct any hypoxia, it will not significantly bronchodilate on its own. It is therefore an adjunct to treatment of an acute asthma attack, but not the main treatment. As mentioned elsewhere in this book, it is important to monitor ABGs in critically ill patients, especially if changes have been made to their treatment or their inspired oxygen concentration.

Nebulisers

The mainstay of acute asthma management is nebulised bronchodilators and oxygen therapy (BTS 2014). High-dose nebulised beta-2 agonists (5mg of salbutamol or terbutaline) should be given as soon as possible. Ideally the nebuliser should be driven with oxygen, not air (BTS 2014), but this should not prevent timely administration of nebulised beta-2 agonists.

While the nebuliser is being administered, the patient should be encouraged to take slow deep breaths where possible and discouraged from talking, to ensure maximal drug deposition. A single 5mg dose of salbutamol may not completely resolve the bronchospasm. The BTS guidelines therefore advise that nebulisers should either be administered at intervals of 15–30 minutes, or the patient should have continuous 5–10mg/hourly nebulisation (BTS 2014). At these high doses, the side effects of tremor and tachycardia are common, but only rarely interfere with the treatment. After this period of stabilisation, salbutamol is commonly given 1–4 hourly, with provision on the drug chart for extra doses as and when necessary.

Combining ipratropium bromide (Atrovent®) with beta-2 agonists is recommended in acute attacks (BTS 2014) but has a lesser role to play in mild attacks or once the patient has stabilised. Ipratropium should initially be given at a dose of 500mcg every 4–6 hours.

There is evidence that magnesium sulphate can improve bronchodilation. BTS asthma guidelines (2014) recommend the administration of intravenous magnesium sulphate (1.2–2g) in either acute severe asthma that has responded poorly to bronchodilators or immediately in a patient diagnosed with life-threatening or near-fatal asthma. It should be given only once, and slowly over a 20-minute period (BTS 2014).

In acute asthma attacks, nebulised drugs should be delivered using oxygen (not air) according to BTS 2014 guidelines. A minimum of 6 litres per minute oxygen flow is required by most nebuliser systems but check your equipment.

Aminophylline does not increase bronchodilation (compared to initiating the above treatment) but has many side effects. Aminophylline should only be used for severe attacks that are unresponsive to treatment, under a senior medical practitioner's supervision (BTS 2014).

Steroids and antibiotics

Steroids reduce mortality if given early in an acute asthma attack (BTS 2014). A dose of 40–50mg of oral prednisolone daily is usually sufficient (a course of at least 5 days or until recovery). If the patient is too unwell to take oral medication, 100mg hydrocortisone intravenously, four times daily, is a good substitute.

Box 15.4 Inhaled and oral steroids in asthma

Steroids are a mainstay in managing both acute and chronic asthma. They down-regulate the troublesome inflammatory pathways, and reduce the expression of some of the more harmful cytokines. Inhaled steroids are typically used over a long period to reduce inflammation and prevent asthma attacks. Examples include budesonide, beclomethasone and fluticasone. During an acute attack of asthma, short courses of oral steroids are used, such as prednisolone. Occasionally, in cases of very severe asthma, intravenous hydrocortisone can be prescribed, until the patient is well enough to take tablets.

Common infections triggering asthma tend to be viral in nature, and antibiotics should not be automatically instigated (BTS 2014). Nevertheless, each patient should be assessed for signs of bacterial infection (such as green sputum or raised temperature) in conjunction with their history, signs and symptoms, and antibiotics should then be considered if appropriate.

C-Circulation

The circulatory system in asthma is not usually a major problem, apart from the sinus tachycardia commonly caused by salbutamol. However, some patients are particularly susceptible, and can develop arrhythmias. The best treatment for these is to ensure that the electrolytes (sodium, potassium, magnesium, calcium and phosphate) are normal and to reduce the dose and/or frequency of salbutamol nebules, if clinically possible. If that fails then, depending on the nature of the rhythm and the blood pressure, amiodarone, digoxin, verapamil or DC cardioversion can be used, as per the Resuscitation Council's *Advanced Life Support Guidelines* (Resuscitation Council UK 2015).

It is good practice to establish intravenous access and take routine bloods (full blood count, urea and electrolytes, CRP and blood cultures) in all acutely unwell patients. Patients having an acute asthma attack are liable to develop hypokalaemia, mainly due to the high doses of salbutamol being administered.

They are also prone to become dehydrated and may therefore need maintenance intravenous fluids with added potassium, until they are able to eat and drink normally (see Chapter 30 for more on electrolytes).

Referral to the intensive care unit

There should be a low threshold for seeking advice from a critical care physician or a chest specialist when it is felt that a patient requires ventilation, or for patients who have severe acute or life-threatening asthma who are not responding to appropriate therapy. Worrying features to look out for are described in Box 15.5.

Box 15.5 Signs of deterioration

- Deteriorating PEFR
- Worsening hypoxia
- Elevated pCO_2
- Acidosis on ABG
- Exhaustion/poor respiratory effort
- Drowsiness or confusion
- Respiratory arrest.

Monitoring the patient

Monitoring a patient with acute asthma is very similar to the close monitoring required for any critically ill patient, as described in Chapter 2. The level and frequency of monitoring depends on the severity of the attack. However, for an acutely unwell asthmatic, the minimum requirement would be to nurse them in an area on the ward that is easily visible.

- Vital signs (respiratory rate, oxygen saturation, heart rhythm, pulse and blood pressure) should ideally be measured continuously or according to hospital policy (usually half-hourly and reducing as the patient stabilises).
- Bloods, specifically potassium, should be monitored daily or more often if very low (<3.0mmol/litre).
- Fluid balance should be recorded hourly. PEF should ideally be done pre- and post-nebuliser. However, it is unlikely that more than four recordings (pre- and post-nebuliser) per day would be of added benefit.

A slow but steady improvement should be seen both acutely and also day to day. Once the patient is stable, usually after 24 hours, the frequency of monitoring can be reduced, along with the frequency of the nebulisers.

HOT TIPS

- Immediately work out the severity of the asthma attack.
- Patients with life-threatening or near-fatal asthma must be moved to a critical care area as soon as possible.
- Administer enough oxygen to maintain the saturations above 94%.

- If your patient requires high-flow oxygen to maintain this saturation (or if saturations are below 92%), perform an arterial blood gas and call for senior help immediately.
- Administer salbutamol (5mg) via a nebuliser on a continuous basis (i.e. one after the other) until there is a clinical improvement with better saturations, reduced respiratory rate and the patient is able to talk in full sentences.
- Administer intravenous magnesium sulphate for acute severe asthma or worse.
- Never administer Bi-PAP on the general ward for an asthmatic patient — seek expert advice if ventilation is required. (For more on Bi-PAP, see Chapter 16.)
- Intravenous aminophylline has no place in the management of the average asthmatic patient.

Conclusion

The patient in the case scenario was given back-to-back salbutamol nebulisers (5mg), with the first containing 500mcg of ipratropium. Her oxygen was increased to 60% via a Venturi mask and her saturations increased to 96%. A repeat arterial blood gas 20 minutes later revealed a PaO_2 of 14kPa, with a low $PaCO_2$ and normal pH. She was also given a dose of 40mg prednisolone. In this case antibiotics were not felt to be necessary. Her PEF improved to 250 litres per minute after four back-to-back nebulisers and her respiratory rate dropped to 25 breaths per minute. She was then able to complete sentences in a single breath and was understandably very flattering about the expert management she received!

References and further reading

Asthma UK (no date). 'Asthma Facts and FAQs'. http://www.asthma.org.uk/asthma-facts-and-statistics (accessed 23 March 2015).

Braun, C.A. & Anderson, C.M. (2011). *Pathophysiology: a clinical approach.* 2nd edn. Philadelphia: Lippincott, Williams & Wilkins

British Thoracic Society (BTS) (2014) & Scottish Intercollegiate Guidelines Network (SIGN) (2014). *British guideline on the management of asthma: a national clinical guideline.* https://www.brit-thoracic.org.uk/document-library/clinical-information/asthma/btssign-asthma-guideline-2014/ (accessed 26 March 2015).

British Thoracic Society (BTS) (2014) & Scottish Intercollegiate Guidelines Network (SIGN) (2014). *British guideline on the management of asthma: a quick reference guide.* https://www.brit-thoracic.org.uk/document-library/clinical-information/asthma/btssign-asthma-guideline-quick-reference-guide-2014/ (accessed 26 March 2015).

Resuscitation Council UK (2015). *Resuscitation Guidelines.* https://www.resus.org.uk/pages/Guide.htm (accessed 11 November 2015).

World Health Organisation (2011). *10 Facts on Asthma.* http://www.who.int/features/factfiles/asthma/en/ (accessed 26 March 2015).

Useful websites

Asthma UK
http://www.asthma.org.uk (Accessed 30 June 2015).

British Thoracic Society
http://www.brit-thoracic.org.uk (Accessed 30 June 2015).

16 Non-invasive ventilation in type 2 respiratory failure

Jayne Fraser

This chapter covers the principles of bi-level non-invasive ventilation. It will enable you to recognise patients who may need non-invasive ventilation (NIV) and explain how to monitor and care for a patient receiving NIV.

Non-invasive ventilation (NIV) enables ventilatory support to be given via a mask into the patient's upper airways, rather than an invasive device that entails inserting a tube into the patient's trachea and bypassing the upper airway (British Thoracic Society 2008). The use of non-invasive ventilation has been recognised as an important tool in the management of type 1 and type 2 respiratory failure and cardiogenic pulmonary oedema; it also offers a means of weaning patients from mechanical ventilation in the critical care environment.

NIV has been reported to reduce hospital mortality and the need for intubation and reduce length of hospital stay (Brochard *et al.* 1995, Plant *et al.* 2000a). It can occur outside the intensive care unit and can therefore save 'precious' intensive care unit beds, at a relatively low cost. Patients are able to eat and drink, to cooperate with physiotherapy, and to communicate with staff and their family because they do not require sedation when receiving non-invasive ventilation.

The Royal College of Physicians, the British Thoracic Society and the Intensive Care Society (2008) have produced comprehensive guidelines for the care of patients receiving NIV. This revised chapter follows these guidelines, as they remain the current recommendations, although they are due to be reviewed in 2015. This chapter considers bi-level non-invasive ventilation in relation to type 2 respiratory failure.

Bi-level non-invasive ventilation

Non-invasive ventilation used in treating patients in type 2 respiratory failure offers bi-level positive airway pressures (Bi-PAP). This gives a pressure at two levels, on inspiration and expiration. Bi-level NIV has a higher pressure on inspiration and lower on expiration. These two pressures are measured in centimetres of water (cmH_2O).

- **Expiratory positive airway pressure (EPAP):** This is the level on expiration. It keeps the alveoli open when the patient breathes out, and has the same function as CPAP (continuous positive airway pressure) and PEEP (positive end expiratory pressure).

- **Inspiratory positive airway pressure (IPAP):** This is the level given on inspiration. The machine senses when the patient breathes in and blows air into the lungs.
- **Pressure support:** This is the difference between IPAP and EPAP (i.e. if IPAP is set at 10cmH$_2$O and EPAP is set at 4cmH$_2$O, then pressure support will be 6cmH$_2$O).

The functions of EPAP, IPAP and pressure support are summarised in Table 16.1.

Table 16.1 Functions of expiratory and inspiratory positive airway pressure (EPAP and IPAP) and pressure support

EPAP	IPAP	Pressure support
Keeps the alveoli partly inflated	Supports inspiratory effort	Reduces the effort of breathing and allows patients to relax and rest
Improves alveolar gas exchange	Improves tidal volume	—
Improves oxygenation	Improves carbon dioxide removal	—
Increases lung volume	—	—

The definitions of forced expiratory volume and forced vital capacity are given in Box 16.1.

Box 16.1

Forced expiratory volume (FEV1): The volume of air that can be exhaled in 1 second. It is reduced in COPD because of the narrowed airways.

Forced vital capacity (FVC): The total volume of air that can be exhaled after a maximal inspiration. It is usually maintained in early COPD, but decreases as the disease progresses.

Age, sex, height and ethnicity all affect FEV1 and FVC. Tables of normal values have been produced and are readily available, as are simple programs designed for use on desktop computers and mobile computer devices. One such program can be found at: http://patient.info/doctor/spirometry-calculator

Patient selection

Non-invasive ventilation should be considered in patients with an acute exacerbation of COPD with a respiratory acidosis. Suggested physiological parameters (Royal College of Physicians 2008) are:

- pH <7.35
- pCO$_2$ >6.0.

First-line treatment

Controlled oxygen therapy – at a flow to maintain oxygen saturations of 88–92% (British Thoracic Society *et al.* 2008) – should be started. This is because a low pH and high carbon dioxide can be a consequence of being given too much oxygen in the ambulance or in the hospital environ¬ment (Plant *et al.* 2000b).

Maximal medical therapy should be prescribed and administered and should consist of (Royal College of Physicians 2008):

- Nebulised salbutamol

- Nebulised ipratropium

- Steroids

- Antibiotics (if there is an indication of new infection)

- Chest x-ray.

The arterial blood gases should then be repeated and if the patient remains acidotic (pH <7.35) then escalation of treatment should be considered. This should occur within the first hour of deterioration or on arrival at hospital.

Case scenario

A 65-year-old man was admitted to the medical assessment unit (MAU) with a six-day history of progressive shortness of breath and a cough productive of thick green sputum. Although his Ventolin inhaler had helped with his breathing initially, it no longer seemed to be making any difference. Normally he was able to walk to his local newsagent without stopping (500 metres) but on the day he came to the MAU he could manage no more than 5 metres. He had been diagnosed with chronic obstructive pulmonary disease (COPD) by his GP around two years previously and had been commenced on a Ventolin and eformoterol inhaler. His last spirometry, eight months earlier, revealed a forced expiratory volume (FEV$_1$) of -1.1 and a forced vital capacity (FVC) of 2.0.

He suffered from at least three chest infections per year, though none had been as bad as this one. He had continued to smoke 10 cigarettes per day and had done so for the last 45 years. The patient was treated with a reduction in his oxygen concentration to 28% via a Venturi mask, and administered nebulised salbutamol and ipratropium.

Routine bloods, including blood cultures, were taken and initial doses of antibiotic (as per local Trust guidelines) and steroids were given intravenously. Despite what appeared to be an initial improvement in his clinical condition, worsening arterial blood gases revealed a pH of 7.25, with a pCO$_2$ of 9.3 kPa. It was also noticed that he had become more drowsy. After consultation with the critical care outreach team and the medical registrar on call, it was decided to commence non-invasive ventilation.

Intubation or NIV?

The Royal College of Physicians guidelines (2008) say that the choice of treatment needs to be made sooner rather than later and patients who are suitable for invasive ventilation should be moved to a critical care area after the first hour if there is no improvement in their arterial blood gas analysis. Those with a pH of <7.25 should be considered for intubation and full ventilation, but if this is not appropriate then NIV may be suitable. However, other patients, who are not suitable candidates for invasive ventilation, should remain in an appropriate designated location where NIV will be prescribed as their ceiling of treatment. Before commencing, a treatment plan should be worked out – in case NIV is not effective in stabilising the patient. This treatment plan should be documented in the patient's notes, paying particular attention to the following:

- The severity of the underlying disease
- The reversibility of the acute illness
- The previous level of disability
- The patient's wishes.

Local guidelines should be in place to help ascertain which patients are suitable for non-invasive ventilation, and also consider the contraindications, as not all are absolute (Plant *et al.* 2000a, Conti *et al.* 2002, Lightowler *et al.* 2003). These are shown in Box 16.2.

Box 16.2 Inclusion and exclusion criteria for NIV

Inclusion criteria
- Primary diagnosis of COPD
- Able to protect airway*
- Conscious and cooperative*
- Potential for recovery to acceptable quality of life (acceptable to the patient)
- Patient's wishes

Exclusion criteria
- Facial trauma, burns, recent facial or upper airway surgery
- Upper gastrointestinal surgery
- Fixed obstruction of the upper airway
- Inability to protect airway
- Life-threatening hypoxaemia
- Haemodynamic instability requiring inotropes or pressers (unless in a critical care unit)
- Severe comorbidity
- Patient moribund
- Confusion, agitation or severe cognitive impairment
- Vomiting
- Bowel obstruction
- Copious respiratory secretions
- Undrained pneumothorax

*Consider NIV if unconscious and endotracheal intubation deemed inappropriate or NIV to be provided in critical care setting.

Non-invasive ventilation is *not* the treatment of choice for patients whose primary diagnosis is heart failure or pneumonia, but it may be used in COPD patients with these complications if escalation to intubation and ventilation is deemed inappropriate.

Starting treatment

Once a patient has been selected as suitable for non-invasive ventilation, the chest x-ray should be reviewed to rule out a pneumothorax. A chest drain may need to be inserted if a pneumothorax is present. Patient cooperation and compliance is crucial to the success of NIV. Patients will often have severe dyspnoea and difficulty speaking and may be exhausted from the effort of breathing. They may be frightened and apprehensive about trying it. All these problems are potentially reversible and can be overcome by giving the patient calm, clear instructions and information. Spending time at the beginning of treatment saves valuable nursing time later on. Many patients find adapting to the mask the most difficult part of the process. However, in recent years the masks available have improved considerably. The patient should be measured up for a mask using the manufacturer's guidelines – do not be tempted to guess the size because an ill-fitting mask can be uncomfortable and may leak excessively or be too tight.

Ideally two healthcare professionals, one of whom is trained to use non-invasive ventilation, should be present to secure the mask and monitor the bi-level NIV machine. Once the patient is comfortable with the mask held against their face, it can be strapped to the head. Do not attach it too tightly (you should be able to move the mask at the chin but not at the nose) and be careful it does not blow into the patient's eyes. The bi-level system on some machines compensates for leakage around the mask itself and also records the amount of leaking.

The pressure of the mask sometimes causes irritation and soreness, especially on the bridge of the nose and the chin, so these areas need to be assessed regularly. A protective dressing can be applied to any areas that begin to look red and sore.

It is of the utmost importance that the patient is comfortable wearing the mask; therefore low pressures are set at first so the patient can get used to the feel of blowing air.

Starting pressures are:

- IPAP: 10cmH2O.
- EPAP: 4cmH2O.
- Pressure support: 6cm.

Please refer to your own Trust guidelines for further information on setting the particular machine you are using. The British Thoracic Society *et al.* (2008) suggest increasing the IPAP by 2cmH$_2$O up to a maximum of 20cmH$_2$O. The British Thoracic Society *et al.* (2008) recommend that NIV should have a prescription chart, and changes to settings should be recorded and patient response assessed.

Humidification, through the bi-level NIV machine, is not usually needed as long as the patient is kept well hydrated, either with oral fluids or with intravenous fluids, usually given during short breaks off the ventilatory support (5–10 minutes). A fluid input and output chart is essential. Refer to the physiotherapist for advice and treatment to help the patient with expectorating any sputum. Nursing care of patients receiving non-invasive ventilation is summarised in Box 16.3.

Monitoring the patient

Close and thorough clinical assessment is of paramount importance when caring for a patient receiving non-invasive ventilation. Physiological monitoring is not a substitute for clinical assessment. The patient should be regularly observed while on the ventilator, and charted according to your individual Trust's guidelines.

Box 16.3
Nursing care of patients receiving non-invasive ventilation

- Ensure consent is gained to initial treatment as per local policy.
- Reassurance – take your time when commencing.
- Measure the patient for the mask – do not guess!
- A full face mask is recommended initially for acute episodes.

- Remember that the mask does not need to be excessively tight.
- Make sure patients have a means of communication and are located near the nurses' station.
- Observe pressure areas on the patient's face for redness and apply a protective dressing if necessary (be particularly careful if a nasogastric tube is present).
- Move the tube regularly.
- Wash the mask with soap and water when washing the patient's face.
- Remember the patient's hydration and nutritional status.
- Patients may have a dry mouth and need mouth care/drinks.
- Give the patient a break if possible for meals, drugs and nebulisers (nasal cannula to give oxygen can be used for periods off NIV).
- Refer to the chest physiotherapist.

The following clinical features should be assessed:

- Chest wall movement
- Coordination of respiratory effort with the ventilator
- Use of accessory muscles
- General assessment (is the patient sweating, clammy or dyspnoeic?)
- Auscultation of the chest
- Patient comfort
- Neurological status (any signs of confusion or tiredness?).

The patient receiving non-invasive ventilation should be on a cardiac monitor with continuous monitoring of their:

- Heart rate and rhythm
- Respiratory rate
- Blood pressure
- Conscious level (use AVPU as in Chapter 2)
- Oxygen saturation (measure via pulse oximetry (SpO_2) continuously for at least 24 hours and aim to keep it at 88–92% with supplemental oxygen therapy; Schwartz *et al.* 2004, British Thoracic Society *et al.* 2008).

These observations should be documented initially every 15 minutes and reduced to at least hourly on the patient's observation chart and an early warning score should also be recorded (see Chapter 1 on critical care outreach). It is important to consider these vital signs alongside the patient's arterial blood gas measurements. The frequency of subsequent measurements will depend on the patient's progress (see Chapter 10 on obtaining and interpreting arterial blood gases).

Once non-invasive ventilation has been commenced, patients should be clinically assessed and arterial blood gases repeated after 1 hour (or after each pressure change) and again at 4 hours and 12 hours. If no improvement is seen and the patient still has a respiratory acidosis after treatment, check the parameters as detailed in Box 16.4. (Remember to use your own hospital's guidelines, as different parameters can be adjusted on different machines.)

Non-invasive ventilation should continue for at least 6 hours (allowing breaks for oral fluids) and as long as possible during the first 24 hours (British Thoracic Society *et al.* 2008).

Arterial blood gas (ABG) analysis should always be interpreted alongside clinical assessment of the patient. Patients often compensate and look worse clinically than the ABGs may indicate. This can lead to a sudden patient collapse if the clinical signs of deterioration are not noted and addressed early.

Box 16.4 Preventing and dealing with treatment failure in NIV
(based on British Thoracic Society *et al.* 2008)

Is the treatment of the underlying condition optimal?
- *Check the medical treatment prescribed and that it has been given.*
- *Consider physiotherapy for sputum retention.*

Have any complications developed?
- *Consider a pneumothorax, aspiration pneumonia, etc.*

PaCO$_2$ remains elevated

Is the patient on too much oxygen?
- *Adjust FiO$_2$ to maintain SpO$_2$ between 88% and 92%; an SpO$_2$ >85% may be required in a minority of patients (British Thoracic Society et al. 2008).*

Is there excessive leakage?
- *Check the fit of the mask.*

Is the circuit set up correctly?
- *Check the connections have been made correctly.*
- *Check the circuit for leaks.*

Is the patient synchronising with the ventilator?
- *Observe the patient.*
- *Consider increasing EPAP.*

Is ventilation inadequate?
- *Observe chest expansion.*
- *Increase IPAP.*

PaCO$_2$ improves but PaO$_2$ remains low
- *Increase FiO$_2$.*
- *Consider increasing EPAP.*

Titrating treatment to blood gas analysis

Box 16.5 can be used as a guide to optimise non-invasive ventilation and ideally reduce the duration of the treatment. However, these pressures are only offered as a guide, and you must adhere to your own hospital's guidelines.

HOT TIP

ABGs, as well as the patient's clinical condition, will guide the practitioner on changing pressure support, IPAP and EPAP levels.

When adjusting pressures, remember to maintain pressure support. If EPAP is increased, IPAP should also be increased. If pressure support is decreased, the work of breathing will get harder.

Box 16.5 Titrating the pressures on the non-invasive ventilator

If no improvement in PCO_2
- Increase IPAP slowly, by 2cm at a time, to a maximum of 20cm (increases pressure support).
- Repeat ABGs to assess effectiveness of pressure changes.
- If no improvement, is the patient having too much oxygen? Consider reducing FiO_2.

If PO_2 remains low and PCO_2 improves
- Increase FiO_2 .
- Increase EPAP (only on expert advice) to a maximum of 8cm.
- Repeat ABGs to assess effectiveness of pressure changes.
- Remember: if EPAP is increased, you should also increase IPAP to maintain pressure support.

If patient shows signs of tachypnoea and fatigue
- Increase IPAP to increase pressure support and reduce the work of breathing.
- Maintain close observation to measure effectiveness of changes.

There may be other parameters that can be adjusted on the non-invasive ventilator but these will depend on the make of equipment being used. All personnel using a non-invasive ventilator should be trained and deemed competent in its usage (the British Thoracic Society *et al.* 2008 suggest the competencies needed). They should also be aware of hospital guidelines. The figures given in this chapter can be used for guidance, but may vary from hospital to hospital.

Weaning

Ideally the patient should remain on bi-level non-invasive ventilation for as long as possible during the first 24 hours; if the patient's condition allows, however, breaks should be given off the machine for meals, drinks and nebulisers. If, after 24 hours, the patient's condition has improved and they are no longer acidotic, the bi-level non-invasive ventilator can be taken off for extended periods of time during the day, and their response assessed. Oxygen can be administered via nasal speculum to maintain oxygen saturations at a level agreed with the medical team. It is important to continue to assess the patient, paying particular attention to their respiratory rate, oxygen saturations and level of consciousness. Some patients may need to continue non-invasive ventilation at night, but often the patient will be able to tell whether they can manage without the machine and will wean themselves.

Conclusion

After 24 hours, the case scenario patient's condition had improved. He was no longer acidotic. The bi-level non-invasive ventilator was taken off for a couple of hours in the morning and again in the afternoon. The following day, the time off the ventilator was extended to 4 hours in the morning and afternoon. During this period of weaning, the patient received oxygen via nasal speculum at 1 litre per minute and this maintained his oxygen saturations at 88–92%.

On the third day, he had non-invasive ventilation at night only. He continued to be assessed, with particular attention given to his respiratory rate, oxygen saturations and level of consciousness, and he reported that he was finding breathing much easier. He remained stable. An ABG was again performed to assess his progress after a period off non-invasive ventilation and no deterioration was noted in his pH or PCO_2. It was decided to stop non-invasive ventilation with a view to recommencing it if he deteriorated further.

Respiratory support in the ward environment is more common in today's health service and has been shown to reduce mortality in patients who are not suitable for invasive ventilation. For further information, please refer to the British Thoracic Society guidance (2008) and the Royal College of Physicians' *Concise Guidance to Good Practice* (2008) and your own hospital's local policy. Critical care colleagues will always be available to assist, such as the critical care outreach team or the intensive care team.

References and further reading

British Thoracic Society, Royal College of Physicians & Intensive Care Society (2008). *The Use of Non-Invasive Ventilation in the management of patients with chronic obstructive pulmonary disease admitted to hospital with acute type II respiratory failure (With particular reference to Bilevel positive pressure ventilation).* https://www.brit-thoracic.org.uk/document-library/clinical-information/niv/niv-guidelines/the-use-of-non-invasive-ventilation-in-the-management-of-patients-with-copd-admitted-to-hospital-with-acute-type-ii-respiratory-failure/ (accessed 4 April 2015).

Brochard, L., Mancebo, J., Wysocki, M. *et al.* (1995). Non-invasive ventilation for acute exacerbation of chronic obstructive pulmonary disease. *The New England Journal of Medicine,* **333**, 817–22.

Conti, G., Antonelli, M., Navalesi, P. *et al.* (2002). Non-invasive vs conventional mechanical ventilation in patients with chronic obstructive pulmonary disease after failure of medical treatment in the ward: a randomised trial. *Intensive Care Medicine.* **28**, 1701–1707.

Lightowler, J.V., Wedzicha, J.A., Elliot, M.W. *et al.* (2003). Non-invasive positive pressure ventilation to treat respiratory failure resulting from exacerbations of chronic obstructive pulmonary disease: Cochrane systematic review and meta-analysis. *British Medical Journal.* **326**, 185–87.

Plant, P., Owen, J. & Elliott, M. (2000a). Early use of non-invasive ventilation for acute exacerbations of chronic obstructive pulmonary disease on general respiratory wards: a multicentre randomised controlled trial. *Lancet.* **355**, 1931–35.

Plant, P., Owen, J. & Elliott, M. (2000b). One year period prevalence study of respiratory acidosis in acute exacerbations of COPD: implications for the provision of non-invasive ventilation and oxygen administration. *Thorax.* **55**, 550–54.

Royal College of Physicians, British Thoracic Society & Intensive Care Society (2008). *Chronic obstructive pulmonary disease: non-invasive ventilation with bi-phasic positive airways pressure in the management of patients with acute type 2 respiratory failure. Concise Guidance to Good Practice Series, No 11.* London: Royal College of Physicians.

Schwartz, A.R., Kacmarek, R.M. & Hess, D.R. (2004). Factors affecting oxygen delivery with bi-level positive airways pressure. *Respiratory Care.* **49**, 270–75.

Useful websites

British Thoracic society
https://www.brit-thoracic.org.uk/ (Accessed 30 June 2015)

Royal College of Physicians
https://www.rcplondon.ac.uk/ (Accessed 30 June 2015)

17 Pulmonary embolism

Gaurav Agarwal

Pulmonary embolism (PE) is defined as a clot (or clots) of blood that compromise circulation in the pulmonary vasculature (Swearingen & Keen 2001). Although there are rarer causes – such as fat and air embolism, which could, strictly speaking, still qualify under the umbrella term PE – we will restrict this discussion to the assessment and management of patients with PE that is due to venous thromboembolism (NICE 2012).

Causes of pulmonary embolism

Venous thromboembolism (VTE) is an umbrella term describing clot (thrombus) formation in the veins. VTE includes deep vein thrombosis (DVT) and pulmonary embolism (PE) (NICE 2012). DVT is the most common cause of pulmonary embolism (NICE 2012). Stasis of blood in the pelvic or large limb veins, microvasculature endothelial injury and hypercoagulability of blood results in the formation of a blood clot. The clot then breaks off and travels to the right side of the heart and so makes its way to the pulmonary vasculature.

Very rarely (if there is an atrial or ventricular septal defect), the clot can travel through to the left side of the heart and into the systemic circulation, resulting in compromised circulation. Some thrombi are associated with organ damage (such as cerebrovascular accident, if the emboli reach the brain).

Other causes of pulmonary embolism

- Right ventricular thrombosis (usually after a myocardial infarction)
- Air (such as traumatic pneumothorax)
- Fat (after major long bone trauma)
- Amniotic fluid (in pregnant women)
- Septic emboli (as in bacterial endocarditis).

History

Probe the patient specifically about the risk factors mentioned below and ask for any family history of coagulation disorders. A sudden onset of pleuritic chest pain and dyspnoea, in the absence of another obvious diagnosis, gives a strong suspicion of PE.

Risk factors

These risk factors comprise the PE Wells Score, which should be undertaken in suspected PE (NICE 2012).

- Clinical DVT, with leg swelling and pain
- Previous proven DVT/PE
- Heart rate >100 beats per minute
- Immobilisation for previous 3 days or surgery in the last 4 weeks
- Haemoptysis
- Malignancy (on treatment, treated in the last 6 months, or palliative).

Other considerations (BTS 2003)

- Pregnancy/post-partum/oral contraceptive pill/hormone replacement therapy
- Recent long-haul air travel.

Symptoms

- Shortness of breath (dyspnoea)*
- Chest pain (pleuritic)*
- Coughing up blood (haemoptysis) *
- Syncope/dizziness/collapse
- Palpitation.

* One of these is present in almost all cases of PE (NICE 2012).

Vital signs

- Tachypnoea
- Tachycardia >100 beats per minute*
- Hypotension*
- Elevated jugular venous pressure (JVP)
- Look carefully for cyanosis*
- Hypoxaemia.*

* May suggest a large PE.

Chest examination

- Pleural rub
- Evidence of small pleural effusion
- Chest x-ray
- Computed tomography pulmonary angiogram (CTPA) (NICE 2012).

Cardiac/neurological/abdominal examination (usually normal)

Look specifically for:

- Immobility in the last 3 days
- Surgery in the previous 4 weeks
- Tender/red/swollen calf

Undertake a PE Well's Score to assess risk (NICE 2012).

Investigations
Chest radiograph
This is often normal. Sometimes a small pleural effusion may be detected. Very rarely there is a wedge-shaped infarct (opacification, with the apex of the wedge being more central and base more peripheral).

Electrocardiogram
This could be normal or it could show sinus tachycardia. There may be evidence of a right-heart strain pattern (right bundle branch block and T wave inversion in V1 to V4). In large PEs, there may be an S-wave in lead I and a Q wave and T-wave inversion in lead III. This is referred to as 'S1Q3T3 pattern'.

Arterial blood gas analysis
Low PaO_2 (due to poor oxygenation) and low $PaCO_2$ (due to 'blowing off' of carbon dioxide) as a result of tachypnoea are common. In large PEs, lactate may be raised due to poor peripheral tissue perfusion, leading to anaerobic metabolism. The alveolar–arterial gradient will be raised by more than 2kPa.

D-dimer test
'D-dimer' is a product formed in the body when a blood clot (such as those found in DVT or PE) is broken down. A laboratory or point-of-care test can be done to assess the concentration of D-dimer in a person's blood. The threshold for a positive result varies with the type of D-dimer test used and is determined locally. The result of the D-dimer test can be used as part of probability assessment when DVT or PE is suspected' (NICE 2012, p. 12)

There is debate about the relevance of D-dimer tests in PE. Yet, if they are used intelligently, they are brilliant for excluding the diagnosis of PEs, provided the clinical probability is low. There is little value in doing a D-dimer test if the clinical probability is moderate or high. In such cases, you should proceed to definitive imaging straight away (NICE 2012).

Emergency imaging
When a patient is haemodynamically unstable, it is difficult to perform definitive imaging studies. Delays can be fatal and echocardiography may be useful to look for right-heart strain. Echocardiography offers the advantage of corroborative evidence before thrombolysis is attempted.

Definitive investigation with computerised tomogram pulmonary angiography (CTPA)
This is a contrast-enhanced study of the pulmonary vasculature that outlines filling defects as a result of emboli.

Ventilation/perfusion scan
If CTPA is unavailable or inaccessible or there is a contrast allergy (NICE 2012), a ventilation/perfusion (V/Q) scan can be done at your hospital's nuclear medicine department. Look for perfusion defects that are not matched with ventilation defects, if there are any. A V/Q scan is not as sensitive a test as CTPA. It often takes longer to perform and is more difficult to interpret, especially if the chest radiograph was abnormal. An indeterminate probability scan should always be followed by a CTPA if the clinical suspicion is high (NICE 2012).

Treatment
Once the diagnosis is suspected, it is mandatory – in the absence of a contraindication – to start treatment-dose heparin. Use of low molecular weight heparin (LMWH) as a single subcutaneous daily

injection (1.5mg/kg) is suggested. Once the diagnosis is confirmed, a vitamin K antagonist (VKA, usually oral warfarin) should be started, in combination with the heparin injections.

Once a stable international normalised ratio (INR) of 2–3 is reached, heparin injections are discontinued and warfarin continued for a period of at least 3 months (NICE 2012). Warfarin treatment often continues longer, and may be life-long in recurrent disease. Careful attention must be paid to monitoring the INR and adjusting the daily dose of warfarin. The GP surgery or anticoagulation clinic services are invaluable in this regard.

HOT TIP

Correctly fitting, below-knee, graduated compression stockings should be advised and normally worn for 2 years. They should be replaced 2–3 times a year, depending on the manufacturer's instructions (NICE 2012).

Occasionally, temporary inferior vena cava filters are required. These are used if there is a failure of anticoagulation or if it is contraindicated. If there has been a massive PE, resulting in haemodynamic compromise, then urgent thrombolysis, using recombinant tissue plasminogen activators, is suggested (BTS 2003, NICE 2012). Rarely, in such situations, pulmonary embolectomy may be required if there is either a failure of or contraindication to thrombolysis. Patients with PE who have haemodynamic instability should be considered for admission to a high dependency unit and/or you may wish to involve the critical care outreach team (or equivalent).

Newer anticoagulants

In recent trials (EINSTEIN-PE 2012), rivaroxaban has shown non-inferiority versus enoxaparin/warfarin in patients with acute symptomatic PE (and/or DVT). Rivaroxaban has the added advantage of being a tablet that does not require regular blood test monitoring and the patient does not have to take low-molecular weight heparin (LMWH) injections when therapy is initiated (NICE 2013). However, there is no specific antidote available (like Vitamin K for warfarin) so its use should be very carefully considered (EINSTEIN-PE 2012). Nevertheless, NICE (2013) have recommended rivaroxaban as a treatment option for DVT and PE.

Prevention

- Prophylactic once-daily subcutaneous LMWH injection
- Removal of agent that increases risk of PE (if feasible)
- Use of correctly fitting, below-knee, graduated compression stockings
- Early mobilisation
- Thrombophilia screen in patients with a family history of thromboembolic disorder (criteria vary so you should follow local haematology department guidelines)

Comprehensive guidance on prevention is available from NICE (2010).

HOT TIP

- An alveolar (A)-arteriolar (a) gradient (A-a) of less than 2kPa in a young, healthy, non-smoking adult woman virtually excludes a PE. Conversely, a gradient of more than 2kPa adds weight to the clinical probability of a diagnosis of PE.

  A-a gradient = FiO_2 (%) - (PaO_2 + $PaCO_2$ x 1.25) kPa
  For example:

  A-a gradient = 21 - (13 + 3 x 1.25) = 4.25kPa

- Allen's test should be performed before an ABG is carried out, to avoid digital ischaemia in case of an anomalous absent radial or ulnar artery (see Box 17.1).

- Low molecular weight heparin is not a clot-buster, but it prevents enlargement of existing clots and inhibits the development of new clots.

Box 17.1 Allen's test (based on Moore & Woodrow 2009, pp. 155–6)

1 Ask the patient to elevate their hand.
2 Occlude both the radial and ulnar arteries and then release the compression on the ulnar artery.
3 The hand should flush pink within 5–7 seconds, indicating that collateral circulation is present.
4 If colour does not return quickly, do not take arterial blood gases from this arm, as circulation to the limb could be compromised.

Case scenario

A 40-year-old woman is admitted to a medical ward with a right leg 'cellulitis' for intravenous antibiotics. She has previously been healthy and has never smoked in her life.

You are the medical foundation year 1 doctor on call for wards, and the ward sister calls you at 2am because the patient has suddenly started complaining of shortness of breath and right-sided pleuritic chest pain. Her blood pressure has dropped to 90/60mmHg and her respiratory rate has increased to 26 breaths per minute. Her SpO2 is 92% on room air and her heart rate is 120 beats per minute. She is apyrexial.

How would you rapidly assess this patient?

Think of the steps you would follow before reviewing the guidance below!

Case scenario review

The patient would be assessed using the ABCDE approach.

A-Airway

Check that the patient's airway is patent.

B-Breathing

The respiratory rate is high. If the patient is cyanosed, initiate high-flow oxygen therapy immediately and perform an arterial blood gas analysis.

C-Circulation

Urgent fluid resuscitation is needed, as well as a portable chest x-ray, and you should consider echo or CTPA. Prescribe thrombolysis (such as recombinant tissue plasminogen activator) as soon as possible. Get a 12-lead ECG. Vital signs observations should be continued half-hourly (or as per hospital policy) initially.

D-Disability

If mentation is altered, the patient might be very hypoxic.

E-Exposure and environment

Ensure that the patient is on a cardiac monitor and in an environment where thrombolysis (if required) is safe. Meanwhile, review the notes to rule out any absolute contraindications to thrombolysis and contact a senior colleague. Consider transfer to a high dependency unit if available.

Conclusion

Pulmonary embolism is a life-threatening complication that needs a high index of suspicion in susceptible patients. Prompt assessment, preventative strategies and treatment are key to the management of this group of patients.

References and further reading

British Thoracic Society (BTS) (2003). British Thoracic Society guidelines for the management of suspected acute pulmonary embolism. *Thorax.* **58**, 470–84.

EINSTEIN-PE (2012). Oral rivaroxaban for the treatment of symptomatic pulmonary embolism. *The New England Journal of Medicine.* **366**, 1287–97. http://www.nejm.org/doi/full/10.1056/NEJMoa1113572 (accessed 28 November 2014).

Kumar, P. & Clark M. (2002). *Clinical Medicine.* 5th edn. London: W.B. Saunders.

Moore, T. & Woodrow, P. (2009). *High Dependency Nursing Care: observation, intervention and support for level 2 patients.* 2nd edn. London: Routledge.

National Institute for Health and Care Excellence (NICE) (2010). *Venous thromboembolism: reducing the risk: Reducing the risk of venous thromboembolism (deep vein thrombosis and pulmonary embolism) in patients admitted to hospital.* http://www.nice.org.uk/guidance/cg92 (accessed 1 July 2015).

National Institute for Health and Care Excellence (NICE) (2012). *Venous Thromboembolic diseases: the management of venous thrombo-embolic diseases and the role of thrombophilia testing (CG144).* http://www.nice.org.uk/guidance/cg144 (accessed 1 July 2015).

National Institute for Health and Care Excellence (NICE) (2013). *Rivaroxaban for treating pulmonary embolism and preventing recurrent venous thromboembolism. NICE technology appraisal guidance 287.* http://www.nice.org.uk/guidance/ta287 (accessed 1 July 2015).

Swearingen, P.L. & Keen, J. (2001). *Manual of Critical Care Nursing: nursing interventions and collaborative management.* 4th edn. Maryland Heights, Missouri: Mosby.

Useful websites

National Institute for Health and Care Excellence (NICE)
http://www.nice.org.uk (Accessed 1 July 2015)

British Thoracic Society
http://www.brit-thoracic.org.uk (Accessed 1 July 2015)

18 Pneumonia

Gaurav Agarwal

This is an acute infection of the lower respiratory tract, often resulting in shadowing on the chest radiograph due to microorganisms, fluid and inflammatory cells (NICE 2014). There is a 5–14% mortality rate among patients requiring hospital admission (NICE 2014). The most common symptoms are fever with chills and rigors, discoloured sputum production, dyspnoea and cough (BTS 2009).

Classification and causes

Community-acquired pneumonia (CAP) (BTS 2004)

This is the most common (default) type of pneumonia. The causative organism is *Streptococcus pneumoniae* in 70% of cases; other causative organisms are *Haemophilus influenzae* and *Staphylococcus aureus* (high mortality with methicillin-resistant *Staphylococcus aureus*, known as MRSA). The so-called atypical pneumonias (presenting with diarrhoea, abnormal liver function tests or no consolidation on the chest radiograph) are caused by *Mycoplasma*, *Chlamydia* and *Legionella*. Viruses such as *influenza*, *varicella* and *cytomegalovirus* (and, rarely, fungi) also cause pneumonia. *Mycobacterium tuberculosis* should be considered if the patient presents with weight loss, malaise and night sweats or has risk factors linked with tuberculosis (BTS 2009).

Hospital-acquired pneumonia (NICE 2014)

This type of pneumonia develops in patients who have been in hospital for more than 48 hours. The organisms responsible, therefore, are those that are more commonly encountered within a hospital rather than in the community. *Staphylococcus aureus* (including MRSA), *Klebsiella*, *Pseudomonas* (which causes green phlegm, green wound discharge, etc.), *Escherichia coli*, *Proteus* and anaerobes are some common causative organisms in this setting.

Aspiration pneumonia

This is common in patients who have lost protection of their airway, (for example, in intoxicated, stroke patients and in neuromuscular disorders such as multiple sclerosis or myasthenia gravis. The anaerobes from the gut or oropharynx cause this type of pneumonia.

Pneumonia in the immunocompromised patient

In diabetics, patients who are post-chemotherapy, HIV patients and in those with malignancies, pneumonia can often be the reason for death if it is not managed aggressively enough early on. Any organism can cause this type of pneumonia but, in addition, consider fungi as a cause, especially if no clinical improvement is noticed after 2 days of standard therapy.

History

The onset is usually over a few days but can be less than a day in immunocompromised patients. The British Thoracic Society (2009) suggests assessing the severity of the pneumonia using the CURB-65 tool (see Box 18.1). This will indicate whether hospital management is required. A CURB-65 score of 2 means that hospital admission should be considered; and a CURB-65 score of >3 has a higher mortality rate and may require critical care admission (BTS 2009).

Symptoms

- Shortness of breath (dyspnoea)
- Pleuritic chest pain
- Fever with chills and rigors
- Coughing up streaks of blood with yellow, green or brown phlegm
- Non-specific systemic symptoms such as anorexia, malaise and nausea
- Confusion (pneumonia is an important cause of confusion in the elderly population).

Vital signs

- Tachypnoea
- Fever
- Tachycardia
- Hypotension
- Cyanosis (look carefully for this)
- Hypoxaemia.

Chest examination

- Inspection (decreased chest expansion on the diseased side)
- Palpation (tenderness on the affected side)
- Percussion (dullness on the affected side)
- Auscultation (bronchial breathing with a gap in between inspiration and expiration, and increased vocal resonance on the affected region of the lung)
- Pleural rub (may sometimes be heard)
- Small pleural effusion (may be evidence of this).

Cardiac, neurological and abdominal examination

- Usually normal.

Box 18.1 Severity assessment CURB-65 tool (NICE 2014)

- **C**–Confusion (score 1 if new onset)
- **U**–Urea (score 1 if >7mmol/litre)
- **R**–Respiratory rate (score 1 if more than 30 breaths per minute)
- **B**–Blood pressure (score 1 if systolic blood pressure <90 mmHg or diastolic <60mmHg)
- **65**–65 years old (score 1 if patient is older than 65).

If the score is <2, the pneumonia is not severe and may be suitable for out-of-hospital management. If the score is >2, the pneumonia should be managed in hospital and will probably need intravenous antibiotics at least for the first 1–2 days. A score of 3–4 suggests that urgent hospital referral is needed (NICE 2014).

Investigations
Chest radiograph
There is patchy consolidation, pleural effusion and (rarely) cavitation. A normal-looking chest radiograph does not exclude the diagnosis of pneumonia – it could be atypical or *Pneumocystis carinii pneumonia* (PCP) so act on history and clinical suspicion rather than just the chest radiograph.

All patients admitted to hospital with suspected CAP should have a chest radiograph performed as soon as possible to confirm or refute the diagnosis. The chest radiograph need not be repeated prior to hospital discharge in those who have made a satisfactory clinical recovery from CAP (BTS 2009)

Blood tests
Carry out a full blood count (neutrophilic leucocytosis is the most common), urea, creatinine, electrolytes (hyponatraemia suggests an atypical infection), liver function tests, C-reactive protein, arterial blood gas analysis and blood cultures. Suspected atypical pneumonia patients should have appropriate serology sent off as well.

Sputum
Send for microscopy and culture or sensitivity. A saline nebuliser may often help to induce sputum.

Arterial blood gas analysis
Often hypoxaemia is evident. Severe hypoxia would merit the use of non-invasive ventilation.

Pleural fluid
This can be invaluable if a diagnostic tap is sent off before antibiotics are started. Check lactate dehydrogenase (LDH), glucose and pH and send some for cultures as well.

Bronchoalveolar lavage
This is useful in an immunocompromised or critical care patient.

Blood cultures
Although not routinely needed, they should be taken in patients who require hospital admission.

Other tests for specific types of pneumonia (BTS 2009)
Tests for Streptococcus pneumonia
Patients with moderate or high-severity CAP should have pneumococcal urine antigen tests performed.

Tests for Legionnaires' disease

Legionella urine antigen tests should be performed for patients with high-severity CAP.

To avoid the spread of Legionella, all patients who are Legionella urine antigen-positive should have respiratory specimens (such as sputum) sent and Legionella culture requested.

Tests for Mycoplasma pneumonia

Where available, polymerase chain reaction (PCR) of respiratory tract samples, such as sputum, should be the method of choice for diagnosing mycoplasma pneumonia. If it is not possible to obtain a respiratory tract sample, a throat swab can be used instead.

Tests for Chlamydophila species

For patients with high-severity CAP, or for suspected psittacosis, *Chlamydophila* antigen and/or PCR detection tests should be used for invasive respiratory samples.

Treatment

Treatment should comprise the following (BTS 2009):

- Oxygen therapy to treat hypoxia (maintain SpO_2 at 94–98%)
- Fluid rehydration (either oral or intravenous, as needed)
- Anti-pyretics and analgesia
- Anti-emetics and other symptomatic therapy (as needed)
- Antibiotics (oral or intravenous depending on the CURB-65 score).

Choice of antibiotics

All patients should receive antibiotics as soon as the diagnosis of pneumonia is confirmed. The choice is often driven by local protocols so please familiarise yourself with your local microbiology guidelines. Often, penicillin should be used as first-line therapy in CAP, and a macrolide in atypical pneumonia. In severe pneumonia, a combination of penicillin and beta-lactamase inhibitor, along with a macrolide, is often advocated.

In severe pneumonia, you must ensure that the intravenous antibiotics are given either by yourself or a colleague the moment you have taken the blood cultures. (Just prescribing on the drug chart does not mean the antibiotic will be given straight away!) The typical duration of a course of intravenous antibiotics is 7 days.

For medical prophylaxis against deep vein thrombosis (unless contraindicated), the patient should be prescribed, for example, dalteparin 5000 units or enoxaparin 40mg once-daily subcutaneous injection.

Monitoring in hospital (BTS 2009)

Temperature, respiratory rate, pulse, blood pressure, mental status, oxygen saturation and inspired oxygen concentration should be monitored and recorded. The frequency of observations will depend on severity but they should be done at least twice-daily.

In patients who are not improving after 3 days of treatment, C-reactive protein should be re-measured and a chest radiograph repeated.

Critical care management of CAP (BTS 2009)

Patients with a CURB-65 of 4–5 should be assessed for admission to a critical care area. NIV or CPAP are not routinely indicated in management of patients with respiratory failure due to pneumonia but can be considered. Steroids are not recommended in high-severity CAP.

Complications

- Pleural effusion (may need a chest drain inserted)
- Empyema (if a chest drain fails to resolve this, a surgical procedure may be required)
- Lung abscess (aggressive longer-duration antibiotic therapy is usually curative)
- Type I respiratory failure, which can then lead on to type 2 respiratory failure (non-invasive or invasive ventilation should be considered in patients with severe disease, particularly those at risk of type 2 respiratory failure).

Prevention (BTS 2009)

- Pneumonia jabs and flu vaccines for all at-risk individuals
- Encouraging and helping people to quit smoking.

- **In COPD patients, watch out for *Moraxella catarrhalis* and *Pseudomonas*.**
- **In immunocompromised patients, think of fungi and *Pneumocystis carinii*.**

Case scenario

A 50-year-old man is admitted to a medical ward with cough and fever, and diagnosed with an upper respiratory tract infection. You are the medical foundation year 1 doctor on call for wards and the ward sister calls you at 8pm because the patient has started coughing up blood-streaked sputum and is very worried.

His blood pressure has dropped to 88/60 mmHg and his respiratory rate has increased to 32 breaths per minute. His SpO2 is 95% on room air and his heart rate is 120 beats per minute. He is apyrexial.

How would you rapidly assess this patient?

Think of the steps you would follow before reviewing the guidance below!

Case scenario review

The patient would be assessed using the **ABCDE** approach.

A-Airway

The patient's airway is patent.

B-Breathing

High respiratory rate. If the patient is cyanosed, initiate high-flow oxygen therapy immediately and perform an arterial blood gas analysis.

C-Circulation

Urgent fluid resuscitation is needed for low blood pressure. A portable chest x-ray is also required.

D-Disability
If mentation is altered, the patient is likely to be very hypoxic.

E-Exposure and environment
Apply 'fan therapy' and 'tepid-sponging' if the patient's temperature is very high. Follow this with definitive treatment of pneumonia if the CURB-65 score is indicative of a severe pneumonia, and inform the senior doctor immediately.

Conclusion

Pneumonia is a serious condition and it is important for clinicians to ensure that patients are followed up post-discharge, are advised to have the influenza and pneumococcal vaccinations and, where applicable, are offered smoking cessation strategies (BTS 2009). Susceptible patients are at risk of future infections, and prevention is key to reducing this risk.

References and further reading

British Thoracic Society (BTS) (2004). *BTS Guidelines for the Management of Community Acquired Pneumonia in Adults – 2004 update* https://www.brit-thoracic.org.uk/document-library/clinical-information/pneumonia/adult-pneumonia/adult-cap-guideline-2001/guidelines-for-the-management-of-community-acquired-pneumonia-in-adults-2004-update/ (accessed 2 July 2015).

British Thoracic Society (BTS) (2009). *BTS Guidelines for the Management of Community Acquired Pneumonia in Adults – 2009 update* https://www.brit-thoracic.org.uk/document-library/clinical-information/pneumonia/adult-pneumonia/a-quick-reference-guide-bts-guidelines-for-the-management-of-community-acquired-pneumonia-in-adults/ (accessed 2 February 2015).

National Institute for Health and Care Excellence (NICE) (2014). *Diagnosis and management of community- and hospital-acquired pneumonia in adults: NICE clinical guideline 191* https://www.nice.org.uk/guidance/cg191 (accessed 2 July 2015).

19 Neurological diseases affecting breathing

Alistair Challiner

Two conditions that may be encountered on acute medical wards are Guillain-Barré syndrome and myasthenia gravis. Both conditions cause muscle weakness, but the important factors to be concerned about are respiratory muscle weakness (causing hypo-ventilation) and loss of control of swallowing reflexes (causing a risk of aspiration and pneumonia).

Both conditions may need admission to the intensive care unit and intubation if symptoms deteriorate. It is therefore essential to know what these signs are, and how to monitor them.

Guillain-Barré syndrome

Guillain-Barré syndrome (GBS) is a demyelinating polyneuropathy that is caused by an immune mediated attack affecting the nerves. The myelin, which covers nerves, is reduced, causing decreased conduction. This leads to inability to move muscles (motor loss).

Two-thirds of patients report a trigger of infections (BMJ 2014), such as influenza, campylobacter or viruses, 1 to 3 weeks prior to onset. Other causes (although rare) include malignancy.

Signs and symptoms

The onset of symptoms is often swift – over a few days. The disease usually starts in the lower legs and symmetrically ascends up the body to affect the arms, leading to reduced mobility (Dimachkie & Barohn 2013). Sensory nerves can be involved, as can autonomic nerves (causing arrhythmias).

In severe cases a flaccid paralysis occurs, including the respiratory muscles. Up to 30% of patients will require mechanical ventilation in an intensive care unit as a result of the disease (BMJ 2014). Neurophysiology studies are used to confirm the diagnosis.

Management

Treatment includes immunoglobulin therapy or plasma exchange. Additional management is supportive and includes prevention of deep vein thrombosis (DVT) and infections, analgesia and vigilance in monitoring respiratory function (in case mechanical ventilation is required).

The symptoms can last for several months and may necessitate prolonged hospital admission. However, 85% of patients make a full recovery over time (BMJ 2014).

Myasthenia gravis

Myasthenia gravis (MG) is an autoimmune disease leading to antibodies that attack the acetylcholine receptors (Shah 2014), where the motor nerve stimulates a voluntary muscle. This causes a weakness that deteriorates the more the muscle is used – leading to increased fatigue and weakness over the course of the day.

Signs and symptoms

The disease usually starts in a distinct area and slowly progresses to affect the whole body over a number of months. Symptoms include drooping of the eyelids, nasal speech and difficulty swallowing. An anti-acetylcholine receptor (AChR) antibody test is used to confirm the diagnosis (Shah 2014).

Management

The main treatment is with drugs called anticholinesterase (AChE) inhibitors, which increase the level of acetylcholine (such as pyridostigmine), but immunosuppression and intravenous immunoglobulin are also used. Excision of the thymus gland in the thorax may be indicated (Shah 2014).

Generally, mortality in MG is low but deterioration can be caused by a worsening of the condition (myasthenic crisis) or by effective over-dosage of the pyridostigmine (cholinergic crisis). Patients admitted to hospital for other reasons may be particularly at risk of an exacerbation of MG due to other drug therapy (such as antibiotics) or stress (Shah 2014). Pyridostigmine causes an increase of acetylcholine by reducing its breakdown. Increased levels of acetylcholine in cholinergic crisis produce a neuromuscular block similar to anaesthetic muscle relaxants. This presents as sweating, fever, salivation, small pupils and muscle weakness, with twitching of the muscles.

Worsening of the condition may increase the risk of respiratory muscle weakness or aspiration, requiring intubation and mechanical ventilation (Shah 2014).

Respiratory muscle weakness

Patients with Guillain-Barré syndrome and myasthenia gravis are at risk of respiratory muscle weakness. Both these conditions may be seen on general wards and need close monitoring as the patient is at increased risk of sudden deterioration, which would need intervention by a specialist team. Simple clinical observations (peak flow, saturations and blood gases) should not be relied upon, as they are not specific or occur too late to determine when mechanical ventilation is necessary.

The most effective way of monitoring patients with respiratory muscle weakness is to measure their forced vital capacity (FVC). This is the volume of air that can be breathed out after taking a maximal deep breath. It is normally in the region of 5–6 litres but when it reduces to 20ml/kg (around 1 litre), admission to a critical care setting is indicated, as ventilation may be required. The patient's FVC should be measured regularly (every 1–6 hours), according to the severity of their condition. Clinical signs, such as being unable to speak or cough, tachypnoea, shallow breaths and exhaustion, are further indications for mechanical ventilation.

A patient who is deteriorating should be transferred to a high dependency unit or intensive care unit for closer observation and readily available mechanical ventilation.

The FVC is measured with a spirometer such as a vitalograph, but these are not normally available in the acute medical environment. It is more common to use a Wright flowmeter, attached to an anaesthetic face mask, usually available from the operating theatre or intensive care unit.

Disordered swallowing or bulbar signs

Signs of this include an abnormal voice (particularly nasal sounding) and difficulty swallowing water or regurgitating water nasally. The risk is aspiration pneumonia. Anaesthetic, or Speech and Language Team (SALT), assessment is required. The patient should be kept nil by mouth, and may require intubation to protect the airway.

Critical illness polyneuropathy

Critical illness polyneuropathy (or myopathy) can result from prolonged intensive care unit admission and may be present in patients discharged from there to the ward (see Chapter 45 on the post-intensive care patient). This condition leads to muscle weakness and wasting and is thought to be an autoimmune response (Hermans *et al.* 2008). The causes are unclear but it is related to immunosuppression, sepsis, and the use of drugs such as muscle relaxants and steroids.

Symptomatically, the patient may have weakness of all limbs and therefore need supportive nursing care, DVT prophylaxis and intensive physiotherapy, which may be key to the swiftness of recovery (Pattanshetty & Gaude 2011). This condition prolongs the patient's hospital stay and can be frustrating for patients and their families but most patients make a full recovery over time.

Conclusion

This chapter provides a brief overview of the neurological conditions affecting breathing that are sometimes seen in acute care wards. Key points to remember are that the patient's airway must be monitored and protected; and their respiratory function and strength must be continually reassessed so that any deterioration can be identified and they can be urgently referred, if necessary.

References and further reading

BMJ Best Practice (2014). *Guillain Barré Syndrome.* http://bestpractice.bmj.com/best-practice/monograph/176.html (accessed 2 May 2015).

Dimachkie, M.M. & Barohn, R.J. (2013). *Guillain-Barré Syndrome and Variants.* http://www.ncbi.nlm.nih.gov/pmc/articles/PMC3939842/ (accessed 2 May 2015).

Hermans, G., De Jonghe, B., Bruyninckx, G. & Van den Berghe, G. (2008). Clinical Review: Critical illness polyneuropathy and myopathy. *Critical Care.* **12**, 238. http://ccforum.com/content/pdf/cc7100.pdf (accessed 2 May 2015).

Pattanshetty, R.B. & Gaude G.S. (2011). Critical illness myopathy and polyneuropathy – A challenge for physiotherapists in the intensive care units. *Indian Journal of Critical Care Medicine.* **15** (2), 78–81. http://www.ncbi.nlm.nih.gov/pmc/articles/PMC3145308/ (accessed 2 May 2015).

Shah, A.K. (2014). *Myasthenia Gravis* http://emedicine.medscape.com/article/1171206-overview (accessed 2 May 2015).

Useful websites

Gullain-Barré Support Group
http://www.guillainbarresupport.org/ (Accessed 2 May 2015)

GAIN – Gullain Barré and associated inflammatory neuropathies
http://www.gaincharity.org.uk (Accessed 2 May 2015)

Myaware – Myasthenia Gravis Association
http://www.myaware.org/ (Accessed 2 May 2015)

▪ A B C D E ▪

Cardiovascular

20 Assessing and managing the cardiovascular system

Ann M. Price

This chapter will focus on the areas of cardiac output, peripheral vascular resistance and heart rate because, in the management of cardiovascular aspects, these are the main areas that are influenced by treatment regimes. The chapter will relate these principles to fluid management, drug therapy and the importance of the electrical conduction of the heart. Subsequent chapters will develop particular areas and give specific management strategies to build on this introductory chapter.

Physiology

The cardiovascular system is made up of the heart and blood vessels and it performs the vital role of transporting blood around the body. This is essential for life, as blood and its components deliver oxygen, nutrients and hormones (among other things) and enable the removal of waste products. The heart pumps approximately 5 litres of blood per minute around the body.

The cardiovascular system is divided into two main areas (Conelius 2014a):

- The pulmonary circulation, which moves blood from the heart through the lungs
- The systemic circulation, which moves blood from the heart to the other tissues and organs of the body.

As the blood passes through the lungs, there is an exchange of gases, including oxygen and carbon dioxide. As blood moves around the body, oxygen and nutrients are delivered to organs and tissues, and waste products are removed in order to be excreted. The components of the cardiovascular system (the heart, arteries, veins and capillaries) enable this transport of blood and they are designed to allow exchange of essential elements between the blood vessels and tissues.

The 'Inner Body' website allows you to interactively explore the cardiovascular system. It includes all the major arteries and veins.

http://www.innerbody.com/image/cardov.html

The heart

The heart, a vital organ within the cardiovascular system, is essential for pumping blood around the system. An understanding of the principles of cardiac output is important for good management of the patient (see Box 20.1). Cardiac output is the amount of blood that the heart pumps in 1 minute. To calculate the cardiac output, the amount of blood pumped in one heartbeat (called 'stroke volume') is multiplied by the heart rate.

The amount of blood the heart can pump with each beat ('stroke volume') depends on the amount of blood returning to the heart and on the strength of the cardiac muscle contraction. If there is poor venous blood flow returning to the heart (as in hypovolaemic shock), the heart will not fill properly and stroke volume will be reduced. Also, if the heart's pumping ability is affected by damage to the cardiac muscle (as in a myocardial infarction), the stroke volume will be reduced even though adequate blood is present. The heart rate is also relevant; the cardiac output may be affected if the rate is reduced or elevated for some reason, or if there is abnormal electrical activity (such as atrial fibrillation) affecting cardiac filling.

Box 20.1 Calculating cardiac output

Cardiac output is the amount of blood that the heart pumps in 1 minute. The cardiac output comprises the amount of blood (in mls) pumped in one heartbeat (called 'stroke volume'), multiplied by the heart rate:

Cardiac output (CO) = stroke volume (SV) x heart rate (HR) over 1 minute

Blood pressure

Pressure is needed within the cardiovascular system to allow blood to flow from the heart to the capillaries. The blood vessels are able to constrict and dilate to ensure that pressure within the system facilitates a good flow. Blood pressure (BP) is a way to measure this flow and is calculated as 'cardiac output' multiplied by 'peripheral vascular resistance' (see Box 20.2).

Remember that blood pressure is affected by the components of cardiac output (such as low blood volume, poor cardiac contraction and heart rate). It is also affected by the resistance within the arteries and veins, such as vasodilation and vasoconstriction. The BP is regulated by a number of neural and hormonal factors so that it remains within parameters that maintain blood flow to the vital organs and tissues (Conelius 2014a).

Box 20.2 Calculating blood pressure

Blood pressure (BP) is determined by the cardiac output and the resistance within the cardiovascular system, known as 'peripheral vascular resistance' (PVR). Thus, blood pressure can also be affected by the components of cardiac output (such as low blood volume, poor cardiac contraction and heart rate). In addition, it is affected by the resistance within the arteries and veins, such as vasodilation and vasoconstriction. The BP is regulated by neural and hormonal factors to ensure that it remains within parameters that maintain blood flow to the vital organs and tissues:

Blood pressure (BP) = cardiac output (CO) x peripheral vascular resistance (PVR)

Heart rate

The heart rate is another key factor affecting the cardiovascular system and circulation of blood. Cardiac conduction is a complex process whereby the heart muscle generates and conducts electrical impulses in a co-ordinated manner so that the heart pumps effectively (Conelius 2014b). Any disruption to this electrical activity can disrupt the co-ordination of the blood flow through the heart and reduce cardiac output. However, the electrical conduction system can also respond to a variety of stimuli to increase the heart rate when cardiac output is low. A full explanation of cardiac conduction is beyond the scope of this book but most anatomy, physiology and pathophysiology books will explore this topic in depth.

The key points to remember are that:

- The right amount of blood is needed to facilitate cardiovascular stability
- The heart needs to pump effectively to ensure that blood is delivered to organs and tissues
- The peripheral vascular system needs to be able to regulate the diameter of the blood vessels in order to maintain blood pressure
- The electrical conduction needs to be sufficient to ensure that a regular rhythm is maintained for efficiency.

The rest of this chapter will examine management of these aspects to improve cardiovascular function in acute illness.

Assessment of patients

Assessment of the patient's circulation has been comprehensively addressed in Chapters 2 and 3. Ideally, it should be fully assessed before initiating treatment. However, when circulatory collapse has occurred, and cardiac arrest or peri-arrest is evident, the *Resuscitation Guidelines* (Resuscitation Council UK 2015) should be followed.

Central venous pressure (CVP) is an important additional assessment strategy and an overview will be included here.

Central venous pressure

A central venous catheter (CVC) is a catheter that is inserted into the inferior or superior vena cava. These two large veins return blood to the right atrium of the heart, and they have the largest blood flow of any veins in the body (Conelius 2014a). Thus, CVP is a way to assess the amount of blood returning to the heart and affecting the stroke volume, as discussed above.

Central venous catheters (CVCs) are dedicated intravenous lines that are inserted for a number of reasons. In acute care, a common indication is to measure the CVP in order to monitor volume changes in a critically ill patient. There are no valves in the vena cava, so the pressure is a direct indication of the pressure in the right atrium of the heart. CVCs are also used to give fluids (particularly if they are required quickly), and to administer drugs and infusions that are not safe to give via peripheral cannulae – for example, vasoactive infusions, hypotonic or hypertonic fluids, or high concentrations of potassium. Parenteral nutrition (PN) is also often infused via a central line. CVCs are also useful for taking repeated blood samples.

Central venous catheters have a high rate of infection (NPSA 2009). However, associated line infection and sepsis can be reduced by incorporating key strategies such as hand hygiene, strict infection precautions, wound site care, careful catheter placement and prompt line removal (Patient Safety First 2015). The insertion of a central venous catheter therefore needs to be performed by a competent professional who is following local and national guidelines (NICE 2002).

The *Royal Marsden Manual* (2015) gives comprehensive, evidence-based guidelines for the care of central venous cannulae, cleaning the insertion site, applying dressings and changing of associated lines. The reader should review this text or their local setting guidelines for line care.

Interpreting CVP results

Central venous pressure is normally monitored through a transducer system and displayed via a monitor. It is vital that staff undertaking this have training regarding the accurate setting up of the system, ensure they can 'rezero' the transducer, align the position accurately, understand the significance of the results and recognise errors (such as poor waveform). If you are unfamiliar with this you may wish to gain local training or contact your critical care outreach service for advice.

The normal range for the CVP is 2–6mmHg when taken from the mid-axillary line, or fourth intercostal space, also called the 'phlebostatic axis' (Cole 2007). See Figure 20.1 for a diagram of the phlebostatic axis.

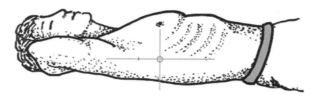

Figure 20.1 *The phlebostatic axis.*

The accuracy of CVP readings in predicting fluid status has been questioned (Kupchik & Bridges 2012) and, therefore, CVP readings must be taken in the context of the patient as a whole. The information below covers areas that should be considered if abnormal CVP measurements are found. However, there are many interventions (such as non-invasive ventilation) that can affect CVP readings.

Staff must ensure that all readings are documented and treatment recorded accurately to assess the response to any interventions. Thus, fluid charts and observations charts are vital.

High CVP

A high CVP may be due to heart failure, pulmonary oedema, fluid overload, a narrowing of the vessels, or an increased intra-thoracic pressure if the patient is receiving, for example, non-invasive ventilation or similar. If unusually high, it may be that the line is occluded or kinked, or pressing against the vessel wall. It may require a flush or repositioning of the line (see *The Royal Marsden Manual*).

Low CVP

A low CVP is usually due to hypovolaemia, or vasodilation due to medication or shock. As part of the ongoing management of a patient with a central venous catheter, goals are usually set regarding a desirable CVP measurement. A physician should set a CVP to aim for (related to national guidance), and fluid should be prescribed in order to reach that goal.

Box 20.3 Key points in nursing care of CVP

Nurses should ensure that:
- Infection control precautions are strictly adhered to
- Local policies regarding dressing and IV line changes are followed
- The CVP measurements are recorded accurately
- The fluid balance and observation charts are completed accurately
- The catheter site is observed for signs of infection
- Removal of the catheter is discussed with senior staff as soon as practical.

CVP is a useful measurement for managing critically ill patients but it has a significant infection risk. The catheter should therefore be removed as soon as the patient's condition allows, to reduce the chance of sepsis.

Management of patients

Management of patients with cardiovascular instability usually involves the following key points:

- Fluid management to maintain adequate blood circulation
- Inotropes to improve cardiac contraction
- Vasopressors or vasodilation drugs to maintain peripheral vascular resistance
- Electrocardiograms and anti-arrhythmic drugs to improve heart regularity.

All these measures affect the cardiac output and blood pressure, and a combination of treatments is sometimes necessary to optimise cardiovascular function. This section will give a brief overview of all these aspects. Specific disease processes will be discussed in detail in subsequent chapters.

Fluid management

Fluid management is a contentious issue and still needs further research (Goldstein 2014). However, for the ward-based healthcare professional, the goal of fluid management is to ensure that cardiac output is maintained and organ perfusion is preserved, particularly to prevent acute kidney injury (Goldstein 2014). Accurate recording of fluid charts is essential – encompassing both input and output, including urine output, stool loss and drains.

In most clinical situations, the first-line treatment for low blood pressure is to give a 'fluid challenge'. This means giving 250–500ml of, normally, crystalloid (such as Hartman's Solution or 0.9% saline) rapidly over about 10 minutes, then assessing whether the blood pressure and urine output improves. Repeated doses may be required until the blood pressure stabilises. However, repeating fluid challenges brings a risk of fluid overload. Ideally, a central venous catheter line should be inserted to measure central venous pressure to prevent this. There is currently some controversy in the literature about the use of excessive fluid challenges. Some studies suggest that increased mortality results if too much fluid is used, and others recommend 'early goal-directed therapy' to achieve certain parameters (Polderman & Varon 2015).

There is also debate as to whether crystalloids (isotonic solutions) or colloids (iso-oncotic solutions) are more effective in fluid management (Arunachalam & MacFie 2015). Colloids, such as hydroxyethyl starch (HES), are thought to expand the circulatory volume up to 80% more than crystalloids but there are many concerns with colloids, such as the effect on coagulation (Arunachalam & MacFie 2015). Other fluids, such as albumin and blood products, may also have a role in certain situations. Whole blood may be used to replace haemoglobin in the anaemic patient, for example, but the risks of blood transfusion are now also recognised. Subsequent chapters will highlight the current guidelines and recommendations for fluid management for the areas discussed.

Inotropes

Inotropic drugs can be defined as 'therapies that enhance myocardial contractile performance' (Francis *et al.* 2014, p. 2069); a number of drugs can be used for this purpose including digoxin, dobutamine and norepinephrine. However, many of these drugs also affect the heart rate and rhythm and can therefore lead to complications. Inotropes may be particularly useful in conditions such as heart failure, where the cardiac contraction is reduced and the stroke volume is affected, thus leading to reduced cardiac output and blood pressure.

Patients receiving these drugs will need close monitoring (particularly when assessing the initial response to the drugs) to assess their blood pressure and any complications involving tachycardia, bradycardia and arrhythmias.

In the critically ill patient, some of these drugs will be administered intravenously and may need observation in a critical care setting (particularly dobutamine and norepinephrine) because of their potent effect. The following chapters will highlight the current guidelines for the use of inotropes within the ward setting. Remember that guidance can be sought from the critical care outreach team (or equivalent) if these drugs are being used in the ward.

Vasopressors and vasodilation

Vasopressors are drugs that lead to vasoconstriction of the vascular system. Some diseases (such as sepsis) result in vasodilation and blood pressure is reduced (Szumita *et al.* 2005). Vasopressor agents include norepinephrine, dopamine and vasopressin. However, most of these drugs are only used in critical care settings because they have potent effects on the circulation, require continuous monitoring and need dedicated central venous access (as extravasation can lead to severe necrosis of tissues, due to the vasoconstriction effect).

Some drugs (such as glycerine trinitrate, GTN) lead to vasodilation. These are often used in heart failure to reduce vascular resistance in order to aid cardiac contraction. The following chapters will highlight situations where vasopressors or vasodilators may be indicated within the ward setting.

Electrocardiograms and anti-arrhythmic drugs

Electrocardiograms (ECGs) record the electrical conduction through the heart in different ways. A 3-lead ECG provides continuous observation of heart conduction via a monitor (there is also a 5 lead ECG version of this). Meanwhile, a 12-lead ECG usually offers a 'snapshot' of the conduction system but gives more detail. Both have their place in monitoring deterioration and assessing abnormalities in the critically ill adult.

Continuous monitoring may be required for patients who are haemodynamically unstable, or for those who have abnormal heart rhythms or who are receiving drugs that may induce dysrhythmias.

A 12-lead ECG will be used to assess a patient, for example, if a heart attack (myocardial infarction) is suspected or to check for arrhythmias or abnormalities. Some conditions require the swift use of an ECG to diagnose and treat a condition. For instance, patients who have an irregular pulse, chest pain or other unexplained symptoms will usually require a 12-lead ECG as a priority. Other critically ill patients will have a 12-lead ECG recorded as a 'baseline' so that any future changes can be identified. In critically ill patients, there is often a strain on the heart and these patients are therefore more prone to myocardial infarctions and arrhythmias.

HOT TIP

ECGs require experienced personnel to undertake the recordings and interpret the results. There are many books available on ECG interpretation if more information is needed.

There are numerous arrhythmias and various causes requiring different treatments. A regular heart rhythm is important to ensure that the cardiac output is maintained and any abnormality should therefore be investigated and treatment prioritised if blood pressure is affected. The following chapters highlight arrhythmias and any drug treatments that are indicated.

Conclusion

The drugs mentioned in this chapter have multiple uses and are often used in combination to gain the effect required for the individual patient. Some of the drugs have multiple effects and serious side effects and they should be used under the supervision of experienced medical practitioners. Always remember that the critical care outreach team can offer advice and should be contacted if more explanation is needed in the above aspects.

The following chapters will indicate situations where certain fluids and drugs may be preferred but healthcare professionals should seek expert advice early if treatment is not achieving desired results.

References and further reading

Arunachalam, L. & MacFie, J. (2015). Colloid versus crystalloid fluid therapy in surgical patients. *British Journal of Surgery*. **102**, 145–47.

Cole, E. (2007). Measuring central venous pressure. *Nursing Standard*. **22**(7), 40–43.

Conelius, J. (2014a). 'Structure and Function of the Cardiovascular System' in S.C. Grossman & C.M. Porth. *Porth's Pathophysiology*. 9th edn. Philadelphia: Wolters Kluwer Health/Lippincott Williams & Wilkins. pp. 712–38.

Conelius, J. (2014b). 'Disorders of Cardiac Conduction and Rhythm' in S.C. Grossman & C.M. Porth. *Porth's Pathophysiology*. 9th edn. Philadelphia: Wolters Kluwer Health/Lippincott Williams & Wilkins. pp. 845–66.

Francis, G.S., Bartos, J.A. & Adatya, S. (2014). Inotropes. *Journal of the American College of Cardiology*. **63** (20), 2069–78.

Goldstein, S.L. (2014). Fluid management in acute kidney injury. *Journal of Intensive Care Medicine*. **29** (4), 183–89.

Kupchik, N. & Bridges, E. (2012). Critical analysis, critical care: central venous pressure monitoring: What's the evidence? *American Journal of Nursing*. **112** (1), 58–61.

National Institute of Health and Care Excellence (NICE) (2002). *Guidance on the use of ultrasound locating devices for placing central venous catheters*. https://www.nice.org.uk/guidance/ta49 (accessed 20 July 2015).

National Patient Safety Agency (NPSA) (2009). *Matching Michigan – reducing central venous catheter related infections*. https://www.nice.org.uk/guidance/conditions-and-diseases/infections/healthcare-associated-infections (accessed 20 July 2015).

Patient Safety First (2015). *Critical Care*. http://www.patientsafetyfirst.nhs.uk/Content.aspx?path=/interventions/Criticalcare/ (accessed 20 July 2015).

Polderman, K.H. & Varon, J. (2015). Do not drown the patient: appropriate fluid management in critical illness. *The American Journal of Emergency Medicine*. **33** (3), 448–50.

Resuscitation Council UK (2015). *Resuscitation Guidelines*. https://www.resus.org.uk/resuscitation-guidelines/ (accessed 29 November 2015).

Szumita, P.M., Enganto, C.M., Greenwood, B. & Wechsler, M.E. (2005). Vasopressin for vasopressor-dependent septic shock. *American Journal of Health System Pharmacology*. **62**, 1931–36.

Useful websites

The Inner Body
http://www.innerbody.com/ (Accessed 2 July 2015)

The Royal Marsden Manual of Clinical Nursing Procedures (2015). 9th edn.
http://www.rmmonline.co.uk/ (Accessed 21 July 2015)

21 Sepsis

Ann M. Price and Sally A. Smith

Sepsis continues to have a high mortality rate despite advances in treatment. The UK Sepsis Trust estimates that 37,000 people die in the UK each year; and, according to the Surviving Sepsis website (2012), sepsis causes millions of deaths worldwide. In 2013 it was recognised that treatment of sepsis, within the UK, needed to become a priority (Parliamentary and Health Service Ombudsman 2013) to save lives and reduce healthcare cost. The Parliamentary and Health Service Ombudsman (2013, p. 5) recognised key signs of SEPSIS as 'Slurred speech; Extreme muscle pain; Passing no urine; Severe breathlessness; 'I feel I might die'; and Skin mottled or discoloured'. There is a clear set of guidelines that should be followed by healthcare professionals when treating sepsis.

This chapter focuses on the initial treatment of severe sepsis within the ward setting. When you have read it, you should be able to: define sepsis, severe sepsis and septic shock; identify the signs and symptoms of sepsis; understand the pathophysiology underpinning sepsis; and describe the initial management of a patient with sepsis.

Definitions

Sepsis is often a progressively worsening condition if left untreated. Three common terms are used to describe it, namely sepsis, severe sepsis and septic shock. The following list is based on updated criteria provided by Dellinger *et al.* (2013):

Sepsis, severe sepsis and septic shock definitions

Sepsis is infection, documented or suspected, and some of the following (Dellinger *et al.* 2013, p. 585):

- Temperature >38.3°C or <36°C
- Tachycardia >90 beats per minute
- Tachypnoea (>20 breaths per minute)

- White blood cells <4 or >12g/litre
- Altered mental state
- Significant oedema or positive fluid balance (>20ml/kg over 24 hrs)
- Glucose >7.7mmol/litre (unless diabetic)
- Hypotension (systolic <90mmHg or decrease in blood pressure by >40mmHg)
- Decreased urine output (<0.5ml/kg/hr despite fluid resuscitation)
- Decreased capillary refill or mottling
- Hyperlactatemia (>1mmol/litre).

Severe sepsis is 'sepsis-induced tissue hypoperfusion or organ dysfunction' (Dellinger *et al.* 2013, p. 586), which presents with the signs of sepsis plus additional organ dysfunction such as hypotension, oliguria, lactic acidosis, hypoxia and coagulopathy.

Septic shock is defined as 'sepsis-induced hypotension persisting despite adequate fluid resuscitation' (Dellinger *et al.* 2013, p. 583).

Causes of sepsis

Many factors should be eliminated when trying to identify the cause of sepsis. The type of infective organism needs to be considered, such as bacteria, virus, fungi or parasite. You will also need to exclude possible causes, such as trauma, pancreatitis, burns, intra-abdominal pathology, pneumonia, urinary tract infection and wound infection (Daniels 2010). However, there are many interventions that can also lead to sepsis such as vascular lines (such as a central venous catheter or a peripheral cannula), procedures (such as surgery) and invasive devices (such as urethral catheters). All these potential causes need to be investigated and excluded. The Surviving Sepsis Campaign (www.survivingsepsis. org, 2012) has produced an easy-to-use version of the severe sepsis screening tool to identify sepsis and its possible causes (see Figure 21.1 on page 171).

Many hospitals have adapted this to suit their own setting and staff should familiarise themselves with their local tools and processes.

Case scenario

A 65-year-old man is admitted with pneumonia. You notice that he is pyrexial, tachycardic and hypotensive. His urine output has reduced to less than 20ml per hour and he has not responded to a fluid challenge. An arterial blood gas shows that he is hypoxic and has a lactate of 2mmol/litre.

The UK Sepsis Trust has a number of resources for ward staff — see http://sepsistrust.org/clinical-toolkit/

(Accessed 20 October 2015).

Chart record – use patient label. Do not remove from chart

Evaluation for Severe Sepsis Screening Tool

Instructions: Use this optional tool to screen patients for severe sepsis in the emergency department, on the medical/surgical floors, or in the ICU.

1. **Is the patient's history suggestive of a new infection?**

    ☐ Pneumonia, empyema
    ☐ Urinary tract infection
    ☐ Acute abdominal infection
    ☐ Meningitis
    ☐ Skin/soft tissue infection

    ☐ Bone/joint infection
    ☐ Wound infection
    ☐ Blood stream catheter infection
    ☐ Endocarditis

    ☐ Implantable device infection
    ☐ Other infection
    _____

    ___ Yes   ___No

2. **Are any two of following signs & symptoms of infection both present and new to the patient? Note: laboratory values may have been obtained for inpatients but may not be available for outpatients.**

    ☐ Hyperthermia > 38.3 °C (101.0 °F)
    ☐ Hypothermia < 36 °C (96.8°F)
    ☐ Altered mental status
    ☐ Tachycardia > 90 bpm

    ☐ Tachypnea > 20 bpm
    ☐ Leukocytosis (WBC count >12,000 µL–1)
    ☐ Leukopenia (WBC count < 4000 µL–1)

    ☐ Hyperglycemia (plasma glucose >140 mg/dL) or 7.7 mmol/L in the absence of diabetes

    ___ Yes   ___No

    If the answer is yes, to both questions 1 and 2, *suspicion of infection* is present:

    ✓ Obtain: **lactic acid**, **blood cultures**, CBC with differential, basic chemistry labs, bilirubin.
    ✓ At the physician's discretion obtain: UA, chest x-ray, amylase, lipase, ABG, CRP, CT scan.

3. **Are any of the following organ dysfunction criteria present at a site remote from the site of the infection   that are NOT considered to be chronic conditions? Note: in the case of bilateral pulmonary infiltrates the remote site stipulation is waived.**

    ☐ SBP < 90 mmHg or MAP <65 mmHg
    ☐ SBP decrease > 40 mm Hg from baseline
    ☐ Creatinine > 2.0 mg/dl (176.8 mmol/L) or urine output < 0.5 ml/kg/hour for 2 hours
    ☐ Bilirubin > 2 mg/dl (34.2 mmol/L)
    ☐ Platelet count < 100,000 µL
    ☐ Lactate > 2 mmol/L (18.0 mg/dl)
    ☐ Coagulopathy (INR >1.5 or aPTT >60 secs)
    ☐ Acute lung injury with PaO2/FiO2 <250 in the absence of pneumonia as infection source
    ☐ Acute lung injury with PaO2/FiO2 <200 in the presence of pneumonia as infection source

    ___ Yes   ___No

If *suspicion of infection* is present AND *organ dysfunction* is present, the patient meets the criteria for SEVERE SEPSIS and should be entered into the severe sepsis protocol.

Date: ____/____/____ (circle: dd/mm/yy or mm/dd/yy)   Time: ____:____ (24 hr. clock)

Version 7.2.13

Figure 21.1 Sepsis screening tool (from www.SurvivingSepsis.org.
Reproduced with permission, Copyright © 2014 Society of Critical Care Medicine)

Pathophysiology

Sepsis is a very complex phenomenon involving the infectious agent, innate immunity and genetic factors (Mitchell & Whitehouse 2010). Pro-inflammatory cytokines, such as tumour necrosis factor alpha (TNF-alpha), interleukins 1 and 6 (IL1 and IL6), play a key role in initiating a systemic inflammatory response (SIRS) (Sagy *et al.* 2013). This causes multiple reactions within the body that lead to the dysfunctions seen in sepsis.

1. Vasodilation of blood vessels leads to hypotension. This limits blood flow to vital organs, causing dysfunction and eventual failure.

2. The vascular endothelium (capillaries) become more permeable, leading to fluid leaking from vascular space into interstitial and intracellular spaces, causing oedema, worsening hypotension and restricting organ perfusion further (Mitchell & Whitehouse 2010). This may also affect the function of the lungs, leading to acute respiratory distress syndrome (ARDS).

3. Initially, the myocardium tries to compensate with a 'hyperdynamic' response to the sepsis (seen as tachycardia and increased cardiac output), but myocardial function is depressed and may progress to cardiac failure (Mitchell & Whitehouse 2010).

4. The clotting cascade is affected in a variety of ways, causing abnormal platelet aggregation and overactive coagulation. This leads to the formation of micro-clots within the circulation that impede blood flow to the vital organs. This can progress to disseminated intravascular coagulation (DIC), which can cause major bleeding problems.

5. The body is unable to utilise energy sources as normal, resulting in metabolic acidosis (seen as lactic acidosis). This means that the cells are starved of energy and metabolise abnormally, leading to cell damage and organ failure (Mitchell & Whitehouse 2010). The body tries to compensate by finding alternative sources of energy, which may lead to high blood sugars and insulin resistance.

6. Acute kidney injury is common. The exact mechanism for this in sepsis is unclear (Mitchell & Whitehouse 2010). However, it leads to poor urine output, accumulation of waste products and increasing oedema.

After approximately 72 hours, the anti-inflammatory processes are thought to become more prominent in the sepsis picture – a process known as compensatory anti-inflammatory reaction syndrome (CARS). This anti-inflammatory response tries to balance the pro-inflammatory reaction initiated in SIRS but means that the immune system is less responsive and makes the patient vulnerable to new infections (Mitchell & Whitehouse 2010).

It is therefore vital that the early signs of sepsis are recognised and treated in order to prevent the sepsis cascade and deterioration to septic shock, which is very difficult to reverse.

Monitoring and management

The Surviving Sepsis Campaign emphasises the importance of treating sepsis swiftly, and they have recently updated their guidelines in line with current evidence (Surviving Sepsis Campaign 2012), Dellinger *et al.* 2013). The steps in the management of sepsis will be outlined here, based on these guidelines, which supersede previous articles published by Dellinger *et al.* in 2004 and 2008. The latest guidelines have been developed internationally and are widely endorsed (Dellinger *et al.* 2013). In addition, the National Institute for Health and Care Excellence has guidelines for the treatment of neutropenic sepsis in cancer patients (NICE 2012).

The management of sepsis is outlined in three key bundles. 'The Sepsis Six' is aimed at swiftly treating suspected sepsis (UK Sepsis Trust). In addition, the 'Severe Sepsis 3-hour Resuscitation Bundle' and the '6-hour Septic Shock', both from the Institute for Healthcare Improvement (2015), are provided for those patients presenting with severe sepsis or septic shock. Ward-based staff should familiarise themselves with their local hospital setting policy detailing the 'Sepsis Six'.

The Sepsis Six

The specific set of actions required within the first hour after onset has been termed 'The Sepsis Six' (Daniels 2008, UK Sepsis Trust) and these are outlined in Box 21.1. The Sepsis Six emphasises the need for oxygen therapy, taking blood cultures, administering antibiotics and fluid challenges, measuring serum lactate and haemoglobin, and completing fluid balance (particularly urine output). These are the immediate actions for someone presenting with sepsis. For further information, please refer to the Surviving Sepsis websites.

Screening for sepsis

Screening every potentially infected seriously ill patient for sepsis is recommended to facilitate early treatment (Dellinger *et al.* 2013) (see Figure 21.1).

Box 21.1 The Sepsis Six

(based on the UK Sepsis Trust, http://sepsistrust.org/wp-content/uploads/2013/10/Gloucester-Sepsis-Six.pdf)

TO BE DELIVERED WITHIN THE FIRST HOUR FOLLOWING THE ONSET OF SEPSIS

1. **Administer high-flow oxygen**: Give 15 litres via non-rebreathe mask and take arterial blood gases. Consider factors affecting breathing (e.g. COPD).

2. **Give intravenous fluid challenges**: Use Hartmann's solution initially at 500–1000mls. Albumin should be considered if large amounts of crystalloid are required. Consider inserting a central venous catheter.

3. **Take blood cultures**: Before starting antibiotics, take bloods from peripheral vein and from any indwelling devices. Consider other investigations to find infection source, such as CT scan and ultrasound.

4. **Give broad-spectrum antibiotics**: Initially administer broad-spectrum antibiotics within 1 hour. Seek microbiology advice.

5. **Measure serum lactate and haemoglobin**: Use arterial blood gas analysis to assess, aiming for Hb 7–9g/dl. Check lactate within first hour. Lactate >2 indicates sepsis, and >4 indicates severe sepsis. Consider other causes of raised lactate.

6. **Measure hourly urine output accurately**: Output target is 0.5ml/hour/kg. Monitor urine output response to fluid challenges. A catheter may be needed if the patient is not fully mobile. A urometer should be used if the patient has a catheter in situ or one is inserted.

Observations: Patients who are at risk of severe sepsis should be continuously monitored, with vital sign recordings taken every 1–2 hours using the local Early Warning Score chart. In case of deterioration, prompt recognition and action is vital.

Recommendations for initial resuscitation and infection issues

Dellinger *et al.* (2013, p.588) further recommended that initial resuscitation during the first 6 hours should aim to achieve:

a Central venous pressure 8–12mmHg

b Mean arterial pressure >65mmHg

c Urine output >0.5ml/kg/hr

d Central venous or mixed venous oxygen saturations of 70% or 65% respectively.

The aim is that high lactate levels should normalise and blood pressure should be stabilised. The above measures may require the patient to be admitted to a level 2 or 3 critical care area, and referral to the critical care team should be considered. If the patient's condition does not improve with these measures, vasopressors (such as norepinephrine) will be needed (IHI 2014).

Diagnosis

Two sets of blood cultures should be taken from the peripheral site and from any invasive lines that have been in situ more than 48 hours, ideally before commencing antibiotics. Other specimens and investigations should be undertaken as indicated (for example, urine, cerebrospinal fluid or CT scan, ultrasound). All these investigations aim to accurately identify the cause of the sepsis.

Antimicrobial therapy

Intravenous broad-spectrum antimicrobials should be commenced within the first hour for severe sepsis and septic shock. The regime should be reassessed daily, and biomarkers (such as procalcitonin levels) may guide the clinician as to when to discontinue therapy.

Antimicrobials should be focused to the most appropriate, once microbiology results are received. Combination therapy should not continue beyond 5 days but targeted therapy may be needed for 10 days (or longer). Antiviral therapy may be needed if indicated.

Controlling the source of infection

Several options should be considered to control the source of the infection: drainage of abscesses; removal of invasive devices; debridement of tissue; and definitive control, usually through surgical intervention (Dellinger *et al.* 2013).

Remember that some causes of sepsis are preventable, and non-essential invasive lines should be removed as soon as possible. Phlebitis scores should be recorded daily, and lines removed or changed when indicated.

Intensive care

Some patients will require admission to a critical care high dependency or intensive care area. Patients who require support (such as mechanical ventilation, vasopressor therapy, sedation, tight glucose control and renal replacement therapy) should be considered for transfer. These specialist interventions are beyond the scope of this chapter. Consider consulting the critical care team about any patient who is in septic shock or does not improve following the administration of these resuscitation care bundle elements (see 'Hot Tips').

Aim of treatment – report quickly if the parameters below are not achieved or they are deteriorating:
- Mean BP >65mmHg
- Systolic BP >90mmHg
- Pulse <100 beats per minute
- Temperature >36<38.3°C
- Urine output >0.5ml/kg/hour

Conclusion

There has been a drive to improve the care of patients with sepsis, with the introduction of measures such as the Commissioning for Quality and Innovation (CQUIN) payment framework (NHS Institute for Innovation and Improvement 2006–2013). However, sepsis, severe sepsis and septic shock are still major causes of mortality in the Western world. Some episodes can be prevented by simple observation and prompt action. Deterioration can be minimised by swift implementation of the sepsis regimen as outlined here, even within the ward setting.

References and further reading

Daniels, R. (2010). 'Defining the Spectrum of Disease' in R. Daniels & T. Nutbeam. *ABC of Sepsis*. Chichester: BMJ/Wiley Blackwell, pp. 5–9.

Daniels, R., McNamara, G., Nutbeam, T. & Laver, K. (2008). *Survive Sepsis Manual.* Sutton Coldfield: Heart of England Foundation Trust.

Dellinger, R.P., Carlet, J.M., Masur, H., *et al* (2004). Surviving Sepsis Campaign: Guidelines for the management of severe sepsis and septic shock. *Critical Care Medicine*. **32** (3), 858–73.

Dellinger, R.P., Levy, M.M., Carlet, J.M., *et al* (2008). Surviving Sepsis Campaign: International guidelines for management of severe sepsis and septic shock. *Critical Care Medicine*. **36**, 296–327; published correction appears in *Critical Care Medicine*. **36**, 1394–96.

Dellinger, R.P., Levy, M.M., Rhodes, A. *et al* (2013). Surviving Sepsis Campaign: International Guidelines for the Management of Severe Sepsis and Septic Shock. *Critical Care Medicine*. **41**, 580–637. DOI: 10.1097/CCM.0b013e31827e83af.

Institute for Healthcare Improvement (IHI) (2015). *Severe Sepsis Bundles.* http://www.ihi.org/resources/Pages/Tools/SevereSepsisBundles.aspx (accessed 29 November 2015).

Mitchell, E. & Whitehouse, T. (2010). 'The Pathophysiology of Sepsis' in R. Daniels & T. Nutbeam (eds). *ABC of Sepsis*. Chichester: BMJ/Wiley Blackwell, pp. 20-24

National Institute for Health and Care Excellence (NICE) (2012). *Neutropenic Sepsis: prevention and management or neutropenic sepsis in cancer patients.* http://www.nice.org.uk/guidance/CG151 (accessed 20 October 2015).

NHS Institute for Innovation and Improvement (2006–2013). *Commissioning for Quality and Innovation (CQUIN) payment framework.* http://www.institute.nhs.uk/commissioning/pct_portal/cquin.html (accessed 20 October 2015).

Parliamentary and Health Service Ombudsman (2013). *Time to Act: Severe Sepsis rapid diagnosis and treatment saves lives.* http://www.ombudsman.org.uk/time-to-act (accessed 20 October 2015).

Sagy, M, Al-Qaqaa, Y. & Kim, P. (2013). Definitions and pathophysiology of sepsis. *Current Problems in Pediatric and Adolescent Health Care*. **43** (10), 260–63.

UK Sepsis Trust (2013). *What is Sepsis?* http://sepsistrust.org/public/ (accessed 20 October 2015).

UK Sepsis Trust (2015). *Sepsis Six Pathway.*
http://sepsistrust.org/ (accessed 20 October 2015).

Surviving Sepsis Campaign (2012). Guidelines'.
http://www.survivingsepsis.org/Guidelines/Pages/default.aspx (accessed 20 October 2015).

Useful websites

Surviving Sepsis
http://www.survivingsepsis.org (Accessed 20 October 2015)

The UK Sepsis Trust
http://sepsistrust.org/ (Accessed 20 October 2015)

Institute for Healthcare Improvement
http://www.ihi.org (Accessed 20 October 2015)

22 Hypovolaemic shock

Tim Collins

C linical shock can be evident in any patient admitted to hospital. The underlying physiology, causes and treatment of this life-threatening condition are often complex and challenging for the healthcare professional. Hypovolaemic shock is a common cause of inadequate tissue perfusion, and results in widespread cellular hypoxia and altered homeostasis. Prompt assessment, recognition and management will improve clinical outcome, as hypovolaemic shock is a significant cause of death both within hospital and in the pre-hospital environment.

This chapter discusses the underlying pathophysiology of hypovolaemia, as well as strategies that can be used to assess and manage this life-threatening condition. It explores the physiology and resultant abnormal homeostasis of hypovolaemic shock; discusses the clinical presentation of a patient suffering from hypovolaemic shock and relates this to the underlying physiology; identifies the potential causes of hypovolaemic shock; and looks at how to assess and manage a critically ill patient presenting with hypovolaemia.

Pathophysiology

The circulating fluid volume of an adult is 70ml/kg (Singh-Radcliff 2013); total blood volume is therefore in the region of 4–5 litres. When circulating fluid volume is reduced, there is a reduction in cardiac output, which results in a low perfusion state, leading to hypovolaemic shock (Garretson & Malberti 2007). This low perfusion state causes widespread cellular hypoxia and lactic acidosis, which will ultimately cause multi-organ failure and death if it is not promptly resolved. Hypovolaemia has many possible causes but it is frequently associated with haemorrhage, which can be classified as either internal or external. Internal haemorrhage may occur following a post-operative bleed, rupture of abdominal aortic aneurysm, abdominal or thoracic trauma, or a traumatic bone fracture. In traumatic bone fractures, Skinner & Driscoll (2013) estimate the following blood loss depending on the site of the fracture:

- Humerus 0.5–1.5 litres
- Pelvis 1–4 litres
- Femur 1–2.5 litres
- Tibia 0.5–1.5 litres.

Internal haemorrhage can be more difficult and complex to diagnose than external haemorrhage, where excessive blood loss is visible and often creates the 'white patient–red floor syndrome' (i.e. you can see the blood loss). External haemorrhages are often related to traumatic injuries or gastrointestinal bleeds. Multiple trauma patients will nearly always present in a hypovolaemic state that quickly progresses to shock, which can result in death. Trauma patients need to be treated promptly and effectively, as trauma is the leading cause of death in young adults (Skinner & Driscoll 2013).

Hypovolaemic shock is not solely caused by haemorrhage. It can also be caused by dehydration and fluid loss from extra-cellular compartments. Conditions that may cause hypovolaemia following fluid loss include: severe diarrhoea and vomiting, excessive nasogastric tube loss, fever, bowel obstruction, burns, pancreatitis, diabetic ketoacidosis, third space fluid shift movements, and inappropriate diuretic therapy. In these situations, lost fluid will mainly consist of plasma rather than whole blood, as in the trauma or haemorrhaging patient (Bench 2004); see below.

Box 22.1 Causes of hypovolaemic shock

- External haemorrhage (e.g. arterial bleed)
- Internal haemorrhage (e.g. ruptured spleen, ruptured internal blood vessel)
- Trauma
- Fracture
- Severe vomiting and diarrhoea
- Bowel obstruction
- Pancreatitis
- Peritonitis
- Burns
- Third space fluid shift movements
- Inappropriate diuretic therapy.

Consequences of hypovolaemia

The reduction in circulatory volume leads to a lower cardiac preload and venous return, which – if severe – will result in hypotension and poor systemic perfusion (Collins & Plowright 2007). In response to abnormal homeostasis, the body will initially instigate compensatory strategies to counteract the fluid loss. This is known as the *compensatory stage* of hypovolaemia. If the fluid loss continues and no action is taken to resolve the condition, the body's compensatory mechanisms will fail, resulting in severe hypotension. This is known as the *de-compensatory* or *progressive stage* of clinical shock (Collins & Plowright 2007).

During the compensatory stage, which occurs with vascular loss of 15–30% of total blood volume, the body will firstly release catecholamines, such as adrenaline and noradrenaline, into the systemic blood circulation (Bersten & Soni 2013). This will bring about peripheral vasoconstriction in an attempt to promote perfusion to the vital aerobic organs such as the brain, heart and lungs. Reduced peripheral circulation follows and the patient will present with cool peripheries, reduced amplitude of distal pulses, delayed capillary refill time (more than 2 seconds) and reduced urine output. These signs and symptoms occur as the body tries to compensate and diverts perfusion away from the non-essential organs (Collins & Plowright 2007). The increased catecholamine release and reduced cardiac output results in tachycardia, which is an attempt to counteract the effects of a reduced preload and cardiac output.

If the hypovolaemia continues, the body's compensatory mechanisms begin to fail and the patient will enter the progressive stage or de-compensated phase of shock. This is where the loss of blood volume has exceeded 30% and the patient's compensatory mechanisms are no longer functioning adequately. There is a dramatic deterioration in the patient's condition and severe hypotension develops. If the patient does not receive immediate treatment, multi-organ failure will develop and death is likely to occur. The four classes of hypovolaemic shock are described in Table 22.1 (below).

Table 22.1 Four classes of hypovolaemic shock
(based on Collins 2000 and Gonce Morton et al. 2003)

Blood loss	Observations
Class 1: Up to 15% blood loss	• Circulatory volume equates to 70ml/kg in adults and 80ml/kg in neonates • Usually few clinical signs, as the body's compensatory mechanisms are activated to cope with the blood loss • Patients who are young and fit can tolerate significant blood loss before their vital signs become abnormal.
Class 2: 15–30% blood loss	• Tachycardia (weak and thready pulse) • Hyperventilation • Vasoconstriction (delayed capillary refill >2 seconds) • Cool or diaphoretic skin • Oliguria (below 0.5ml/kg/hr) • Concentrated urine • Confusion and agitation • Poor peripheral pulses • SvO_2 <60% • Haemodynamics: low cardiac output and high systemic vascular resistance (SVR) • Low stroke volume and high stroke volume variation • Reduced central venous pressure (CVP) • Elevated lactate. *N.B. Changes in all observations except for blood pressure.*
Class 3: 30–40% blood loss	• Dramatic deterioration in all vital signs • Severe tachycardia and hypotension develops as above • Reduced oxygen saturations • Oliguria leading to anuria • Mental stupor • SvO_2 <55% • Metabolic acidosis.
Class 4: Above 40% blood loss	• Immediate threat to life • Cardio-respiratory arrest impending • Drastic surgery and treatment required.

Assessment and management of patients in hypovolaemic shock

As with any critically ill patient, the standard **ABCDE** approach should be utilised when assessing a patient suspected of hypovolaemic shock. The patient should be attached to continuous monitoring of their heart rate, oxygen saturations, and non-invasive blood pressure. Vital signs (including respiratory rate and urine output) and any other fluid losses (such as blood loss, vomit and drains) should be recorded. Fluid input must also be recorded, and balance calculations made every 4 hours. The frequency of vital sign recordings must be assessed on an individual basis, but they should be at least hourly in the acute phase, and must include a 'track and trigger' (early warning) score. A patient requiring aggressive fluid resuscitation must not be left unattended until they are more stable.

If experienced personnel are available, a central venous catheter should be inserted. This will allow direct measurement of the patient's CVP and will provide a route for drug and fluid resuscitation. A recent meta-analysis by Marik & Cavallazzi (2013), involving 43 studies, concluded there was no data to support the widespread practice of using CVP to guide fluid therapy. However, the central venous catheter still provides benefits, with multiple access for drugs and fluids during resuscitation. In a critical care area, consider inserting an arterial line to allow continuous recording of blood pressure and the option of taking regular arterial blood gases and other blood samples.

Treatment involves optimising ventilation and oxygenation by administering oxygen therapy, correcting the cause of the hypovolaemia, and fluid resuscitation. Urgent surgery in the operating theatre may be needed if bleeding is suspected. It is imperative that early referral is made to senior surgical and anaesthetic personnel, including referral to the critical care outreach team. It is essential that early aggressive treatment and assistance is obtained for patients suffering from hypovolaemic shock, as cell damage and death can occur rapidly in this life-threatening condition. See Table 22.3.

Signs and symptoms of hypovolaemia

- Rapid, weak and thready pulse
- Tachypnoea
- Delayed capillary refill (over 2 seconds)
- Cold, pale, diaphorectic peripheral digits (vasoconstriction)
- Weaker peripheral pulses
- Oliguria (reduced below 0.5ml/kg/hour and concentrated)
- Confusion and agitation
- Reduced Glasgow Coma Score (see Chapter 34) or AVPU (see Box 2.1, p. 12)
- There may be visual signs of blood loss
- Excessive blood loss from wound drains
- Abdomen may be hard, distended and painful
- History of recent surgery or trauma (fractures)
- Blood results will show falling haemoglobin
- Arterial blood gases will show metabolic acidosis
- Elevated lactate level (normal <1.5)
- Low central venous pressure

- SvO_2 <60%
- Cardiac output measurements will show low cardiac output and high systemic vascular resistance
- Low stroke volume and high stroke volume variation (SVV)
- Reduced oxygen saturations (poor signal may be associated with vasoconstriction)
- Hypotension (late sign)
- Decreased pulse blood pressure.

Management plan

The management of patients with hypovolaemia focuses on restoring circulatory volume and correcting the cause of the fluid loss. All shocked patients should be given high-flow oxygen via a non-rebreathe face mask, with the aim of improving arterial oxygen-carrying capacity and oxygen delivery (DO_2) to the tissues (Bersten & Soni 2013). If respiratory or airway compromise is present then early intubation should be considered, particularly if a patient is becoming confused and agitated. This is most likely to be due to hypoxia, which would impede vital fluid resuscitation and haemodynamic monitoring. (See Figure 22.1 on page 182 for a summary of hypovolaemic shock.)

Fluid resuscitation

Optimising preload and increasing circulatory fluid volume is paramount for patients, and several litres of fluid may be required to achieve this. In uncomplicated hypovolaemia (such as dehydration from extra-cellular fluid losses), the instigation of intravenous (IV) fluid therapy may quickly correct the hypovolaemia. However, in cases of haemorrhage, the correction of shock can be a far more complex and challenging process. It also needs to be remembered that an increase in blood pressure may not mean that the bleeding has stopped.

It is widely accepted that the fluid used to correct any deficit should be the type of fluid lost (Roth, Garcia & Chaudhry 2005). NICE (2013) advocates giving 500ml fluid boluses of crystalloid solutions containing sodium in the range of 130–154mmol/litre. Crystalloid fluid resuscitation involving uncomplicated hypovolaemia (such as extra-cellular fluid losses, including vomiting and diarrhoea) may replace missing fluid and essential electrolytes. However, caution needs to be exercised because the additional sodium load associated with a potential hyperchloremic acidosis may worsen an underlying metabolic acidosis resulting from the hypovolaemia.

In the case of bleeding patients, a blood transfusion will be required. This often involves administering packed red blood cells (RBC), which will increase the haemoglobin (Hb) and subsequent oxygen-carrying capacity (Bersten & Soni 2013). It is best to aim for an Hb maintained between 7 and 9g/dl, compared to a more traditional level of 10–12g/dl in a bleeding or critically ill patient (Rossaint *et al.* 2010).

Transfused blood usually takes the form of packed red blood cells to provide oxygen-carrying capacity, and does not contain essential clotting factors and fluid. As blood is lost and replaced with packed cells and IV fluids, a dilutional coagulopathy will develop, as clotting factors bleed out. It is therefore essential to consider administering fresh frozen plasma (FFP) and platelets in a haemorrhaging patient; otherwise the coagulation deficiencies will prolong and worsen any haemorrhage. All hospitals have a policy on massive blood transfusion, which should be implemented with an acute bleeding patient. All healthcare professionals should be aware of how to access their hospital's policy on major haemorrhage.

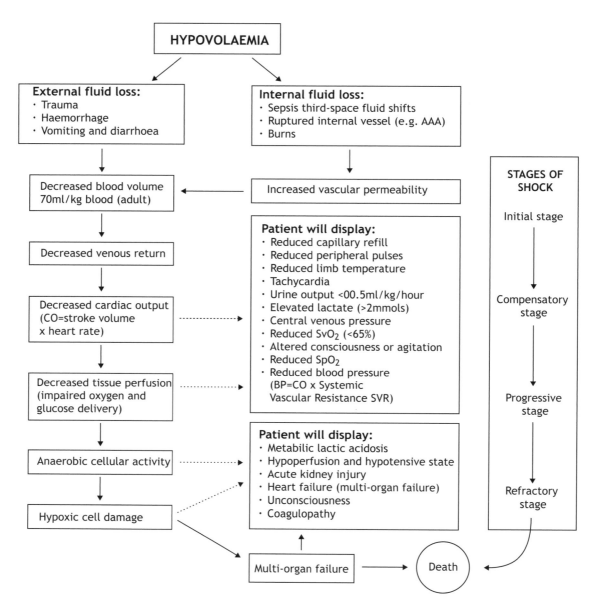

Figure 22.1 Summary of hypovolaemic shock

For a bleeding patient, it is essential to combine red blood cells and clotting factors with an IV fluid to enhance the circulating fluid volume (Bersten & Soni 2013). Over the last few decades, there has been considerable discussion concerning what type of fluid should be used for fluid resuscitation and this is often referred to as the 'colloid versus crystalloid debate' (Alderson *et al.* 2003). This debate continues to rage, as some practitioners believe that colloids (gelatins, starches, albumin) are more effective in hypovolaemia, as they have a higher molecular weight (>30kDa) than crystalloids (normal saline). This means they stay in the intravascular compartment for longer, enhancing available circulatory volume by increasing intravascular oncotic pressure (Woodrow 2011).

The alternative argument is that crystalloids are cheaper and have fewer adverse side effects than colloids and, as there is no conclusive research showing that colloids improve survival, crystalloids will suffice (Alderson *et al.* 2003). The NICE intravenous fluid therapy guidelines (2013) advocate that an IV crystalloid solution containing sodium in the range of 130–154mmol/litre should be used for fluid resuscitation. This includes the use of 0.9% sodium chloride and Hartman's solution. NICE (2013) states that tetrastarch fluids should not be used and that 4–5% human albumin solution may be considered in sepsis. Despite the debate, it cannot be stressed enough that aggressive IV fluid resuscitation, whether using a colloid or a crystalloid, is essential for any patient suffering from hypovolaemia.

Fluid challenge

A fluid challenge is required for any patient suspected to be suffering from hypovolaemia and displaying the signs and symptoms listed previously. A fluid challenge may be with either a crystalloid or colloid but it needs to be administered quickly and have a significant volume to help counteract the signs of volume depletion. If the signs and symptoms of hypovolaemia are seen, a fluid challenge of 500ml of an IV crystalloid (such as normal saline or Hartman's) is given over less than 15 minutes (see Figure 22.2 on when to give a fluid challenge) (NICE 2013). If the patient has myocardial impairment as the cause for hypotension, then the fluid challenge should be reduced to 250ml (Smith 2003, Collins & Plowright 2007). It is important to remember that the most common cause of hypotension is hypovolaemia, and a fluid challenge is vital for restoring organ perfusion (Cecconi *et al.* 2011).

Following the fluid challenge, the practitioner should reassess the patient's heart rate, capillary refill, blood pressure and urinary output. If there is little or no improvement, a further fluid challenge is required. This process may need to be repeated, as patients may need several fluid challenges to re-establish effective perfusion. Regular assessment for the signs of fluid overload should be undertaken – for instance, auscultation of the lungs for crepitations – as this will limit further IV fluid boluses.

Ideally, fluid challenges should be aided by measuring improvements to patients through haemodynamic monitoring. This may be possible through cardiac output monitoring but is normally available in intensive care units or operating theatres. Haemodynamic moitoring should include:

- Stroke volume variation
- Stroke volume
- Cardiac index
- Arterial blood pressure with arterial line waveform monitoring
- Central venous pressure.

Central venous pressure can be used to measure preload pressure but, as previously discussed, Marik & Cavallazzi (2013) state that CVP is not reliable to guide fluid therapy too. It is recommended that CVP is not used alone as an assessment of fluid resuscitation and that other parameters (such as heart rate, blood pressure and urine output) are used in conjunction with CVP measurements to assess response to fluid resuscitation. Remember, if the cause of the fluid depletion is haemorrhage, you should administer blood and clotting products and ensure early referral to the surgical team (see Figure 22.2, page 184).

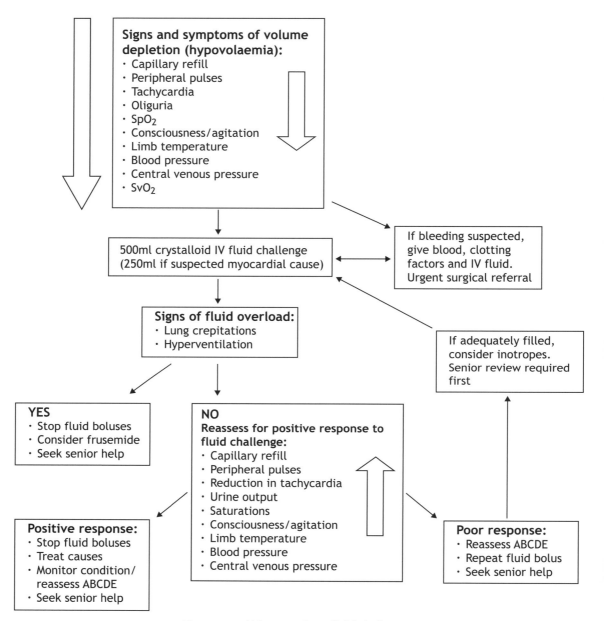

Figure 22.2 When to give a fluid challenge.

Conclusion

Patients suffering from hypovolaemia should be assessed using the **ABCDE** approach and early treatment is essential. Treatment involves maximising oxygen delivery, fluid resuscitation and haemostasis, and may or may not involve urgent surgery in the operating theatre. All patients with hypotension should be considered to be hypovolaemic until proven otherwise and an IV fluid challenge should be administered.

References and further reading

Alderson, P., Schierhout, G., Roberts, I. & Bunn, F. (2003). Colloids versus crystalloids for fluid resuscitation in critically ill patients. *The Cochrane Database of Systematic Reviews*. 3.

Bench, S. (2004). Assessing and treating shock, a nursing perspective. *British Journal of Nursing*. **13**, 715–21.

Bersten, A. & Soni, N. (2013). *Oh's Intensive Care Manual*. 7th edn. London: Butterworth Heinemann.

Cecconi, M., Singer, M. & Rhodes, A. (2011). The fluid challenge. *Annual Update in Intensive Care and Emergency Medicine*. **1**, 332–39.

Collins, T. (2000). Understanding shock. *Nursing Standard*. **14** (49), 35–41.

Collins, T. & Plowright, C. (2007). 'Identifying and managing a life-threatening situation' in McArthur-Rouse & Prosser (eds). *Assessing and Managing the Acutely Ill Adult Surgical Patient*. London: Blackwell.

Garretson, S. & Malberti, S. (2007). Understanding hypovolaemic, cardiogenic and septic shock. *Nursing Standard*. **21**, 46–55.

Gonce Morton, P., Fontaine, D., Hudak, C. & Gallo, B. (2003). *Critical Care Nursing, A Holistic Approach*. 8th edn. Philadelphia: Lippincott.

Marik, P. & Cavallazzi, R. (2013). Does the central venous pressure predict fluid responsiveness? An updated meta-analysis a plea for common sense. *Critical Care Medicine*. **7**, 1774–1881.

National Institute for Health and Care Excellence (NICE) (2013). *Intravenous Fluid Therapy in Adults in Hospital. Clinical Guideline 174*. http://www.nice.org.uk/guidance/cg174 (accessed 6 July 2015).

Rossaint, R., Bouillon, B., Cerny, V. *et al.* (2010). Management of bleeding following major trauma: A European guideline. *Critical Care*. **14**, R52.

Roth, M., Garcia, F. & Chaudhry, A. (2005). First aid: bleeding and hypovolaemic shock. *Student British Medical Journal*. **13**, 139–41.

Singh-Radcliff, S. (2013). *The Five Minute Anaesthesia Consult*. Philadelphia: Lippincott Williams & Wilkins.

Skinner, D. & Driscoll, P. (2013). *ABC of Major Trauma*. 4th edn. London: Wiley Blackwell.

Smith, G. (2003). *ALERTTM: A Multiprofessional Course in Care of the Acutely Ill Patient*. University of Portsmouth Learning Media Development

Woodrow, P. (2011). *Intensive Care Nursing*. 3rd edn. London: Routledge.

23 Cardiogenic shock

Russell Canavan

Cardiogenic shock is defined as reduced cardiac output, leading to tissue hypoperfusion. It differs from hypovolaemic shock in that the circulating volume is adequate. The shock is caused by the heart itself not pumping blood effectively.

By the end of this chapter, you should understand the pathophysiology and causes of cardiogenic shock; know how to assess a patient with cardiogenic shock; and understand the management of cardiogenic shock in the ward.

Mortality rates

Mortality rates from cardiogenic shock are initially high during acute hospital admission (Kim *et al.* 2012, Morici *et al.* 2015) but those who survive generally have a good quality of life. Important new advances have radically improved the prognosis and have reinforced the need for timely intervention.

Most cases of cardiogenic shock are caused by acute myocardial infarction. Although overall mortality has decreased with the introduction of percutaneous coronary intervention (PCI), mortality remains high in those patients who develop cardiogenic shock (French *et al.* 2011). The New York Heart Association (McCormick 2007) has a well-recognised grading system (see Table 23.1). The majority of patients survive with grade 1 heart failure (minimal) and are therefore able to enjoy a good quality of life.

Definition and causes

Cardiogenic shock is defined as a low cardiac output state, leading to inadequate tissue perfusion in the presence of adequate left ventricular filling (Braun & Anderson 2011). It ranges from a mild hypoperfusion to a profound shock (Holger *et al.* 2015) and is sometimes known as a low output state or acute circulatory failure. The European Society of Cardiology (2012) notes that there are many terms for different types of heart failure, which can be confusing.

The most common cause is acute myocardial infarction. Other causes include pericardial, myocardial and endocardial (valvular) disease, pericardial tamponade or dissecting aneurysm.

Although it does not fulfil the above definition for cardiogenic shock, pulmonary embolism is often considered in the same category. This is also true for right ventricular infarction, in which the problem is primarily poor left ventricular filling, but clinically appears as the pattern of cardiogenic shock.

Table 23.1 New York Heart Association classification

(Used with permission – Criteria Committee of the New York Heart Association. *Nomenclature and Criteria for Diseases of the Heart and Great Vessels*. 9th edn. Boston: Little Brown and Co. 1994.)

Class	Patient symptoms
Class I (mild)	• No limitation of physical activity • Ordinary physical activity does not cause undue fatigue, palpitation or dyspnoea (shortness of breath)
Class II (mild)	• Slight limitation of physical activity • Comfortable at rest, but ordinary physical activity results in fatigue, palpitation or dyspnoea (shortness of breath)
Class III (moderate)	• Marked limitation of physical activity • Comfortable at rest, but less than ordinary activity causes fatigue, palpitation or dyspnoea
Class IV (severe)	• Unable to carry out any physical activity without discomfort • Symptoms of cardiac insufficiency at rest • If any physical activity is undertaken, discomfort is increased

Case scenario

A 50-year-old man with type 2 diabetes mellitus is admitted with chest pain. He is sweaty and unwell.

A–Airway

He is maintaining his airway.

B–Breathing

His respiratory rate is raised, at 28 breaths per minute, and his oxygen saturation is 85% FiO_2 0.21 increasing to 96% FiO_2 0.85. Auscultation revealed bi-basal crepitations to mid-zones.

C–Circulation

Pulses are barely palpable peripherally and his blood pressure is 85/40mmHg. Capillary refill time is 5 seconds.

D–Disability

He is alert and orientated.

E–Exposure

He is overweight and sweaty but there are no specific findings. He has an Early Warning Score requiring referral to the medical team and intervention.

Pathophysiology

In all cases of cardiogenic shock there is a failure to eject blood from the heart, leading to hypotension and, therefore, inadequate cardiac output (Braun & Anderson 2011). The preload of the heart increases as blood accumulates that has returned to the heart but is not able to be pumped forward. This may be reflected as a high central venous pressure (CVP) due to impaired ejection of blood from the heart during systole.

Increased afterload due to vasoconstriction (resistance to ventricular systole), plus the increased preload, further complicates the patient's cardiac status. This pump failure means there is impaired perfusion of peripheral tissues and major organs. The sympathetic nervous system is activated, due to the reduction in blood pressure, and perfusion leads to an increase in heart rate and vasoconstriction (cool peripheries) in an effort to improve stroke volume (Braun & Anderson 2011).

Assessment

This clinical pattern is common to a number of other disorders, and must be differentiated from other shocks, such as hypovolaemic, anaphylactic and septic shock (see Chapters 21, 22 and 24).

Shock is defined as cardiogenic where there is a clear cardiac cause (Holger *et al.* 2015). Patients in cardiogenic shock are cold peripherally and they are also sweaty. They have low blood pressure, often a tachycardia, dyspnoea (secondary to pulmonary oedema), and may have chest pain or dysrhythmias (Braun & Anderson 2011), and be anxious and fatigued. Of particular note is the raised jugular venous pressure (JVP) or CVP, which differentiates cardiogenic shock from other forms of shock.

Clinical assessment may miss the features of pulmonary embolus and right heart failure. It is important to identify or exclude these causes of shock, which may complicate the picture of cardiogenic shock.

A full clinical assessment is important (Scott & MacInnes 2006); a chest x-ray is useful to detect pulmonary oedema and an enlarged heart; arterial blood gases will assess acid-base balance and hypoxaemia; and a 12-lead ECG will help to identify abnormalities such as dysrhythmias, acute coronary syndrome and embolism. Echocardiography is key to assessing the patient although it may not be available at the onset. However, echocardiograms can identify treatable conditions such as mitral regurgitation (secondary to chordal rupture) or a ventriculo-septal defect (VSD).

In the ward setting, it is imperative that the patient is placed on a cardiac monitor. The patient's heart rate, blood pressure, respiratory rate and oxygenation need to be recorded at regular intervals. It may be difficult to obtain an accurate oxygen saturation trace, due to peripheral shutdown; but an ear probe may help. High-flow oxygen should also be administered.

Treatment

Treatment involves administering high-flow oxygen via a non-rebreathe mask to improve hypoxaemia and breathlessness; reducing preload and JVP through use of diuretics or nitrates; treating hypotension with inotropes (see Table 23.2); and giving analgesia to reduce pain and anxiety. Diuretics need to be used with caution as they can reduce blood pressure further and, if the underlying cause is not addressed, can lead to dehydration. Diuretics (such as Furosemide) have an immediate venodilator effect, reducing preload. However, later diuresis may contribute to circulating volume loss, reducing cardiac output.

Once the immediate concerns (airway, breathing and circulation management) have been addressed and the patient has been stabilised, early assessment by a cardiologist with early reperfusion, in the form of PCI, coronary artery bypass grafts or thrombolysis, has been shown to significantly improve survival (Morici *et al.* 2015). Early correction of surgical lesions (VSD or chordal rupture) may also give a favourable outcome.

As a temporary measure, inotropes can help to improve cardiac output but they do not improve the long-term outcome if the underlying condition is not treated. There is little evidence to differentiate between choice of inotrope. However, dobutamine causes less of a chronotropic (increase in heart rate) response and is often favoured. Milronone has the added advantage of being a vasodilator and can reduce preload and afterload. Nitrates can improve coronary perfusion, and reduce preload (venodilator). This means that they reduce the work of a failing heart, thus improving ischaemia, but they need to be used with caution (NICE 2014), as they can reduce the blood pressure further.

Table 23.2 Terms and definitions (based on McKinley & Robinson 2001)

Inotropes	• Affect heart's contractility • *Positive* inotropes increase contractility (e.g. dobutamine, epinephrine) • *Negative* inotropes decrease contractility (e.g. lidocaine)
Chronotropes	• Affect heart rate • *Positive* chronotropes increase heart rate (e.g. atropine, isoprenaline) • *Negative* chronotropes decrease heart rate (e.g. verapamil, digoxin, adenosine, beta-blockers)
Preload	• The amount of fluid returning to the ventricle • Drugs that reduce preload include diuretics, nitrates and morphine • Fluids increase preload
Afterload	• The amount of resistance that the ventricle is pumping against • Drugs to decrease afterload (vasodilation) include amrinone and hydralazine • Drugs to increase afterload (vasoconstriction) include norepinephrine

In diffuse coronary artery disease, the intra-aortic balloon pump (IABP) can improve peripheral perfusion and also improve diastolic filling of the coronary arteries. It is an invasive device that acts in a similar way to inotropic support but also increases coronary artery perfusion. A balloon catheter is inserted via the femoral artery into the aorta. The balloon rapidly inflates during diastole, triggered by the ECG, increasing pressure and flow into the coronary arteries. At systole, the balloon rapidly deflates, reducing afterload and the work of the heart.

The balloon is inflated with helium, which has a very low density and therefore passes in and out of the balloon faster than air would (Krishna & Zacharowski 2009). The IABP is a specialised treatment that may be available in peripheral hospitals to stabilise patients for transfer to specialist centres. It can thus be used to support a failing heart until definitive reperfusion therapy or surgery can be carried out.

A left ventricular assist device is a surgically implanted device used in specialist centres. It increases the left ventricular output mechanically and is often used as a bridge to transplant. It buys the patient time when they are on the waiting list for a heart transplant. Again, early referral for assessment of suitability is needed, and a left ventricular assist device is not always useful in the acute situation.

Conclusion

Cardiogenic shock is most commonly associated with acute myocardial infarction and is characterised by shock, adequate blood volume and vasoconstriction. Definitive treatment, such as reperfusion therapy or cardiac surgery, is aimed at resolving the cause. Initial management is resuscitation, following **ABCDE** principles, and the use of drugs (such as inotropes and venodilators) and mechanical therapies (such as IABP) prior to definitive management.

References and further reading

Braun, C.A. & Anderson, C.M. (2011). *Pathophysiology: A Clinical Approach.* 2nd edn. Philadelphia: Lippincott, Williams & Wilkins.

European Society of Cardiology (2012). Guidelines for the treatment of acute and chronic heart failure. *European Heart Journal.* **33**, 1787–1847. doi:10.1093/eurheartj/ehs104

French, J.K., Armstrong, P.W., Cohen, E., Kleiman, N.S., O'Connor, C.M., Hellkamp, A.S., Stebbins. A., Holmes, D.R., Hochman, J.S., Granger, C.B. & Mahaffey, K.W. (2011). Cardiogenic shock and heart failure post-percutaneous coronary intervention in ST-elevation myocardial infarction. *American Heart Journal.* **162** (1), 89–97.

Hochman J.S, Sleeper L.A., Webb, J.G., Sanborne, T.A., White, H.D., Tally, J.D., Buller, C.E., Jacobs, A.K., Slater, J.N., Col, J., McKinley, S.M. & LeJemtel, T.H. (1999). Early revascularization in acute myocardial infarction complicated by cardiogenic shock. Shock Investigators. Should we emergently revascularize occluded coronaries for cardiogenic shock. *New England Journal of Medicine.* **341** (9), 625–34.

Holger, T., Ohman, E.M., Desch, S., Eitel, I. & de Waha, S. (2015). Management of cardiogenic shock. *European Heart Journal.* **36** (20), 1223–30.

Kim, U., Park, J., Kang, S., Kim, Y., Park, W., Lee, S., Hong, G., Shin, D., Kim, Y., Jeong, M., Chae, S., Hur, S., Song, I., Hong, T., Chae, I., Cho, M., Jang, Y., Yoon, J., Seung, K. & Park, S. (2012). Outcomes according to presentation with versus without cardiogenic shock in patients with left main coronary artery stenosis and acute myocardial infarction. *The American Journal of Cardiology.* **110** (1), 36–39.

Krishna, M. & Zacharowski, K. (2009). Principles of intra-aortic balloon pump counterpulsation. *Continuing Education in Anaesthesia Critical Care and Pain.* **9** (1), 24–28. doi: 10.1093/bjaceaccp/mkn051

McCormick, S. (2007). 'Classifications of Heart Failure'. http://heartfailurecenter.com/hfcheartfailureclassifications.shtm (accessed 21 April 2015).

McKinley, M.G. & Robinson, C.F. (2001). 'Shock' in M.L. Sole, M.L. Lamborn & J.C. Hartshorn. *Introduction to Critical Care Nursing.* 3rd edn. Philadelphia: W.B. Saunders.

Morici, N., Sacco, A., Paino, R., Oreglia, J.A., Bottirole, M., Snnie, M., Nichelatti, M., Canova, P., Russo, C., Garascia, A., Kulgmann, S., Frigerio, M. & Olivia, F. (2015). Cardiogenic shock: how to overcome a clinical dilemma. Unmet needs in emergency medicine. *International Journal of Cardiology.* **186**, 19–21.

National Institute for Health and Care Excellence (NICE) (2014). Acute Heart Failure: Diagnosing and managing acute heart failure in adults. *Clinical Guideline 187.* https://www.nice.org.uk/guidance/cg187 (accessed 3 April 2015).

Port, C.M. (2003). *Essentials of Pathophysiology: Concepts of Altered Health States.* Philadelphia: Lippincott, Williams & Wilkins.

Ren, X. (2014). *Cardiogenic Shock.* http://emedicine.medscape.com/article/152191-overview (accessed 6 April 2015).

Scott, C. & MacInnes, J. (2006). Cardiac assessment: putting the patient first. *British Journal of Nursing.* **15** (9), 502–508.

Useful websites

Heart Failure Society of America
http://www.hfsa.org/hfsa-wp/wp/patient/ (Accessed 8 July 2015)

British Heart Foundation
http://www.bhf.org.uk/ (Accessed 8 July 2015)

24 Anaphylactic shock

Ann M. Price

Anaphylaxis is the term used for a severe life-threatening, generalised or systemic hypersensitivity reaction with the release of histamine (Resuscitation Council 2012). It becomes anaphylactic shock when the patient's haemodynamic status is compromised, leading to airway and/or breathing and/or circulation problems, often with skin and mucosal change. It is thought that the incidence of anaphylaxis is increasing but that recognition of the signs and symptoms can still be poor (Resuscitation Council 2012).

This chapter discusses potential causes of anaphylaxis in hospitalised patients; identifies signs and symptoms, using **ABCDE** assessment; and outlines key treatment priorities.

Causes

Anaphylaxis is thought to be an allergic response that may be immunologically mediated, non-immunologically mediated, or idiopathic (no identified cause) (NICE 2011). There are numerous potential causes of a severe allergic reaction (Resuscitation Council 2012) but the common ones include certain foods, insect venoms, and some drugs (including antibiotics) and latex. Within the hospital setting, patients are exposed to numerous potential triggers. Recent examples include amiodarone (Serhan Özcan *et al.* 2014), thrombolytics (Zarar *et al.* 2014) and transfusions (Abe *et al.* 2014). Thus, there are various and rare causes of anaphylaxis that could be missed in the ward setting.

Signs and symptoms

Staff should be alert for the signs and symptoms of anaphylaxis because of the wide range of causes. Symptoms are sudden and develop rapidly, usually over several minutes. Patients can therefore deteriorate very quickly and need swift intervention (NICE 2011).

Assessment, using the **ABCDE** approach, may identify the following (Resuscitation Council 2012):

- Airway (pharyngeal or laryngeal) oedema – stridor or hoarseness may be present
- Breathing difficulties including bronchospasm – wheezing, tachypnoea, cyanosis, SpO$_2$ <92%

- Circulation – hypotension and/or tachycardia, pale, clammy
- Disability – the patient may become distressed or confused or lose consciousness
- Exposure – patients may have facial swelling, rashes and itching but these signs are not present in all anaphylactic reactions (Resuscitation Council 2012)
- A small number of patients may have vomiting or abdominal pain.

Case scenario

Jane is a 29-year-old woman, who was admitted following an appendectomy. She has returned to the ward, where she is given intravenous antibiotics (second dose). She suddenly starts to complain that she is having difficulty breathing and feels very unwell. An audible wheeze is evident and she has a rapid pulse. Anaphylaxis is suspected.

Treatment priorities

Anaphylaxis is life-threatening so prompt treatment is essential. Within the ward setting, you need to raise a 'medical emergency' call (as per local policy) so that expertise in airway management and treatment regime is swiftly obtained.

The Resuscitation Council (2012) recommends the following priorities:

- Use the **ABCDE** approach to identify problems
- Call for help early
- Treat the greatest threat to life first.

Do not delay initial treatment trying to diagnosis cause.

- **Use the ABCDE approach to identify problems.**
- **Call for help early.**
- **Treat the greatest threat to life first.**

According to the Resuscitation Council (2012), treatment should follow these steps:

1. Lay the patient flat and raise their legs.

2. Give adrenaline (epinephrine) intramuscularly (IM), or intravenously if skilled staff are available. The adult dose is 500 micrograms (0.5ml of 1:1000 solution). This can be repeated every 5 minutes as needed. Note that pre-filled syringes usually contain 1:10,000 concentration = 100mcg/ml. (Adrenaline works by stopping histamine release and may abort the progress of anaphylaxis. It is therefore very important in treatment of severe cases.)

3. Ensure that the airway is patent and give high-flow oxygen.

4. Intravenous fluid challenge – 500–1000ml Hartman's solution or 0.9% saline for an adult patient.

5. Chlorphenamine (antihistamine), 10mg (adult dose) – IM or slow IV.
6. Hydrocortisone (steroid), 200mg (adult dose) – IM or slow IV.

- Lay the patient flat.
- Administer IM or IV adrenaline (epinephrine).
- Give high-flow oxygen.
- IV fluid challenge.
- Give IM or IV chlorphenamine.
- Administer IM or IV hydrocortisone.

Monitoring

Patients suspected of anaphylaxis should be monitored closely, including blood pressure, pulse oximetry and continuous ECG. NICE (2011) recommends recording the time of onset, symptoms, and circumstances prior to the anaphylactic episode. Patients should be monitored for at least 6 hours after an anaphylactic reaction, and may be hospitalised for longer.

Further advice

Further investigations and treatment may be needed, considering the precipitating allergen and comorbidities (such as asthma). After the reaction, patients may be prescribed antihistamine and steroid therapy, usually for three days – to reduce symptoms (such as urticaria).

Some patients may have a recurrence of symptoms within 72 hours (called a biphasic reaction). All anaphylactic patients should be advised to seek medical advice urgently if their symptoms return. Patients may be referred to a specialist allergy service to investigate triggers and offer preventative advice.

Conclusion

Anaphylaxis is an emergency situation that requires staff to act swiftly to prevent death. Staff need to be aware that allergic reactions can occur in unpredictable circumstances and, although relatively rare, anaphylactic patients need a prompt response and expert help.

The Resuscitation Council (2012) provides a clear algorithm that can be utilised for emergency treatment of anaphylaxis.

References and further reading

Abe, T., Shimada, E., Takanashi, M., Takamura, T., Motji, K., Okazaki, H., Satake, M. & Tadokoro, K. (2014). Antibody against immunoglobulin E contained in blood components as causative factor for anaphylactic transfusion reactions. *Transfusion.* **54** (8), 1953–60.

National Institute for Health and Care Excellence (NICE) (2011). *Anaphylaxis: assessment to confirm an anaphylactic episode and the decision to refer after emergency treatment for a suspected anaphylactic episode. Clinical Guideline 134.* https://www.nice.org.uk/guidance/cg134 (accessed 8 July 2015).

Resuscitation Council UK (2012). *Emergency Treatment of Anaphylactic Reactions.* http://www.resus.org.uk/pages/reaction.htm (accessed 8 July 2015).

Serhan Özcan, K., Zengin, A., Tatlisu, A., Aruğarslan, E. & Nurkalem, Z. (2014). Anaphylactic shock associated with intravenous amiodarone. *Journal of Cardiology Cases.* **9** (2), 61–62.

Zarar, A., Khan, A.A., Adil, M.M. & Qureshi, A.I. (2014). Anaphylactic shock associated with intravenous thrombolytics. *American Journal of Emergency Medicine.* **32** (1), 113.e3-113.e5

25 Management of the critically ill patient with malignancy

Angus Turner

Patients with malignancy who become critically ill require special consideration if they are to be managed correctly. That said, the principles of assessment, resuscitation and referral are the same as when dealing with other groups of patients and are described in full elsewhere. The aim of this chapter is not to be an exhaustive text on all critical illnesses related to malignancy. Instead, it will cover the common scenarios and highlight the areas that often cause anxiety and confusion.

Critically ill patients with malignancy cover a vast range of issues – from specialist oncological, through to general medical, surgical and ethical. It is not unusual to become involved on the ward with these patients when emotions are running high, when adequate information is not available, when key senior personnel are not contactable, and when proper communication has not occurred and decisions need to be made.

To make matters more challenging, treatment and prognosis are continually changing and improving for many malignancies. Specialists in treating malignancy are at risk of becoming frustrated when communicating with other disciplines that are, understandably, not up to date. In the worst-case scenario, this lack of knowledge can be perceived as prejudice.

Assessing and understanding the situation
Malignancy

The term 'malignancy' includes all malignant solid tumours (cancers and sarcomas) and haematological malignancies (leukaemias and lymphomas) (Braun & Anderson 2011). You cannot manage a critically ill patient with malignancy, or communicate properly, unless you understand the language that will be used to describe them.

Palliative

'Palliative' means different things to different people. The term needs special attention because it is commonly used in two very different contexts: 'palliative care' and 'palliative therapy'.

Palliative care

This refers to an approach in which the primary aim is to relieve symptoms and improve quality of life. This might include some 'palliative therapy' (see below). When the palliative care team becomes involved, there has been a recognition that the patient is not going to survive their illness. This is invariably in the context of a limited life expectancy, which may be as short as a few hours or as long as a few months. It is generally accepted that a critical illness in these patients should be treated as a terminal event, and should be managed with symptom control rather than resuscitation.

The National Council for Palliative Care (2015) notes that palliative care is now extended beyond cancers and includes other diseases too; but this is beyond the scope of this chapter.

Palliative therapy

This means that a patient is receiving active 'anti-cancer' treatment (such as chemotherapy, radiotherapy or surgery) with the aim of improving their quality of life by relieving their symptoms. It has been accepted that the treatment will not be curative. The life expectancy, in this instance, varies tremendously from a few weeks to many years. A good example is the palliative treatment of bone metastasis from breast cancer – a situation that may be stable for many months.

The prognosis for patients receiving palliative therapy can be the same as for patients without a malignancy. In other words, the presence of an 'incurable cancer' should not necessarily be a bar to full active treatment, including organ support on the intensive care unit.

Know the patient, know the disease

Patients with malignancy who become critically ill are more difficult to manage. In addition to the usual problems of their critical illness and comorbidities, their malignancy adds a number of very important variables that impact significantly on management. As well as the usual thorough history and examination, it is vital to seek out as much information as possible from all sources.

Diagnosis and stage

Different malignancies behave in different ways. Although this seems obvious, it is important to get it right. For instance, the difference between squamous cell and small cell cancer of the lung has important implications for its assessment, treatment and prognosis. Similarly, stage IA Hodgkin's disease behaves very differently to stage IVB. The Cancer Research UK website provides more detail about the stages of cancer.

Treatment received and response

The amount of treatment received by a patient can be an important indicator for prognosis. For example, a patient with acute myeloid leukaemia with neutropenic sepsis after the first cycle of chemotherapy, prior to a bone marrow transplant, has a good prognosis. However, the prognosis is grave with the same critical illness following rescue chemotherapy, after the transplant has failed.

Prognosis and level of communication

A knowledge of the expected prognosis is an essential tool to help tailor appropriate therapy (such as admission to the intensive care unit). Although the prognosis might be known to the specialists treating the patient's malignancy, this information must also be readily available to all professionals managing the critical illness. The prognosis needs sensitive discussion with the patient who has mental capacity (and include family and friends, with the patient's permission). It is surprising how often the prognosis is not appreciated by the patient or their friends and family. Insight into this is important to avoid awkwardness during discussions.

Functional status and general health and comorbidities

It is important not to lose sight of a 'holistic' approach to treating critically ill patients with malignancy. A good example would be a patient with congestive cardiac failure and a poor exercise capacity, presenting with tumour lysis syndrome and renal failure after chemotherapy for lymphoma. This patient probably has a worse prognosis from the concomitant illnesses than from the malignancy and its complications. A proper history must be taken, including a full systems review and exercise tolerance and functional capacity.

Acute oncology services

In 2008, the National Confidential Enquiry into Patient Outcome and Death (NCEPOD) report, *Systemic Anti-Cancer Therapy: For better, for worse?*, looked into deaths within 30 days of receiving systemic anti-cancer therapy and identified significant concerns regarding the quality and safety of patient care, both at an organisational and clinical level. Delays in admission, delays in prescribing and administering antibiotics, lack of assessment by senior staff, poor communication between teams, lack of documentation, lack of oncology input and lack of clear policies were just a few of the concerns identified. The subsequent National Chemotherapy Advisory Group report (2010), *Chemotherapy Services in England: Ensuring quality and safety,* highlighted the need for an acute oncology service (AOS) in every hospital.

Acute oncology focuses on managing patients with a new acute diagnosis and also on those patients who have complications of their cancer diagnosis and treatment. Although patients are often treated in specialist oncology centres, they are more likely to present to their local hospital when acute problems develop. The National Cancer Action Team stipulate in their *Manual for Cancer Services* (2011) that acute oncology protocols should be available in the chemotherapy and radiotherapy units, A&E departments, acute medical admissions wards and oncology in-patient wards. Although there is significant consensus across the UK about the management of oncology emergencies, no national guidelines are available. When caring for a patient who is acutely unwell with their cancer, you should contact the AOS in your local setting as part of your routine care.

HOT TIPS

When managing critically ill patients with malignancy:

- Have all the relevant information about the patient, their malignancy, treatment, functional status and general medical condition to hand.
- Ensure that communication has occurred, and decisions are made, at an appropriately senior level. Involving the consultant staff is mandatory in all but the most exceptional cases.
- Move quickly and push for help and decisions. If in doubt, play safe and call for assistance (from more senior personnel, the critical care outreach team or the intensive care team). If help is not forthcoming, most hospitals now have a 'peri-arrest' or 'medical emergency' call system. Use this if you cannot get the help you need in any other way.

Common critical illnesses in patients with malignant disease

Specific critical illness scenarios affecting patients with malignant disease need specialist knowledge to diagnose and treat. Most oncology and haematology units will have protocols in place to deal with these situations. However, the initial assessment and resuscitation needs to be performed using the same principles that apply to other patient groups.

Neutropenic sepsis

This is a medical emergency, usually seen in patients being treated for a haematological malignancy. It is defined as an absolute neutrophil count of 0.5 x 10⁹/litre or lower, with a pyrexia of over 38°C, or clinical signs of septicaemia or site of infection. Specialist advice must be sought immediately, along with ongoing management of the septicaemia. Neutropenic sepsis is the most common problem resulting in critical illness in patients with malignancy (NICE 2012).

Cardiovascular failure

Sepsis is the most important cause of cardiovascular collapse in this context and should always be considered, if not treated speculatively. However, there are other specific causes of cardiovascular collapse that should also be considered:

- Dehydration, especially in the presence of diarrhoea, which can occur with some chemotherapy regimens (e.g. 5-fluocytosine)
- Pericardial tamponade
- Myocardial failure, which can be a result of disease infiltration or chemotherapy (e.g. anthrocyclines).

Respiratory failure

There are many routes by which a patient with malignancy can develop respiratory failure. These include:

- Pulmonary infection
- Pulmonary oedema
- Pleural effusions and/or massive ascites
- Airway obstruction.

The route to respiratory failure may also involve neurological causes such as:

- Malignancies of the brain, leading to compromise of the respiratory centre or post-ictal respiratory depression
- Cervical cord compression
- Secondary to opioid analgesia.

Patients with malignant disease have a worse prognosis than other groups if they are treated with invasive artificial ventilation. It is therefore very important to ensure that all potentially reversible factors have been dealt with. Examples include draining pleural effusions, treating infection, using steroids or epinephrine nebulisers to ease airway obstruction, and targeted fluid balance. Non-invasive positive pressure ventilation (NIV) is becoming more sophisticated and more widely available and confers a better prognosis. In many situations NIV should be the first-line therapy if respiratory support is needed. For more about this, see Chapter 16 (Larché *et al.* 2003).

Renal failure - Tumour lysis syndrome

This syndrome occurs due to massive tumour breakdown following chemotherapy, or even steroid therapy for bulky sensitive malignancies, especially leukaemias and lymphomas; occasionally it can occur prior to therapy. The cell breakdown causes the patient to become acidotic, hyperkalaemic, hyperuricaemic, hyperphosphataemic and hypocalcaemic, and renal failure frequently occurs. Prompt resuscitation and specialist treatment, coupled with appropriate referral for renal dialysis, means that the prognosis is often good (Davidson *et al.* 2004).

Remember, of course, patients with malignant disease will also present with unrelated medical and surgical problems (for instance, patients with cancer will still suffer myocardial infarctions or appendicitis) and their malignancy will need consideration, either to limit therapy appropriately in advanced, incurable disease, or to be excluded as an insignificant consideration because their disease has a potentially good prognosis.

The role of the intensive care unit in treating critically ill patients with malignant disease

The decision whether or not to refer a patient with malignant disease to the intensive care unit (ICU) can be easy, or it can be fraught with dilemmas. In cases where the patient is so unwell that any delay could compromise their chances of survival, it should be possible for any member of the team to assess and refer them. Examples of such cases are critical airway obstruction and severe neutropenic sepsis. When the situation allows, it is important that a proper full history is taken, information gathered and senior input obtained prior to referral to the intensive care unit. Although this is occasionally regarded as unnecessary, such an approach avoids exposing the patient to inappropriate, dangerous or invasive interventions.

A trial of ward-based therapy is also possible after a proper assessment, again avoiding unnecessary intervention; this could be with the support of the intensive care unit and/or outreach teams. Figure 25.1 shows an algorithm of referral guidelines that could be considered when caring for critically ill patients with malignancy who may need referral to the intensive care unit.

While every case must be judged on its own merits, some guidelines are useful. The ones illustrated here are used at our own hospital and have been found to work well when audited. They are based on the following considerations:

- Mortality from multi-organ failure is as high as 90%, even in patients without malignant disease.
- Multi-organ failure results in a prolonged stay on the intensive care unit (sometimes lasting several weeks), and a period of recuperation that lasts several months.
- Single organ failure confers a good prognosis, even in patients with advanced malignant disease. Therefore, treatment of single organ failure may be appropriate in the context of good palliative therapy.

It is not always possible to reliably assess acutely critically ill patients. If it is difficult to make a confident assessment, it is reasonable to admit the patient for a trial of support in the intensive care unit. A regular review should be made every 48 hours. This is an opportunity to withdraw or continue organ support in the face of objective clinical deterioration or improvement (Thiéry *et al.* 2005). See Figure 25.1 for sample guidelines relating to the intensive care unit.

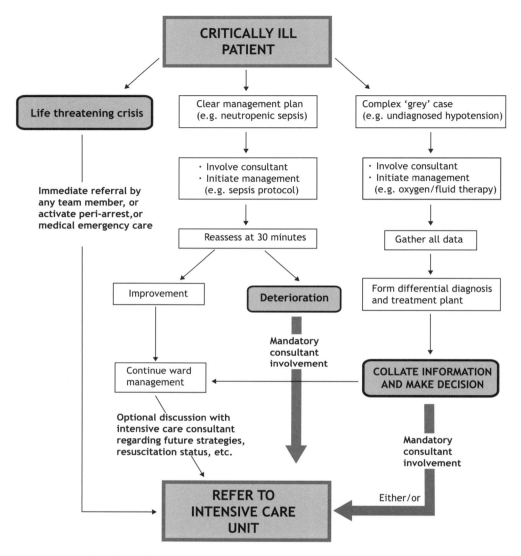

Figure 25.1 *Algorithm for referral of critically ill patients with malignancy to the intensive care unit.*

Box 25.1
Sample guidelines for considering admission to intensive care

Consider ward management if:
- The patient is clearly too well for intensive care
- The patient's condition has deteriorated, meaning that intensive management is unlikely to succeed

Admit to intensive care if:
- There is established failure of 1–2 organs.
- There is a realistic chance of cure or prolonged survival (over 6 months) from the underlying malignancy.

The patient should *not* be admitted if:
- The underlying prognosis is <3 months
- There is established failure of 3+ organs.

If in doubt:
- Admit the patient for a trial period of intensive care therapy.

In any event, you should regularly review the patient's progress or deterioration.

You should also have a clear plan with regard to limitation of therapy in the face of increasing organ failures.

N.B. Bone marrow failure, as manifest by low white cell count, anaemia and low platelet count, is usually due to the effect of chemotherapy. In this context, it should not be counted as 'organ failure' as it is predictably reversible without specific therapy (although granulocyte colony-stimulating factor can be used to enhance recovery).

Case scenarios

Consider the following scenarios.

Case scenario 1

You are attending a 65-year-old man with a diagnosis of advanced squamous cell carcinoma of the tongue, with local spread to cervical lymph nodes. He had radical surgery 18 months ago but the tumour has recurred and he has been treated with a full dose of radiotherapy to the affected lymph nodes. His last dose of radiotherapy was 1 week ago.

Over the past 24 hours, he has developed stridor. The peripheral oxygen saturations are 65% on high-flow oxygen. His blood pressure is 130/80mmHg, his heart rate is 110 beats per minute and his respiratory rate is 40 breaths per minute.

He has a good urine output and normal renal function. There is no other significant past medical history and he played 18 holes of golf twice a week prior to his diagnosis.

Discussion of scenario 1

This man has respiratory failure secondary to airway obstruction by recurrent cancer. Despite the fact that treatment of single organ failure has a good prognosis on intensive care, it will not be possible to treat this cancer because a full dose of palliative radiotherapy has already been given and there is no further surgical option. The prognosis, even in the absence of airway obstruction, is certainly less than 3 months; therefore the current situation should be treated as a terminal event.

Management plan

If not already aware, the consultant oncologist must be informed of the patient's deteriorating condition. Admission to intensive care is inappropriate and the onus must be on palliative care, symptom control, and achieving as comfortable and dignified a death as possible. An urgent referral to the palliative care team should be made. Initial symptom control can be started with titrated doses of intravenous diamorphine, at 1mg increments every 5–10 minutes to relieve distress. Intravenous steroids (dexamethasone 8mg) and nebulised epinephrine (0.5mg) will temporarily reduce the element of airway obstruction caused by oedema, and help to gain control of the situation. Appropriate discussions with the patient and family need to take place. Consider a 'do not resuscitate' order.

Case scenario 2

A 35-year-old woman is on the haematology ward with neutropenia following the first dose of chemotherapy for acute myeloblastic leukaemia. She is pyrexial at 38.5°C and has had 24 hours of broad-spectrum antibiotics for a chest infection, confirmed clinically and on x-ray. She now has a blood pressure of 75/30mmHg, a heart rate of 120 beats per minute, a respiratory rate of 35 breaths per minute and a poor urine output.

Arterial blood gases show a PaO_2 of 10kPa on FiO_2 0.6 and a $PaCO_2$ of 4.0kPa. The base excess is –8.2, with a serum lactate of 6.0mmol/litre. Her platelet count is 20×10^9/litre, her haemoglobin concentration 85g/litre and her white blood cell count is 1.0×10^9/L (absolute neutrophil count 0.01×10^9/L).

Discussion of scenario 2

The prognosis for acute myeloblastic leukaemia is potentially very good. However, this woman is at very high risk of progressing rapidly into established multiple organ failure due to septic shock. There is a window of opportunity to reverse the process, with prompt, targeted treatment on the intensive care unit. Ideally, this should involve the consultant haematologist, but referral to intensive care must not be delayed by this – minutes count.

On the other hand, failure to escalate her treatment in a timely manner will probably result in deterioration to multiple organ failure, which would result in her requiring invasive positive pressure ventilation and other organ support measures, such as haemofiltration or dialysis. The prognosis, should this situation occur, is extremely poor and such measures should only be undertaken after significant discussion between senior medical and nursing staff, relatives, and (if possible) the patient.

Management plan

This patient should be urgently reviewed and initial treatment with high-flow oxygen, fluid resuscitation through a large-bore cannula and an urgent antibiotic review should be immediately commenced. Simultaneously, an urgent referral to intensive care must occur and senior haematology assistance be requested. Admission to an intensive care or high dependency unit is mandatory.

Fluid resuscitation (guided by invasive haemodynamic monitoring, such as arterial line, central venous line ± cardiac output monitor), cardiovascular support with inotropes and vasopressors, respiratory support with non-invasive ventilation (NIV) and urgent review of her antibiotic regimen by a consultant microbiologist should take place. With these measures, a rapid improvement in her septic shock can be achieved. Haematology input will be required with regard to supporting the low platelet count, anaemia and optimising bone marrow recovery (for example, with granulocyte colony stimulating factor).

Conclusion

Patients suffering from malignant disease and presenting with acute critical illnesses create a unique set of challenges that require knowledge, insight and experience. It is not possible for any one discipline to possess all the skills needed to provide the highest quality of care; therefore, a multidisciplinary team approach is central to a successful outcome. Inherent in this process is the application of thorough basic clinical skills, good communication between specialties, and the prompt involvement of senior medical personnel. Novel therapies have resulted in an improved outlook for many malignancies. With objective and prompt intensive care input, highly satisfactory outcomes can be achieved in a variety of difficult clinical scenarios.

References and further reading

Braun, C.A. & Anderson, C.M. (2011). *Pathophysiology: A Clinical Approach.* 2nd edition. Philadelphia: Lippincott, Williams & Wilkins

Cancer Research UK (no date). *Stages of cancer.* http://www.cancerresearchuk.org/about-cancer/what-is-cancer/stages-of-cancer (accessed 29 April 2015).

Davidson, M.B., Thakkar, S., Hix, J.K., Bhandarkar, N.D., Wong, A. & Schreiber, M.J. (2004). Pathophysiology, clinical consequences and treatment of tumor lysis syndrome. *American Journal of Medicine.* **116**, 546–54.

Larché, J., Azoulay, E., Fieux, F. *et al* (2003). Improved survival of critically ill cancer patients with septic shock. *Intensive Care Medicine.* **29** (10), 1688–95.

National Cancer Action Team (2011). *Manual for Cancer Services: Acute Oncology – Including Metastatic Spinal Cord Compression Measures (version 1.0).* London: NHS.

National Chemotherapy Advisory Group report (2010). *Chemotherapy Services in England: Ensuring quality and safety.* London: NHS.

National Council for Palliative Care (NCPC) (2015). *Palliative Care Explained.* http://www.ncpc.org.uk/palliative-care-explained (accessed 29 April 2015).

National Confidential Enquiry Into Patient Outcome and Death (NCEPOD) (2008). *Systemic Anti-Cancer Therapy: For better, for worse?* http://www.ncepod.org.uk/2008sact.htm (accessed 10 July 2015).

National Institute for Health and Care Excellence (2012). *Neutropenic sepsis: prevention and management of neutropenic sepsis in cancer patients. Clinical Guideline 151.* https://www.nice.org.uk/guidance/cg151 (accessed 29 April 2015).

Thiéry, G., Azoulay, E., Darmon, M. *et al* (2005). Outcome of cancer patients considered for intensive care unit admission: a hospital-wide prospective study. *Journal of Clinical Oncology.* 23 (19), 4406–13.

Useful websites

National Cancer Research Institute
http://www.ncri.org.uk/ (Accessed 11 July 2015)

Cancer Research, UK
http://www.cancerresearchuk.org (Accessed 11 July 2015)

BASO – The Association for Cancer Surgery
http://www.baso.org/ (Accessed 11 July 2015)

26 Tachyarrhythmias in the acutely ill

Kuno Budack

Arrhythmias are very common in the acute setting. They can be the cause (primary problem) or simply a symptom of an underlying disease. Tachyarrhythmias in the acutely ill are a common problem.

By the end of this chapter, you should be able to recognise an arrhythmia, and be aware of the appropriate investigations and treatment needed to give your patient the best chance.

Cardiac output

Cardiac output is stroke volume (volume ejected with each heartbeat) multiplied by heart rate in 1 minute, and is measured in litres per minute.

Box 26.1 Cardiac output

Cardiac output (CO) = stroke volume (SV) × heart rate (HR)

A patient will try to maintain an adequate cardiac output through several responses; one of them is to increase heart rate (see Figure 26.1). The heart is sensitive to adrenergic influences, making arrhythmias familiar sequelae in the unwell patient. Tachyarrhythmias are divided into *narrow* complex (supraventricular) and *broad* complex (ventricular or supraventricular with aberrant conduction). On identification of an abnormal heart rate or rhythm, urgent help is needed. It may be safer to put out an emergency call, as per your Trust's policy, but ideally the responder needs to be someone with advanced life support (ALS) training. The initial management should follow the latest Resuscitation Council UK (2015) guidelines.

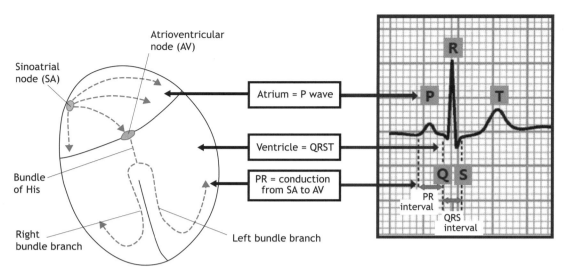

Figure 26.1 Normal conduction of the heart.

Narrow-complex tachycardia

Narrow-complex refers to the width of a QRS complex on a standard 12-lead ECG at 25mm per second. Anything less than 0.12 seconds (three little squares) is deemed to be *narrow* (Resuscitation Council, 2015). By far the most common tachyarrhythmia in the unwell patient is a sinus tachycardia (see Figure 26.2).

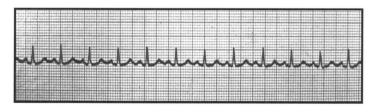

Figure 26.2 ECG of sinus tachycardia.

Abnormal tachycardias include:

- Atrial fibrillation/flutter (AF)
- Supraventricular tachycardia (SVT/AV nodal re-entry tachycardia)
- Wolfe–Parkinson–White (WPW) syndrome.

Possible causes of tachycardia in the acutely ill patient are listed in Box 26.2.

Box 26.2 Possible causes of tachycardia

1 Anything that makes you unwell such as:

- Surgery
- Infection
- Poorly controlled pain
- Trauma.

2 **Hyperthyroidism**
   - Always check thyroid-stimulating hormone
   - If hyperthyroidism is suspected, treatment may be different.

3 **Electrolyte imbalances**
   - Always check electrolytes, particularly potassium
   - Magnesium is less important but consider replacement when indicated.

4 **Structurally abnormal heart**
   - Previous myocardial infarction
   - Heart failure
   - Valvular heart disease.

5 **Drugs**

Atrial fibrillation

Atrial fibrillation is the most common pathological narrow-complex tachycardia and is irregularly irregular in nature. An irregular, narrow-complex tachycardia is atrial fibrillation until proven otherwise. Predisposing factors are shown in Box 26.3.

Box 26.3 Predisposing factors for atrial fibrillation

- Age: prevalence increases with age
- Gender: men have a higher prevalence than women
- Abnormal heart structure
- Medical conditions: hypertension, hyperthyroidism, acute illness, drugs
- Lifestyle: intake of alcohol, coffee, drugs

Atrial fibrillation is an irregular narrow-complex tachycardia (see Figure 26.3). In atrial fibrillation, no P-waves are visible.

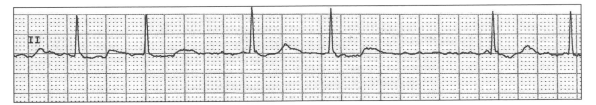

Figure 26.3 ECG of atrial fibrillation.

Atrial *flutter* is often irregular, but can have a block to conduction that makes it look like a regular narrow-complex tachycardia. Atrial flutter shows a typical *saw-tooth* pattern (see Figure 26.4).

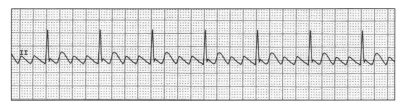

Figure 26.4 ECG of atrial flutter.

The annual risk of stroke attributable to atrial fibrillation increased from 1.5% in Framingham Study participants aged 50 to 59 years to 23.5% for those aged 80 to 89 years (Wang *et al.* 2003). The total mortality rate is approximately doubled in patients with atrial fibrillation compared with those in normal sinus rhythm, and is linked with the severity of underlying heart disease. Current guidelines recommend use of the CHA_2DS_2-VASc Score (Congestive heart failure/left ventricular dysfunction, Hypertension, Age ≥75 [doubled], Diabetes, Stroke [doubled] – Vascular disease, Age 65–74, and Sex category [female]) to assess risk of stroke in atrial fibrillation (Camm *et al.* 2012); see Table 26.1.

Table 26.1 Annual stroke risk according to CHA_2DS_2-VASc score
(based on MDCalc 2015)

C Congestive cardiac failure history	1 point
H Hypertension	1 point
A Age	(<65yrs) – 0 points (65–74) – 1 point (>75) – 2 points
D Diabetes mellitus	1 point
S Stroke/TIA/Thromboembolysis	2 points
V Vascular disease (MI, PVD)	1 point
Sex category	1 point if female

The score goes from 0 to 9, with the risk of stroke increasing as the score increases.

When managing unwell patients with atrial fibrillation, the main aim is to treat the cause. Other management and treatment issues are related to the arrhythmia itself and the prevention of thromboembolism.

Supraventricular tachycardia
Supraventricular tachycardia is a regular narrow-complex tachycardia (see Figure 26.5).

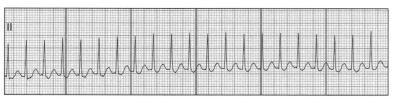

Figure 26.5 ECG of supraventricular tachycardia.

Wolfe-Parkinson-White syndrome (WPW) (accessory pathway)

Accessory pathways can, in theory, cause any arrhythmia. However, the WPW syndrome is easily recognisable on a resting ECG with controlled rate by a short PQ interval with the typical delta wave (see Figure 26.6).

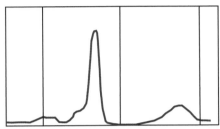

Figure 26.6 ECG of Wolfe–Parkinson–White syndrome, highlighting delta wave.

Narrow-complex tachycardia

Diagnosis

The diagnosis of a narrow-complex tachycardia is based solely on the ECG. This can sometimes be difficult, so call someone with experience early on. An easy guide is that every irregular narrow-complex tachycardia is atrial fibrillation, and every regular narrow-complex tachycardia is supraventricular tachycardia (SVT) until proven otherwise.

Assessment

The **ABCDE** approach should be used: give oxygen (if indicated), insert a cannula, monitor the ECG, blood pressure and SPO2, and record a 12-lead ECG. Consider electrolyte abnormalities.

Treatment

Always treat the cause. For example, good analgesia reduces the sympathetic overdrive and may terminate a tachycardia. With severe sepsis, it is virtually impossible to terminate a tachyarrhythmia until the underlying sepsis is improving.

- If the patient is haemodynamically *unstable* (blood pressure <90mmHg, confused, chest pain or heart failure), consider synchronised cardioversion irrespective of the type of tachyarrhythmia, whether narrow or broad (Resuscitation Council 2015); sedation may be indicated and specialist help should be sought (e.g. from an anaesthetist).
- If the patient is haemodynamically *stable* (with blood pressure >90mmHg, conscious, no chest pain or heart failure), assess whether the tachycardia is regular or irregular (adenisone can be used for this in non-asthmatic patients). Regular narrow complex tachycardias may respond to vagal manoeuvres or adenosine (Resuscitation Council 2015).
- Irregular narrow-complex tachycardias (usually atrial fibrillation) may respond to beta-blockers (e.g. atenolol), digoxin or amiodorone (Resuscitation Council 2015).
- If the tachycardia is not controlled, expert advice should be sought (Resuscitation Council 2015).
- If the tachycardia is still not controlled, consider elective DC cardioversion (synchronised).

The Resuscitation Council (2015) has an adult tachycardia algorithm with pulse, which should be used to guide management.

Broad-complex tachycardia

'Broad-complex' refers to the width of a QRST complex on a standard 12-lead ECG at 25mm per second. Anything more than 0.12 seconds (three little squares) is deemed 'broad'. A heart rate of more than 100 beats per minute is considered tachycardic. This includes ventricular tachycardia (VT) and supraventricular with aberrant conduction. Fortunately these are much rarer than narrow-complex tachycardia. A true VT is a peri-arrest arrhythmia with a high morbidity and mortality. You should treat every broad-complex tachycardia as VT in the acute onset situation until proven otherwise. See Box 26.4 for possible causes of broad-complex tachycardia.

Box 26.4 Possible causes of broad-complex tachycardia

- Ischaemic heart disease
- Electrolyte disturbances
- Structurally abnormal heart (heart failure, valvular disease, other cardiomyopathies, cardiac surgery)
- Drugs
- Bradyarrhythmias (a complete heart block can trigger VT as an escape rhythm)

The incidence of VT is not well quantified because of the clinical overlap of VT with ventricular fibrillation (VF). Examination of sudden death data provides a rough estimate of VT incidence. Most sudden cardiac deaths are thought to be caused by VT or VF (Koplan & Stevenson 2009). However, many patients have non-fatal VT and some sudden deaths are associated with bradycardia, rather than VT/VF. Incidence of VT increases in patients with coronary artery disease.

Diagnosis

Again, the diagnosis of a broad-complex tachycardia is based solely on the ECG. It can sometimes be difficult, so call in an expert early on to aid diagnosis. As a guide, regular broad-complex tachycardias are usually VT, whereas irregular broad-complex tachycardias could be atrial fibrillation with bundle branch block (BBB) or a polymorphic VT (such as torsades de pointes) (Resuscitation Council 2015).

A broad-complex tachycardia is VT until proven otherwise.

The likelihood of a broad-complex tachycardia being VT (see Figure 26.7) and not atrial fibrillation with bundle branch block (see Figure 26.8) is increased when:

- The QRS complexes are very broad
- There is a gross cardiac axis shift
- There is concordance in the chest leads (the R waves are all upwards or all downwards)
- There are capture beats (an 'own' complex captured among the VT beats)
- A fusion beat (a bizarre QRS complex made up of an 'own' and a VT beat)

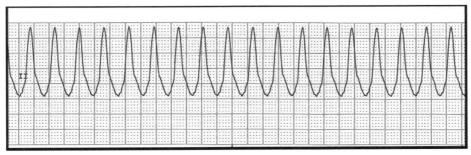

Figure 26.7 ECG of ventricular tachycardia.

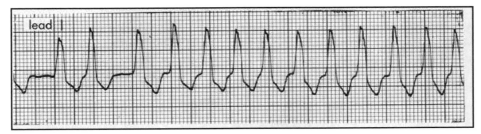

Figure 26.8 Atrial fibrillation with bundle branch block (note the irregularity).

Assessment

The **ABCDE** approach should be used: give oxygen, insert a cannula, monitor the ECG, blood pressure and SPO2, and record a 12-lead ECG. Consider electrolyte abnormalities.

Treatment

- If the patient is haemodynamically *unstable* (blood pressure <90mmHg, confused, chest pain or heart failure), consider urgent synchronised cardioversion; sedation may be indicated and specialist help should be sought (e.g. anaesthetist). Amiodorone may be administered after three synchronised shocks if the arrhythmia continues (see Resuscitation Council 2015 algorithm).

- If the patient is haemodynamically *stable* (i.e. none of the above), assess if the rhythm is regular or irregular. Irregular rhythms should be referred for expert help; regular rhythms (ventricular tachycardiac) give amiodarone (note: intravenous amiodarone should be given into a central, large vein) (Resuscitation Council 2015).

The Resuscitation Council has an adult tachycardia algorithm with pulse (Resuscitation Council 2015), which should be used to guide management.

HOT TIPS

Every patient with a tachycardia should:
- **Have this documented on an ECG**
- **Have their electrolytes checked**
- **Have their underlying condition treated primarily**

- Every patient with a tachycardia who is haemodynamically unstable (hypotension, heart failure, chest pain, reduced consciousness) should be cardioverted as a matter of urgency, regardless of the type of tachycardia.
- Get help from an ALS provider, and more senior help as required.

Conclusion

Tachyarrhythmias are termed 'peri-arrest' because they can deteriorate to cardiac arrest. You need to quickly determine whether a patient is stable or unstable. If they are unstable, synchronised DC cardioversion is the treatment of choice – irrespective of the type of tachyarrhythmia. It is important to call the cardiac arrest or medical emergency team so that you can get expert help quickly. If the patient is haemodynamically stable, then medical treatment is appropriate. The arrhythmia is nevertheless deemed a 'peri-arrest arrhythmia' and expert help should be sought early on.

References and further reading

Camm, A.J., Lip, G.Y.H., De Caterina, R., Savelieva, I. *et al* (2012). Focused update of the ESC Guidelines for the management of atrial fibrillation. An update of the 2010 ESC Guidelines for the management of atrial fibrillation. Developed with the special contribution of the European Heart Rhythm Association. *Europace.* **14** (10), 1385–1413
doi: http://dx.doi.org/10.1093/europace/eus305 (accessed 12 July 2015).

Koplan, B.A. & Stevenson, W.G. (2009). Ventricular tachycardia and sudden cardiac death. *Mayo Clinic Proceedings.* **84** (3), 289–97
doi: 10.1016/S0025-6196(11)61149-X

MDCalc (2015).
http://www.mdcalc.com/cha2ds2-vasc-score-for-atrial-fibrillation-stroke-risk/ (accessed 29 November 2015).

Resuscitation Council (2015). *Peri-arrest arrhythmias.*
https://www.resus.org.uk/resuscitation-guidelines/peri-arrest-arrhythmias/ (accessed 29 November 2015).

Resuscitation Council UK (2015). *Adult Advanced Life Support.*
https://www.resus.org.uk/resuscitation-guidelines/ (accessed 29 November 2015).

Wang, T.J., Massaro, J.M., Levy, D. *et al* (2003). A risk score for predicting stroke or death for individuals with new-onset atrial fibrillation in the community: The Framingham Heart Study. *Journal of the American Medical Association.* **290**, 1049–56.

Useful websites

American Heart Association
http://www.heart.org/HEARTORG/ (Accessed 13 July 2015)

Resuscitation Council UK
http://www.resus.org.uk (Accessed 29 November 2015)

27 Cardiac chest pain

Kuno Budack

Chest pain is a very common complaint and may be the cause of a patient being unwell or a direct result of another condition. It is often one of the more difficult situations to deal with in an acute setting. The differential diagnoses are varied and it is impossible to investigate for all possibilities.

The aim of this chapter is to provide you with knowledge about the assessment needed; the possible causes of cardiac chest pain; and the initial treatment for the patient who complains of chest pain.

Background

It is vital to take a swift but thorough history and carry out a physical examination. This will usually give a fair idea of the likely cause of the chest pain. In fact, the right questions, a good examination and a few tests will be able to establish the most likely diagnosis quickly. However, a doctor should be called in early for any patient with chest pain.

HOT TIP

In most cases, the diagnosis will be based on:
- A good history
- A physical examination
- A few tests.

With an acutely ill patient presenting with chest pain, the main concern is that the pain may have a cardiac origin. Acute myocardial infarction will therefore need to be considered initially. Table 27.1 identifies other possible causes of chest pain that need to be excluded.

Table 27.1 Possible causes of chest pain (based on Karnath *et al.* 2004)

Type of chest pain	Possible causes
Cardiovascular	Angina pectoris Acute myocardial infarction Valvular disease Pericarditis Aortic dissecting aneurysm
Pulmonary	Pneumonia Pulmonary embolism Pneumothorax
Gastrointestinal	Reflux oesophagitis Peptic ulcers Pancreatitis Cholecystitis
Musculoskeletal	Costochondritis Trauma/fracture Rheumatoid arthritis Cervical/thoracic disc compression
Miscellaneous	Anxiety Herpes zoster (shingles) Tumours

Case scenario

You are called to see a 65-year-old man on a medical ward who has developed chest pain. On arrival you note that he is anxious, sweaty and has central chest pain. He is able to talk to you. His respiratory rate is 26 breaths per minute and his blood pressure is 160/80mmHg. He has a tachycardia of 120 beats per minute and his saturations are 96%.

Pathophysiology

Chest pain can have a variety of causes, as outlined above. It is important to identify the type, severity, position and any radiation of pain, its duration and any other associated symptoms. The patient should be asked to describe the pain and whether anything makes the pain better or worse.

HOT TIP

Refresh your understanding of the anatomical structures and functions of the heart, coronary blood supply, responses to stress and the development of atheroscleroma.

Pathophysiology of Heart Disease (available at: http://www.scribd.com/doc/217196087/Pathophysiology-of-Heart-Disease#scribd) is a freely available online resource or you can access any pathophysiology textbook.

In the acutely ill patient, any chest pain should be treated as potentially of cardiac origin. When a patient is acutely ill, the body is under increased stress. This may mean that the heart has an increased workload and so needs a greater oxygen supply. If the coronary arteries are compromised because of atherosclerotic plaques, the added workload on the heart can lead to myocardial ischaemia and chest pain (angina). In severe cases, a myocardial infarction may be precipitated.

Assessment and monitoring

Assessment of the patient in the case scenario should follow the ABCDE method.

A-Airway

In this patient, the airway is patent, as he is able to speak.

B-Breathing

His respiratory rate is slightly fast. The use of oxygen therapy is controversial in chest pain (Meier *et al.* 2013) but NICE (2010a) recommends that oxygen therapy should be considered if the O_2 saturation is less than 94%. Respiratory rate should be recorded half-hourly and saturations should be measured. Remember that the patient is sweaty and may be peripherally shut down, so peripheral saturations may not be accurate. If there is any suspicion that the chest pain has a respiratory cause, then a chest x-ray may be indicated.

C-Cardiovascular

The patient's blood pressure (BP) is raised and he is tachycardic. Continuous ECG monitoring should be commenced and observations of blood pressure and heart rate should be recorded half-hourly. Temperature readings should be taken. A history should also be taken; suggested 'questions to ask' are listed in Box 27.1.

A physical assessment (including palpation, percussion and auscultation) should be undertaken. The patient's pulse should be felt and assessed for strength (bounding or weak), capillary refill can be assessed, and jugular venous pressure can be estimated. The heart should be auscultated for evidence of any murmurs and the lungs for signs of pulmonary oedema (see Chapter 13 on acute heart failure).

It may be useful to measure blood pressure on both arms to help exclude aortic dissection. A 12-lead ECG should be done as a priority and reviewed by a knowledgeable professional. A venous cannula should be inserted and blood tested for glucose and urea and electrolytes and a full blood count as well as cardiac enzymes (troponin I or T) (NICE 2010a).

Box 27.1 Questions to ask patients with acute chest pain

Where exactly do you feel the pain?
- Lateral pains are unlikely to be due to an acute cardiac event or aortic dissection.
- Back pain is unlikely to be of cardiac origin but an aortic dissection is possible.

What does the pain feel like?
- 'Tight' suggests cardiac pain.
- 'Sharp' suggests inflammation (pleurisy, infection).
- 'Tearing' suggests dissection.

Does the pain spread anywhere?
- Associated arm or jaw pain suggests the heart.
- Radiation to the back suggests aortic dissection.

What makes the pain worse?
- Anything triggered from the outside (inspiration, pressure) points away from the heart and aorta (but does not exclude them).
- Pain related to exertion suggests angina.
- Pain after a meal could be gastrointestinal (reflux, cholecystitis, pancreatitis).

What helps the pain?
- Glyceryl trinitrate (helps angina and reflux).
- Sitting up (eases pericarditis).

Do you get anything else with the pains?
- Sweating and giddiness are alarm signs.

D-Disability

Analgesia should be given to relieve the pain (this is probably why his blood pressure is high). Morphine is often used, but glycerine trinitrate (GTN) tablets or sublingual spray may be indicated if the patient has a history of angina. Both morphine and GTN work by dilating the coronary arteries and improving oxygen supply to the heart muscle. Morphine has the added benefit of reducing anxiety (NICE 2010a). Aspirin 300mg may be considered if there are no contraindications (NICE 2010a).

Assistance is required from a senior person or the outreach team to review the need for a specialist bed, such as on the coronary care unit. For ST-elevation myocardial infaction (STEMI), referral to the appropriate specialist is essential. The patient will need assessment for coronary percutaneous intervention (PCI) or thrombolysis, depending on local services (see NICE 2010b, NICE 2013).

The patient's level of consciousness should be assessed because deterioration or increased confusion can indicate a worsening condition, and possibly an imminent cardiac arrest. Suggest keeping the patient 'nil by mouth' if a non-cardiac cause is suspected.

E-Exposure and environment

The priority for these patients is to reduce their distress. However, it is also important to examine the patient fully for any possible injuries, peripheral oedema (which may indicate heart failure) or signs of peripheral vascular disease (which can indicate concurrent cardiovascular disease).

Investigations

ECG

- Look for ischaemia (ST depression, ST elevation, new left bundle branch block).
- Helps with diagnosis of pericarditis (widespread saddle-shaped ST segment elevation in most leads).
- Helps with diagnosis of pulmonary embolism (SIQIIITIII) or right heart strain (right axis shift, incomplete or complete right bundle branch block, anterior T-wave inversion).

Chest x-ray

- Check for pneumothorax.
- Helps with diagnosis of pneumonia.
- Might point towards aortic dissection (mediastinal widening).

Blood tests

- Full blood count (to look for anaemia and signs of gastric bleeding).
- Urea and electrolytes (to look for imbalances, particularly of potassium).
- Troponin (a sensitive test of myocardial injury if raised above normal).
- Amylase (to exclude pancreatitis).
- Glucose (to look for undiagnosed diabetes).
- Arterial blood gases (to exclude respiratory problems, see Chapter 10).

Echocardiogram

- Useful when a new murmur has been detected.
- Can help with diagnosis of aortic aneurysm if the ascending aorta or the aortic root is involved.

Management

Treatment of chest pain will depend on the final diagnosis. This chapter concentrates on the management of chest pain caused by underlying ischaemic heart disease. Firstly, an ECG should be taken within minutes of arrival in the emergency department and this should be interpreted by a knowledgeable healthcare professional.

The decision as to whether someone requires immediate attention is based on only three types of ECG changes:

- ST elevation (see Figure 27.1)
- New onset left bundle branch block (see Figure 27.2)
- True posterior MI (see Figure 27.3).

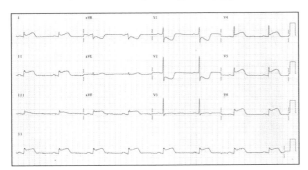

ST elevation in at least 2 consecutive leads
Inferior = leads II, III, aVF
Anterior = leads V1–V3
Lateral = lead I, aVL, V5–V6

Figure 27.1 ST elevation.

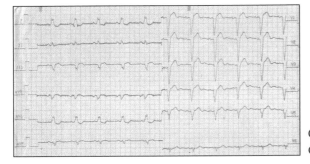

QRS complex ≥120ms (3 little squares)
Complex in V1 is downgoing (looks like a 'V' or 'W')

Figure 27.2 New onset left bundle branch block.

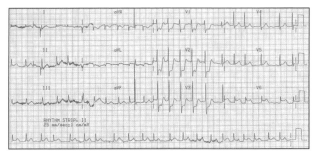

Dominant R wave in V1 or V2
Deep horizontal ST depression in aVL
Do an ECG that goes further round the back
(V7–V9)

Figure 27.3 *True posterior MI.*

If the patient has symptoms that suggest a cardiac event and he has any of the above ECG changes (NICE 2010a, NICE 2013):

- Manage the pain with morphine or diamorphine and GTN
- Load antiplatelet therapy with 300mg aspirin and 600mg clopidogrel (or prasugrel or ticagrelor)
- Start anticoagulation with fondaparinux 2.5mg OD
- Liaise urgently with the primary percutaneous coronary intervention (PCI) centre; the patient should have PCI within 90 minutes
- Consider thrombolysis in patients who cannot have a primary PCI in a timely manner
- The decision on early beta blockade depends on the patient's clinical status – stable patients (with normal blood pressure and heart rate and without clinical heart failure) would probably benefit. Those who have any of the above can wait.

If the ECG does not show any of the three ECG changes mentioned above but does show ST or T wave changes, diagnosis of an acute coronary syndrome is possible (either unstable angina or a non-ST segment elevation MI). In this case:

- Manage the pain with morphine or diamorphine and GTN
- Load antiplatelet therapy with 300mg aspirin (Note: Do not give clopidogrel yet)
- Start anticoagulation with fondaparinux 2.5mg OD.

Now assess the patient's risk using the Global Registry of Acute Coronary Events (GRACE Risk Calculator), either online or using their app (http://www.gracescore.org). This assesses acute coronary syndrome risk, based on age, heart rate, systolic blood pressure, creatinine and Killip class (measures evidence of heart failure on a scale of 0–4) to assess heart failure. The calculator also requires an ECG assessment of ST-deviation, and a troponin level as well as a creatinine level. You should wait for these tests before initiating further ischaemic treatment. The GRACE score estimates mortality over differing time periods. In hospital a score of 1 is low risk, 2 is medium risk and 3 is high risk and may help guide treatment.

Conclusion

Chest pain is a common problem in the acutely ill adult and can lead to potentially life-threatening complications if the cause is not identified swiftly and treated appropriately.

References and further reading

Karnath, B., Holden, M.D. & Hussain, N. (2004). Chest pain: differentiating cardiac from noncardiac causes. *Hospital Physician.* **40** (4), 24–27, 38.

Meier, P., Ebrahim, S., Otto, C.M. MD & Casas, J.P. (2013). Oxygen therapy in acute myocardial infarction – good or bad? [editorial]. Cochrane Database of Systematic Reviews. **8**, ED000065. dx.doi.org/10.1002/14651858.ED000065

National Institute for Health and Care Excellence (NICE) (2010a). *Chest pain of recent onset: Assessment and diagnosis of recent onset chest pain or discomfort of suspected cardiac origin. Guideline 95.*
http://www.nice.org.uk/guidance/cg95 (accessed 23 February 2015).

National Institute for Health and Care Excellence (NICE) (2010b). *Unstable angina and NSTEMI: The early management of unstable angina and non-ST-segment-elevation myocardial infarction. Guideline 94.*
http://www.nice.org.uk/guidance/CG94 (accessed 23 February 2015).

National Institute for Health and Care Excellence (NICE) (2013). *Myocardial infarction with ST-segment elevation: The acute management of myocardial infarction with ST-segment elevation. Guideline 167.*
https://www.nice.org.uk/guidance/cg167 (accessed 23 February 2015).

Useful websites

GRACE Risk Calculator
http://www.gracescore.org/WebSite/WebVersion.aspx
(Accessed 14 July 2015)

28

Acute abdomen

Russell Canavan and Ann M. Price

Approximately half of all acute surgical admissions present with abdominal pain (ASGBI 2014). Thus the acute abdomen is relatively common and presents a special challenge, as it includes a number of clinical conditions. Often it requires a definitive intervention (for example, surgery), which may be high risk in the acutely ill patient. A methodical approach to resuscitation and timing of a procedure is essential to optimise the patient's chances of survival. The detailed acute abdomen is the subject of other books. This chapter gives a typical case example and points to some pitfalls in managing a patient with an acute abdomen.

When you have read this chapter, you should be aware of the main causes of an acute abdomen; and be able to assess the patient, and plan and initiate treatment.

Background

The acute abdomen is not a diagnosis in itself but is part of a nebulous group of medical, surgical and gynaecological conditions that require hospitalisation. Often the cardinal feature of the admission is abdominal pain.

Case scenario

A 46-year-old obese woman attended the emergency department. She arrived vomiting, with sudden-onset central abdominal pain that radiated through to her back. On arrival she was assessed according to the **ABCDE** approach.

A–Airway
She was alert and talking (complaining of pain).

B–Breathing
She had a respiratory rate of 24 breaths per minute, with saturations of 100% on air. She had a clear chest on auscultation.

C–Circulation

She was dehydrated and flushed. Her pulse was bounding, with a rate of 110 beats per minute and she had a blood pressure of 90/40mmHg.

D–Disability

She was alert and orientated. Her capillary blood glucose came back as 9.8 mmol/litre.

E–Environment and exposure

Exposing the patient revealed no abnormality.

Abdominal examination was performed:

- Inspection: her abdomen was tense but essentially normal.
- Percussion: gave no suggestion of any enlarged organs or ascites.
- Palpation: proved difficult as she was voluntarily guarding. However, she was noted to be diffusely tender and her abdomen was soft when distracted. She had no palpable organs.
- Auscultation: active bowel sounds could be heard.

Mechanism of condition and therapy

This woman was clearly unwell with an acute abdomen. The ABCDE approach showed she reached three of the criteria for sepsis (see more about sepsis in Chapter 21), which are likely to be secondary to an abdominal cause. Therefore, she needs urgent assessment and appropriate treatment to prevent any further deterioration.

You will need to consider the causes of an acute abdomen and consider which of these are relevant in this woman (see Table 28.1). Although this is a long list, most of the conditions are fairly straightforward to diagnose and their treatment is well established. The pathophysiology of the acute abdomen is varied, depending on the cause, and you should refer to other texts for further details (such as NICE guidelines on a variety of conditions).

As surgical teams are often asked to manage these patients, it is important not to miss medical conditions that can mimic a surgical abdomen. These include diabetic ketoacidosis, acute myocardial events, biochemical abnormalities and sickle cell disease.

Assessment and management

A thorough assessment is required. Box 28.2 describes the assessment required in acute abdomen. Pregnancy must be excluded in all women of childbearing age. Box 28.3 describes bowel sounds and their possible causes.

Irrespective of the cause of the pain, the patient's immediate needs are fluid resuscitation, analgesia and antibiotics. Two large-bore cannulae should be inserted and fluid should be given according to the response of the heart rate, blood pressure and urine output. Continuous monitoring would be the gold standard, with hourly observation of vital signs and fluid input and output; ideally a urinary catheter will be needed (refer to NICE 2007). A central venous line should be considered if the patient's condition does not improve swiftly. If available, a high-dependency bed may be required so that close observation is possible.

Table 28.1 Causes of acute abdominal pain (based on Cole *et al.* 2006)

Liver	Hepatitis Liver abscess Budd–Chiari syndrome Hepatic ischaemia
Gynaecological	Ectopic pregnancy Ovarian cyst Salpingitis Pelvic inflammatory disease Fibroids
Pancreatobiliary	Cholangitis Cholecystitis Pancreatitis Biliary leak/perforation
Peritoneum	Primary peritonitis Secondary peritonitis
Urogenital	Acute retention Obstructive uropathy Testicular torsion
Gastrointestinal	Gastritis Bowel obstruction Gastroenteritis Peptic ulcer disease Hernia Volvulus Diverticulitis Ischaemic bowel Appendicitis Intersusception Perforation
Medical	Diabetes mellitus Addison's disease Herpes zoster
Spleen	Rupture Infarction
Haematological	Sickle cell disease Malaria

Box 28.1 Assessment in acute abdomen (based on Cole *et al.* 2006 and ASGBI 2014)

Past medical history and history of present complaint
This should highlight previous episodes of abdominal pain and their outcome. Current history (e.g. rate of onset, precipitating factors) may aid diagnosis. Predisposing factors should become evident (e.g. alcohol, foreign travel, family history).

Physical observation
This includes the **ABCDE** approach and incorporates inspection, percussion, palpation and auscultation of the abdomen using the 4- or 9-quadrant method. Remember to ask about the type and frequency of stools and vomiting, and examine skin turgor.

Haemodynamic
Include blood pressure, heart rate, respiratory rate, urine output, temperature and capillary refill time.

Blood tests
Full blood count (for low haemoglobin and high white cell count), urea and electrolytes (for renal impairment and electrolyte imbalances), clotting, liver function tests, amylase, blood glucose, blood cultures, arterial blood gases, and others as indicated (e.g. pregnancy test).

Others as indicated
Urinalysis, ECG, endoscopy, CT scan, MRI, X-ray, ultrasound.

A tense or distended abdomen means that the diaphragm cannot function properly, causing 'splinting'; this can lead to respiratory problems so oxygen therapy and respiratory assessment is important.

The choice of analgesic varies with the cause of the abdominal pain; opiates (such as morphine) are thought to cause spasm of the sphincter of Oddi and may increase pain in biliary problems. However, in the acute phase controlling pain with analgesia and assessing response using a pain score will guide treatment, and ASGBI (2014) suggest that opiates do not affect the assessment at this stage. Patient-controlled analgesia (including epidurals) can be useful for abdominal pain and referral to the acute pain team or anaesthetist; if pain is poorly controlled, this type of analgesia should be considered.

Early aggressive (usually intravenous) antibiotics are crucial and should be instigated with consideration of the likely cause of the pain, local hospital antibiotic policy and, when needed, input from the consultant microbiologist. Once appropriate microbiological investigations have been carried out, such as stool and urine specimens, wound swabs and blood cultures, if antibiotics are not being effective then specialist advice should be sought.

Box 28.2 Bowel sounds

Absent sounds: possibly caused by gastrointestinal paralysis (e.g. ileus or peritonitis).

Overactive or tinkling sounds: possibly caused by gastrointestinal obstruction.

NB: The usefulness of bowel sounds in the acute situation is controversial but Li *et al.* (2012) recommend assessing bowel sounds in critically ill patients.

It is not uncommon for these patients to aspirate if they are vomiting. A large-bore nasogastric tube can be life-saving in this situation (size 14 Fr is suggested). Nasogastric tubes also help to ensure accurate fluid balance because the amount of vomitus can be underestimated (see Chapter 40 on placing a nasogastric tube). If the patient is actively vomiting they should be made 'nil by mouth'; and you should instigate anti-emetics and review the effect. If a patient is to remain nil by mouth or has a poor oral intake it will be important to consider their nutritional requirements (see Chapter 39 for more on meeting nutrition in the acutely unwell patient).

The woman in our clinical scenario was critically unwell and needed hourly monitoring of her vital signs, including her urine output. She remained hypotensive and needed central venous pressure monitoring. In the acute abdomen, there is often a definitive procedure that can be carried out to alleviate the problem, so when the patient is stable enough they should be sent for this.

In the case of the woman in our scenario, the bloods revealed that she had an acute pancreatitis with deranged liver enzymes. Using the Glasgow criteria, she was classified as severe pancreatitis (see Box 28.3). Abdominal ultrasound demonstrated a dilated common bile duct and the presence of gallstones. Within 72 hours of admission, she underwent an endoscopic retrograde cholangiopancreatography (ERCP), during which the gallstones were removed. Following her recovery, she was booked for a laparoscopic cholecystectomy (NICE 2010).

Review an anatomy and physiology book to locate key organs in the abdomen, including the spleen, liver, stomach, small and large intestines, ovaries, uterus, kidneys, bladder and aorta. You should also review the 4 or 9 quadrants of the abdomen used in physical assessment.

Early referral to senior clinicians is of paramount importance with patients who remain hypotensive despite fluid resuscitation. See Chapter 2 for more on assessing and monitoring the acutely unwell patient.

Box 28.3
Pancreatitis scores according to Ranson and Glasgow criteria
(based on Felstead 2007)

Ranson criteria (three or more factors indicates severe disease)

Age >55 years

>10% decrease in haemoglobin

White cell count >16,000mm^3

Urea >16mmol/litre

Calcium <2 mmol/litre

Glucose >10mmol/litre

Fluid loss >6 litres

Glasgow criteria (three or more factors indicates severe disease)

Age >55 years

White cell count >15,000 mm^3

Urea >16mmol/litre

Calcium <2mmol/litre

Glucose >10mmol/litre

Albumin <32g/litre

NB: Some organisations use adapted versions of these scores so please refer to local guidance.

Conclusion

The acute abdomen is a common cause for admission to hospital. Most of these patients will have a correctable condition that needs swift diagnosis and treatment to ensure a good outcome. Early aggressive resuscitation using the **ABCDE** approach in the unwell patient, with careful monitoring, can significantly improve outcome. There are a few pitfalls but they can be easily avoided.

References and further reading

Association of Surgeons of Great Britain and Ireland (ASGBI) (2014). *Commissioning guide: Emergency General Surgery (acute abdominal pain).* Publisher: ASGBI

Cole, E., Lynch, A. & Cugononi, H. (2006). Assessment of the patient with acute abdominal pain. *Nursing Standard.* **20** (39), 67–75.

Felstead, I. (2007). 'Upper gastrointestinal surgery' in F.J. McArthur-Rouse & S. Prosser (eds). *Assessing and Managing the Acutely Ill Surgical Patient.* Edinburgh: Blackwell Publishing.

Li, B., Wang, J. & Ma, Y. (2012). Bowel sounds and monitoring gastrointestinal motility in critically ill patients. *Clinical Nurse Specialist.* **26** (1), 29–34.

National Institute for Health and Care Excellence (NICE) (2007). *Acutely ill patients in hospital: Recognition of and response to acute illness in adults in hospital. CG 50.*
http://www.nice.org.uk/guidance/cg50/chapter/1-Guidance (accessed 22 April 2015).

National Institute for Health and Care Excellence (NICE) (2010). *Pancreatitis – acute: Clinical Knowledge Summaries.*
http://cks.nice.org.uk/pancreatitis-acute#!scenario (accessed 22 April 2015).

Useful websites

Association of Surgeons of Great Britain and Ireland
http://www.asgbi.org.uk/ (Accessed 15 July 2015)
British Society of Gastroenterology
http://www.bsg.org.uk/ (Accessed 15 July 2015)

29 Oesophageal varices

Russell Canaven and Ann M. Price

Patients with oesophageal varices are at risk of large upper gastrointestinal bleed (a GI bleed). When they bleed, they present in an alarming way and have a high mortality (NICE 2012). A methodical approach to their management can relieve the anxiety of both the patient and the staff managing the patient. Recent advances in the treatment of varices have had a significant impact on the outcome of the disease and should be incorporated in its treatment. NICE clinical guidance 141 (2012) offers detailed guidance on the management of oesophageal varices.

At the end of this chapter you will be confident in diagnosing variceal haemorrhage and managing variceal haemorrhage.

Background

The portal circulation is normally a low-pressure (1–6mmHg) system (Bosch *et al.* 2015) that carries 1500ml blood per minute from the spleen, stomach, small and large bowel to the liver. If the blood flow is restricted before, within or after the liver, then the pressure in the system will rise. Portal-systemic shunting occurs, and leads to the development of varices. In some patients their underlying liver disease may not be apparent until their first bleed.

HOT TIP

Carry out a review of the anatomy and physiology of the upper gastrointestinal tract.

The Khan Academy Website has videos about this. See https://www.khanacademy.org/science/health-and-medicine/human-anatomy-and-physiology or review any anatomy and physiology books available in your library. Revise the position of the liver, spleen, gall bladder and portal circulation, the oesophageal veins, and the pre-, intra- and post-hepatic obstruction. Identify the structure and function of each aspect.

Case scenario

A 43-year-old man is referred for assessment of 'coffee ground' vomiting. Shortly after arrival, he vomits approximately 1 litre of fresh red blood and is assessed according to the **ABCDE** approach.

A–Airway

He is agitated but talking to you.

B–Breathing

His respiratory rate is 30 breaths per minute.

C–Circulation

His pulse is 120 beats per minute and is regular. He has a blood pressure of only 80/50mmHg. His peripheries are cold and his capillary refill time is 5 seconds.

D–Disability

He is alert but confused.

E–Exposure and environment

There is nothing to note when the patient is exposed.

An abdominal examination is conducted:

- **Inspection:** This gentleman is pale and has multiple spider naevi (defined as small blanching vascular skin lesions that fill centrally; they can be a normal finding but in association with other features imply chronic liver disease). He has abdominal distension and pedal oedema. Some distended veins are noted on his abdomen. You note that he has several tattoos.
- **Palpation:** He has no palpable organomegaly.
- **Auscultation:** He has normal bowel sounds.
- **Percussion:** He has evidence of shifting dullness on palpation.

For more on bowel sounds and their possible causes, see Box 28.2 in the previous chapter.

Pathophysiology and aetiology

In our case scenario, the clinical examination showed clear signs of portal hypertension. Portal hypertension, and the development of oesophageal varices, is a complex topic. It is thought to be a combination of increased vascular volume, alterations in vasodilation and resistance within the portal system that lead to development of collateral veins and varices (Bosch *et al.* 2015). The most likely explanation for the presentation is that this man has portal hypertension, resulting in an acute variceal bleed. (See Box 29.1 for causes of portal hypertension.)

In most cases, the pathology is hepatic cirrhosis and this carries additional problems (Bosch *et al.* 2015). In the developed world, the most common cause of this has been alcoholic liver disease, but the demographics are changing. As a result of our modern lifestyle, many patients are now being seen for non-alcoholic fatty liver disease (NAFLD), which can also lead to cirrhosis.

Box 29.1 Causes of portal hypertension (based on Cole *et al.* 2006)

Pre-hepatic: portal vein disease (such as thrombosis)
Hepatic: liver disease (such as liver cirrhosis, chronic hepatitis, toxins)
Post-hepatic: hepatic vein disease (such as Budd-Chiari syndrome, right heart failure)

Liver cirrhosis

Cirrhosis can be defined as the histological development of regenerative nodules surrounded by fibrous bands in response to chronic liver injury, which leads to portal hypertension and end-stage liver disease (Schuppan & Adfha 2008). In the most common scenario, the patient will have liver cirrhosis as well as a problem with bleeding varices or portal hypertension. The cirrhotic patient may have deranged synthetic and metabolic functions of their liver, possibly including hepatorenal complications (Gines 2004).

Liver function tests

Liver function tests include those for aspartate aminotransaminase (AST), alkaline phosphatase (ALP) and bilirubin (conjugated and total). These are usually elevated in liver disease (British Liver Trust). There is retention of free body water in patients with liver cirrhosis, which leads to a dilution of serum sodium, causing a relative hyponatraemia. This can lead to cerebral oedema and its sequelae.

Hepatic encephalopathy

Hepatic encephalopathy is a syndrome observed in patients with cirrhosis. It is defined as a spectrum of neuropsychiatric abnormalities in people with liver dysfunction, after exclusion of other known brain disease. It is characterised by personality changes, intellectual impairment and a depressed level of consciousness. Grading of the symptoms of hepatic encephalopathy is performed according to the so-called West Haven classification system (Wolf 2014), as shown in Box 29.2.

Box 29.2 The stages of hepatic encephalopathy (based on Wolf 2014)

Stage 0:
- Minimal hepatic encephalopathy
- Undetectable changes in personality or behaviour
- Little effect on memory, concentration, intellectual function and coordination
- Asterixis is absent.

Stage 1:
- Minor lack of awareness
- Short attention span and reduced ability to perform mental tasks
- Changes in sleep pattern
- Euphoria, depression or irritability
- Mild confusion
- Asterixis detectable.

Stage 2:
- Lethargy
- Disorientation
- Inappropriate behaviour
- Slurred speech
- Obvious asterixis
- Increased difficulty in performing mental tasks
- Obvious personality changes
- Can be disorientated.

Stage 3:
- Somnolent but rousable
- Unable to perform mental tasks
- Marked confusion, disorientation and amnesia
- Possible outbursts of rage
- Incomprehensible speech.

Stage 4:
- Coma that may be unresponsive to painful stimuli.

Liver proteins and metabolism

The liver has a major role in the synthesis of various proteins. The most useful of these for the clinician in the acute situation is the albumin, and clotting factors. These can be measured and are prognostic when evaluated in combination with other markers. Albumin is usually low and prothrombin time may be prolonged (British Liver Trust). The Childs–Pugh–Turcotte classification (see Table 29.1) is used to predict severity of liver disease in these patients. The scores for all the criteria are added up to predict a patient's life expectancy, prior to acute deterioration.

Table 29.1 Childs–Pugh–Turcotte classification (Schuppan & Adfhal 2008)

Parameter	Score 1	Score 2	Score 3
Ascites	None	Moderate	Severe
Encephalopathy	None	Mild	Severe
Prothrombin time (above normal)	<4 secs	4–6 secs	> 6 secs
Serum bilirubin	<35µmol/litre	35–50µmol/litre	> 50µmol/litre
Serum albumin	>35g/litre	30–35g/litre	< 30g/litre
Scoring system Record the score for each criterion and add them all up to predict a patient's life expectancy, prior to acute deterioration. Childs–Pugh A: Score 5–6 (life expectancy 15–20 years) Childs–Pugh B: Score 7–9 (life expectancy 4–14 years) Childs–Pugh C: Score 10–15 (life expectancy 1–3 years)			

Various metabolic functions are carried out in the liver, and a basic understanding of these is useful when looking after patients with liver problems. An example of this is the importance of the liver in glucolysis. This can lead to hypoglycaemia in the context of liver failure – an important clinical finding in liver patients who are agitated, drowsy or confused.

The liver is also key in the metabolism of many drugs, which should be checked in the appendix of the *British National Formulary* prior to administration. If the metabolic function of the liver deteriorates, the waste products of metabolism can build up and cause hepatic encephalopathy (Wolf 2014). This problem can be exacerbated by opiates and sedatives, which are also metabolised by the liver. Reversible causes of portal hypertension should be identified and treated as a matter of urgency when the patient is stable.

Assessment

History

It is particularly important to get the diagnosis of chronic liver disease. There are many clues that can help give the likely diagnosis.

- Alcohol: not only whether they drink but how much and for how long; confirm the amount with a third party if possible.

- Age: neonates, children, teenagers, adults, middle-aged people and elderly people all have differing causes of liver diseases.
- Ethnicity: certain ethnic groups have specific liver conditions associated with them (Bosch *et al.* 2015).
- Past medical history: for example, lupus and liver disease.
- Associated symptoms: for example, skin rashes and arthralgia.
- Viral risk factors: for example, living abroad, blood transfusions, injecting drug use history, unprotected sex, being a healthcare worker and having tattoos.
- Drugs: prescribed, non-prescribed, social and herbal.

Look

Assess the patient's colour and pallor. They may be losing blood. This may also elicit an assessment of their hydration status (for example, do they have a dry tongue?). Inspect for stigmata of chronic liver disease (see Box 29.3). Although sensitive, features of chronic liver disease are often non-specific (Braun & Anderson 2011).

Box 29.3 Stigmata of chronic liver disease

- Clubbing
- White nails
- Palmar erythema
- Spider naevi
- Facial telangiectasia
- Gynaecomastia
- Parotidomegaly
- Testicular atrophy
- Hepatic encephalopathy
- Ascites
- Irregular liver surface
- Tender liver edge
- Splenomegaly
- Caput medusa

Listen (auscultate)

Occasionally a venous hum or arterial bruit can be heard over the liver in patients with cirrhosis or hepatocellular carcinoma. Bowel sounds will be normal.

Feel (palpate)

Splenomegaly is a key feature. Although it is present in many conditions, it is highly suggestive of cirrhosis in the presence of liver disease. Feel for a liver edge. Is it thickened or irregular?

Note the presence of ascites by testing for shifting dullness (see Box 29.4). The presence of shifting dullness confirms the presence of fluid (normally ascites) in the abdomen. This is a common feature in liver disease (Braun & Anderson 2011).

Box 29.4 How to test for shifting dullness

- Place the patient flat and relaxed, with their arms by their side. Let any fluid settle in the flanks and explain to the patient what you are doing.
- Percuss in the mid-line of the abdomen. The note should be resonant.
- Move laterally, percussing continuously, until a dull note is reached. Mark this spot.
- Move the patient through 90° so they are lying on their side. The spot that was dull should now become resonant (i.e. the dull spot has moved with the fluid).
- Confirm the result by repeating the process in reverse, starting with the patient on their side.

Assessment tools

NICE (2012) recommends the use of the Blatchford Score to assess bleeding risk for patients presenting with suspected oesophageal varices. The Rockall Score is recommended for patients post-endoscopy to monitor response (NICE 2012).

Versions of the assessment scores are available online.

The Blatchford Score is available at:
http://www.mdcalc.com/glasgow-blatchford-bleeding-score-gbs/

The Rockall Score calclator is available at:
http://www.bsg.org.uk/rockall-score-calculator.html

Monitoring

Although there is no agreed way of monitoring liver patients during an acute bleed, there is a need for close supervision:

- Every 15 minutes: pulse, blood pressure, oxygen saturation monitoring
- Every hour: temperature, central venous pressure (if present), urine output.

The organisation's Early Warning Score should be utilised and escalation policy followed. The initial priority is to control bleeding. Once the patient is stabilised and the bleeding has stopped, then all the above measurements can be taken every hour. When in liver failure, the patient is at risk of hypoglycaemia so capillary blood glucose should also be monitored.

Fluid management

In the acute setting, it is not uncommon for the patient to be intravascularly depleted while the extravascular compartment is grossly overloaded. In this situation, central pressure monitoring can be useful (see Chapter 20 on central venous catheters). Initial resuscitation of the patient with fluids is vital, as the patient may have lost significant amounts of blood and is likely to require blood transfusion. Variceal bleeds often involve large blood loss; many units of packed red cells may therefore be needed, further depleting clotting factors and platelets. NICE (2012) gives guidance on whether to replace these factors when the patient is actively bleeding.

Each hospital should have a protocol for massive blood transfusions to guide them on replacement of clotting factors and platelets. Advice from a haematologist can be invaluable in these situations. NICE (2012) suggests that over-transfusion may be counter-productive. Careful assessment and management of fluid status will therefore be required.

NB: *There is some suggestion that raising the portal pressure with over-transfusion may contribute to varices continuing to bleed (McCormick et al. 1999, Duggan 2001).*

Endoscopy

NICE (2012) recommends the early use of endoscopy (once the patient is more stable) to control and prevent further bleeding. The first consideration of endoscopy is the loss of protection of the airway. When the patient is starved for endoscopy this is not a problem, but in acute haematemesis the stomach is full and aspiration is a real concern.

Intubation to protect the airway should be considered when considering endoscopy in the context of upper gastrointestinal bleeding. Endoscopy is diagnostic in most cases. During the endoscopy, elastic bands can be placed on the veins in a sequential fashion to stop the bleeding, or clips or stents may be used. Varices can also be injected with agents that induce sclerosis and obliteration of the varice, in combination with other treatments (NICE 2012).

Drugs in the acute setting

Terlipressin and somatostatin analogues

These are used initially to lower portal pressure and, therefore, control haemorrhage. They can be used as an adjunct to endoscopic therapy and should be continued for 72 hours. The drug of choice is terlipressin because it has the additional effect of protecting against hepatorenal failure (NICE 2012).

Broad-spectrum antibiotics

Many cirrhotic patients presenting with upper gastrointestinal haemorrhage have concurrent infection precipitating their bleed (Thalheimer *et al.* 2005). Early treatment with antibiotics has been shown to reduce mortality.

Other drugs

The value of laxatives and prokinetics and proton inhibitors in the acute phase is limited (NICE 2012). Using these would necessitate discussion with a specialist.

Specialist help

Early help from a gastroenterologist can be helpful. Most are very keen to hear about patients with a variceal bleed and they can assist in patient management using the following techniques.

Balloon tamponade

Balloon tamponade involves a long tube (often called a Sengstaken–Blakemore tube) that is inserted into the oesophagus. The balloon is then inflated to put pressure on the bleeding varices to prevent further bleeding. NICE (2011) suggests this can be used when other methods have failed, are unavailable or inappropriate. Traction on the tube pulls on the varices and stems the bleeding.

Prolonged use of the balloon can lead to pressure necrosis (Dib *et al.* 2006) and it is advisable for patients to be placed in a critical care area for this treatment so that trained personnel can monitor the airway and the device.

The patient's airway needs to be protected, as aspiration is a risk – so the patient's level of consciousness must be considered. Intubation and ventilation are sometimes needed to protect the airway.

Shunting

In specialist centres, shunts may be available and NICE (2012) recommends the use of shunts if bleeding cannot be controlled by other methods. Shunts connect the portal and systemic circulation, reducing the portal pressure that causes the bleeding. A transjugular intrahepatic portosystemic shunt (TIPS) is positioned via the internal jugular, under screening. It is placed along the hepatic vein and pushed through to the portal vein, effectively forming a liver bypass, and lowering the portal pressure. However, bypassing the liver may precipitate hepatic encephalopathy or right heart failure, and there are other problems related to the shunt (Dib *et al.* 2006).

Transplant

One final option is to perform a liver transplant, if the patient meets the necessary criteria. This can be considered by your local centre (NICE 2012).

Conclusion

Oesophageal varices present some very specific challenges. Issues concerning immediate resuscitation should be borne in mind when treating these patients. Close monitoring, aggressive fluid resuscitation, control of clotting abnormalities, early intervention with endoscopy and use of terlipressin are key interventions in the initial stages. Additional physical interventions, such as transjugular intrahepatic portasystemic shunt (TIPS), need specialist input to assess their value.

References and further reading

Bosch, J., Groszmann, R.J. & Shah, V.H. (2015). Evolution in the understanding of the pathophysiological basis of portal hypertension: How changes in paradigm are leading to successful new treatments. *Journal of Hepatology.* **62** (1) supplement S121–130.

Braun, C.A. & Anderson, C.M. (2011). *Pathophysiology: A Clinical Approach.* 2nd edn. Philadelphia: Lippincott, Williams & Wilkins.

British Liver Trust (no date). *Liver Function Tests.* http://www.britishlivertrust.org.uk/liver-information/tests-and-screening/liver-function-tests/ (accessed 25 April 2015).

Dib, N., Oberti, F. & Calès, P. (2006). Current management of the complications of portal hypertension: Variceal bleeding and ascites. *Canadian Medical Association Journal.* **174** (10), 1433–43.

Duggan, J.M. (2001). Transfusion in gastrointestinal haemorrhage. If, when and how much? *Alimentary Pharmacology and Therapeutics.* **15**, 1109–13.

Gines, P., Cardenas, A., Arroyo, V. & Rodes, J. (2004). Current concepts: Management of cirrhosis and ascites. *New England Journal of Medicine.* **350** (16), 1646–54.

McCormick, P.A., Jenkins, S.A., McIntyre, N. *et al.* (1995). Why portal hypertensive varices bleed and bleed: A hypothesis. *Gut.* **36**, 100–103.

National Institute for Health and Care Excellence (NICE) (2011). Stent insertion for bleeding oesophageal varices. *Interventional Guideline* **392**. https://www.nice.org.uk/guidance/ipg392 (accessed 25 April 2015).

National Institute for Health and Care excellence (NICE) (2012). *Upper Gastrointestinal Bleeding. Clinical Guideline 141.* http://www.nice.org.uk/guidance/cg141 (accessed 25 April 2015).

Schuppan, D. & Afdhal. N.H. (2008). Liver cirrhosis. *The Lancet.* **371**, 883–51.

Thalheimer, U., Triantos, C.K., Samonakis, D.N., Patch, D. & Burroughs, A.K. (2005). Infection, coagulation and variceal bleeding in cirrhosis. *Gut.* **54** (4), 556–63.

Wolf, D.C. (2014). *Hepatic Encephalopathy.* http://www.emedicine.com/med/topic3185.htm (accessed 25 April 2015).

Useful websites

British Liver Trust
http://www.britishlivertrust.org.uk (Accessed 17 July 2015)
British Society of Gastroenterology
http://www.bsg.org.uk (Accessed 17 July 2015)

30 Electrolytes

Philip Woodrow

This chapter outlines some of the more significant electrolytes and micronutrients in the body, explaining what they do, the significance of abnormally high or low levels, and common treatments. This chapter also discusses the metabolite glucose, and the pathophysiology of diabetic ketoacidosis.

Once you have read this chapter, you should be able to list common acute electrolyte abnormalities, recognise them in your patients, identify their likely causes and which of these abnormalities should be treated, and suggest the most appropriate way to treat them.

Background

Electrolytes are elements or compounds that, in solution, dissociate into ions, making them capable of conducting electrical currents (Braun & Anderson 2011). Electrolytes therefore affect skeletal and cardiac muscle conduction and contraction. Electrolytes also regulate movement of substances between plasma, interstitial fluid and intracellular fluid. Electrolyte imbalances can cause:

- Cardiac dysfunction
- Skeletal muscle dysfunction
- Fluid imbalances.

In healthy people, normal daily intake and production balances loss. Illness may disrupt normal balance, either through abnormal intake or absorption, or through abnormal loss. Restoring and maintaining electrolyte balance is fundamental to health.

The electrolytes discussed in this chapter are:

- Sodium
- Potassium
- Calcium
- Magnesium
- Phosphate
- The metabolite glucose is also discussed.

With the single exception of sodium, plasma levels of all electrolytes are relatively low. Higher levels are found elsewhere in the body, often in the intracellular fluid. Low levels are caused by one or more of the following:

- Dilution
- Loss
- Failure of supply or production.

High levels are caused by one or more of the following:

- Dehydration (haemoconcentration)
- Failure to clear
- Excessive intake or production.

Electrolytes can be divided into two main groups: positively charged cations and negatively charged anions. As cations are positively charged, their symbols have one or more positive (+) signs (e.g. potassium K+) (Braun & Anderson 2011). All the electrolytes discussed in this chapter are cations. This chapter follows the recently introduced Pathology Harmony reference ranges, which are now used in nearly all UK laboratories.

Case scenario

A woman is admitted to the medical assessment unit with a diagnosis of diabetic ketoacidosis. Laboratory blood results show widespread abnormalities, including:

- Glucose 43.2mmol/litre
- Sodium 162mmol/litre
- Potassium 2.3mmol/litre
- Magnesium 0.65mmol/litre
- Phosphate 0.6mmol/litre

She is polyuric (passing large volumes of urine). An intravenous infusion of 1 litre 0.9% saline and a fixed rate insulin infusion (FRIII) are in progress.

After reading this chapter, identify the likely cause and significance of her electrolyte abnormalities.

Sodium (Na⁺)

The normal range of sodium is 133–146mmol/litre.

Sodium is the main extracellular cation. Bound to chloride as salt, it creates an osmotic pull ('where salt goes, water follows'). Hormones – aldosterone (from the adrenal gland) and natiuretic peptides (from the heart) – regulate renal sodium loss. Normally, nearly all filtered sodium is reabsorbed. Unless there are chronic disorders, the *quantity* of serum sodium is usually stable, but its *concentration* is affected by blood volume (water).

Hypernatraemia (acute, high sodium)

This is usually caused by dehydration, when the normal quantity of sodium is concentrated in a smaller volume (Reynolds *et al.* 2006, Fisher & Macnaughton 2006). Dehydration should be treated by rehydration.

Hyponatraemia (acute, low sodium)

This is usually caused by:

- Water overload, especially with renal failure (Reynolds *et al.* 2006, Sargent 2005).

It may also be caused by:

- Dehydration (fluid shifts – intracellular fluid is potassium-rich but sodium-poor)
- Salt deficiency or excessive loss.

Persistent hyperkalaemia and hyponatraemia, in the context of large cumulative fluid balance deficits, is likely to be caused by fluid shifts.

Neurological symptoms often appear with sodium below 130mmol/litre (Overgaard-Steensen 2010), which may progress to encephalopathy (<120mmol/litre).

Hyponatraemia may be treated by:

- Giving salt (e.g. 0.9% saline intravenous infusion; healthy kidneys will conserve salt while excreting excess water)
- Fluid restriction (e.g. 1000ml per day).

Causes of hyponatraemia should be carefully assessed to identify appropriate treatment. For example, restricting fluids in an already dehydrated patient is likely to cause further deterioration and renal failure (Sargent 2005).

Potassium (K⁺)

The normal range of potassium is 3.5–5.3mmol/litre.

Most potassium loss is via urine (normally, about 90%), the remainder being lost in stools. Abnormal urine output (oliguria or polyuria) is the most common cause of potassium imbalance in hospitalised patients. Except for furosemide, most diuretics either spare potassium or have potassium added.

Potassium is used for muscle conduction, including that of the myocardium. Hyperkalaemia can cause cardiac over-excitability, while hypokalaemia can cause under-excitability. Either may cause dysrhythmias, ectopic beats and infarction. Because potassium affects cardiac conduction, target levels are usually above 4mmol/litre if patients have any cardiac history.

Potassium affects the T waves on ECGs:
- Peaked T waves usually indicate hyperkalaemia
- Shallow T waves suggest hypokalaemia

Hyperkalaemia (high potassium)

Unlike plasma, intracellular fluid is potassium-rich, normally containing about 150mmol/litre (Barrett *et al.* 2010). Therefore trauma, injury or fluid shifts may cause hyperkalaemia, as potassium moves from the intracellular compartment. Intracellular fluid shifts usually occur either as a result of dehydration (including fluid restrictions) or during storage of blood for transfusion. Hillman and Bishop (2004) suggest that plasma levels in stored blood reach 30mmol/litre after 35 days. If furosemide is given concurrently with blood transfusions, this potassium infusion is matched by increased renal loss of potassium. See Box 30.1 for the main causes of hyperkalaemia.

HOT TIP

Erythrocyte recovery may cause rebound hypokalaemia within 24 hours (Isbister 2014), so blood levels of potassium should be checked the day after transfusion.

Box 30.1 The main causes of hyperkalaemia

- Oliguria
- Major trauma or massive injury
- Fluid shifts
- Large blood transfusion
- Excessive intake or infusion
- Constipation

HOT TIP

The Renal Association (2014) *Emergency Management of Hyperkalaema in Adults* **guidelines suggest the following drug doses:**
- **10 units soluble insulin (often Actrapid) in 50ml 50% glucose over 15 minutes**
- **Intravenous 10% calcium chloride 10ml, given through large vein over 5—10 minutes.**

Other preparations are available; see the full guideline or your local policy for recommendations.

Hyperkalaemia should be treated by removing potassium from plasma. If urgent (i.e. plasma levels >6mmol/litre), intravenous insulin and glucose is usually used. Glucose and insulin transports plasma potassium into the intracellular fluid, thus averting immediate risk of cardiac arrest. Recommended doses are detailed in the *Emergency Management of Hyperkalaema in Adults* guidelines (Renal Association 2014) or refer to your local policy. However, the potassium remains in the body, and may later return into the plasma. Calcium gluconate or calcium chloride is often given concurrently with insulin and glucose to stabilise cardiac conduction. Intravenous calcium can precipitate dysrhythmias in patients taking digoxin.

Less severe hyperkalaemia (<6mmol/litre) is usually treated with oral or rectal calcium resonium (Chapagain & Ashman 2012). However, calcium resonium reduces serum potassium relatively slowly (2–3 hours).

A few small-scale paediatric studies recommend using salbutamol to reduce serum potassium; while this will work, its safety in adults is questionable, so it is not recommended.

Hypokalaemia (low potassium)

This is usually caused by polyuria, especially furosemide-induced polyuria (Higgins 2013). Anything increasing cell uptake of potassium, such as salbutamol (Rang *et al.* 2007), can cause hypokalaemia. See Box 30.2 for the main causes of hypokalaemia.

Box 30.2 The main causes of hypokalaemia

- Polyuria
- Malnutrition
- Drugs (insulin, salbutamol)
- Profuse vomiting or diarrhoea

Mild hypokalaemia (3–3.5mmol/litre) can be reversed by giving oral (or nasogastric) potassium (e.g. Kay-Cee-L® or Sando-K®). Potassium supplements can taste bitter, so many patients prefer them dissolved in a strongly flavoured drink.

If patients are unable to take or absorb oral or nasogastric drugs, or their hypokalaemia is severe (<3mmol/litre), intravenous potassium is used. Various concentrations of intravenous potassium are currently produced, but strong potassium concentrations (e.g. 40mmol in 100ml or 20mmol in 10ml) should only be used in critical care areas (National Patient Safety Agency 2002). Where these are used:

- 20mmol ampoules should be further diluted before use
- Patients should have their ECG continuously monitored
- Sufficient staff should be available, with sufficient knowledge of ECG monitoring, to detect significant cardiac changes promptly
- Quick access to a blood gas analyser, or another means of measuring serum potassium, is advisable.

For most clinical areas, intravenous potassium infusions are restricted to 20 or 40mmol/litre. Because oliguria reduces potassium excretion, potassium should be replaced cautiously in oliguric patients.

Calcium (Ca^{++}, also written Ca^{2+})

The normal total range of calcium is 2.2–2.6mmol/litre (laboratory samples).
The normal ionised level is about 1.2mmol/litre (blood gas analysers).

Most body calcium (99%) is in the bones and teeth (Braun & Anderson 2011). The bone–blood balance is regulated by hormones – calcitonin and parathyroid hormone. Calcium is excreted in the urine. Plasma calcium enables cardiac and skeletal muscle conduction, nerve conduction and clotting. Normally about half of plasma calcium is protein-bound, and therefore inactive. Only the ionised, or free, calcium is physiologically active.

Protein binding is affected by various factors, including the amount of protein available (usually measured by albumin levels) and by acid–base balance, whereby acidosis reduces protein binding. Laboratories normally measure total blood calcium, but blood gas analysers measure ionised calcium. Because abnormal blood protein concentrations affect the total ionised balance, laboratories may also *correct* blood calcium measurements, adjusting them to reflect physiological activity from ionised calcium.

Hypercalcaemia (high calcium)

This is usually caused by hyperparathyroidism, especially from tumours (Higgins 2013). Hypercalcaemia can cause dysrhythmias (especially supraventricular tachycardia), cardiac arrest and muscle spasticity. Hyperparathyroidism usually necessitates parathyroidectomy (NICE 2014).

Hypocalcaemia (low calcium)

This is relatively rare, and is usually due to failure of calcium-regulating hormones (Higgins 2013). Hypocalcaemia can impair cardiac and skeletal muscle conduction, resulting in dysrhythmias (especially blocks and escape ectopics and rhythms) and muscle weakness. Severe hypocalcaemia may cause tetany. Where sufficient calcium cannot be obtained through diet, calcium may be given in various oral or intravenous preparations.

Frequent ectopic beats and dysrhythmias may be caused by potassium or calcium imbalances.

Magnesium (Mg^{++}, also written Mg^{2+})

The normal range of magnesium is 0.7–1.0mmol/litre.

Less than 1% of the body's magnesium is in plasma (Parikh & Webb 2012), but serum magnesium is important as a calcium antagonist for:

- Reducing the heart rate
- Relaxing the smooth muscle, causing vasodilatation (reducing blood pressure) and bronchodilatation.

Magnesium is also used in the cells, for adenosine triphosphate (ATP) storage and production. Although the kidneys filter magnesium, nearly all of it (98%) is normally reabsorbed. Renal losses are regulated by parathyroid hormone (Chalmers 2008).

Hypermagnesiumaemia (high magnesium)

This is relatively rare, but plasma levels exceeding 3mmol/litre can cause bradypnoea, potentially precipitating respiratory arrest. High levels in acute illness are usually caused by renal failure (Astle 2005).

Hypomagnesiumaemia (low magnesium)

This is relatively common, occurring in 7–11% of hospitalised patients (Parikh & Webb 2012). Risk factors for hypomagnesiumaemia include:

- Poor diet (including 'nil-by-mouth')
- Polyuria (including drug-induced)

- Critical illness
- Long-term PPI use (Drug Safety Update 2012)
- Alcoholism.

Hypomagnesiumaemia may cause tachydysrhythmias, hypertension and muscle weakness (Astle 2005, Ormerod *et al.* 2010). Magnesium is a key drug for torsades de pointes (Resuscitation Council 2015), and is sometimes used for other dysrhythmias. Its place in treating migraine, alcohol withdrawal, delirium or seizures remains unclear (Kaye & O'Sullivan 2002).

HOT TIP

Intravenous magnesium can cause bradycardia and hypotension, so the patient should be monitored frequently for both these conditions during infusions.

Phosphate (PO_4^{3-})

The normal range of phosphate is 0.8–1.5mmol/litre.

Most of the body's phosphate (85%) is in the bones. Phosphate, another micronutrient, is essential for cell energy (adenosine triphosphate) (Ormerod *et al.* 2010). It is also:

- The main intracellular buffer, and is therefore crucial for intracellular acid–base balance
- Used for nerve conduction (Ormerod *et al.* 2010)
- Used to regulate 2, 3-diphosphoglycerate (2, 3 DPG), the chemical in red blood cells that facilitates oxygen dissociation from haemoglobin (Ormerod *et al.* 2010).

Freely filtered by kidneys, most phosphate is reabsorbed, regulated by parathyroid hormone. As with many electrolytes, loss is increased with polyuria, including furosemide-induced loss (Taylor *et al.* 2004).

Hyperphosphataemia (high phosphate)

This is extremely rare, and seldom problematic.

Hypophosphataemia (low phosphate)

This can cause muscle weakness, dysrhythmias, delirium, immunocompromise and other problems (Ormerod *et al.* 2010). With malnourishment, nutrition should commence slowly; otherwise refeeding syndrome can cause life-threatening hypophosphataemia and hypokalaemia (Mehanna *et al.* 2008).

Hypophosphataemia can be treated by giving phosphate, either orally (e.g. Phosphate-Sandoz®) or intravenously (e.g. Addiphos® or another polyfusor). Polyfusors, but not necessarily Addiphos, should be infused slowly (over 12–24 hours) into a large (preferably central) vein. Phosphate has no known compatibility with any other drug, so it should not be mixed with any other drug when being infused.

Phosphate and magnesium affect muscle strength, so check that the patient's levels are normal before mobilising or rehabilitating them.

Glucose ($C_6H_{12}O_6$)

The normal non-diabetic, fasting range of glucose is 4.0–5.9mmol/litre (DiabetesUK website 2012).

Glucose is a metabolite – not an electrolyte. It is the main source of cell energy and it is transported from blood into the cells by insulin. In the cells, the mitochondria metabolise glucose aerobically to produce adenosine triphosphate (ATP), the main source of cell energy.

Hypoglycaemia (low glucose)

This usually occurs when diabetics take medication but have insufficient sugar in their diet. Blood glucose below 1mmol/litre is a medical emergency (Keays 2014). Mild hypoglycaemia may be reversed with diet or oral glucose (e.g. Hypostop® or glucagon), but severe hypoglycaemia requires 20ml intravenous 50% glucose.

Hyperglycaemia (high glucose)

In a healthy person, insulin production varies to maintain normoglycaemia. Hyperglycaemia occurs if insufficient insulin is produced to achieve this. It may be caused by a relative deficiency of insulin production or excessive resistance to insulin function. Although diabetes is usually a chronic condition, transient hyperglycaemia may be caused by stress ('the fight or flight response'), which frequently occurs during severe illness (Cely *et al.* 2004). Hyperglycaemia can be caused by drugs, especially cardiac drugs.

Tight glycaemic control (Van Den Berghe *et al.* 2001) is no longer recommended, as it can cause fatal hypoglycaemia (Cooper-DeHoff *et al.* 2010) but keeping glucose within normal limits is recommended.

Diabetic ketoacidosis (DKA)

This results from severe hyperglycaemia and deficient insulin, which lead to metabolic acidosis and osmotic diuresis (Braun & Anderson 2011). DKA usually occurs in type 1 diabetes and is characterised by:

- Ketonaemia (ketosis): ≥3mmol/litre or >++ on urine dipsticks
- Hyperglycaemia (>11mmol/litre)
- Acidaemia.

The management of diabetic ketoacidosis guidelines from the Joint British Diabetes Societies (JBDS) Inpatient Care Group (2013) emphasise focusing on ketonaemia rather than hyperglycaemia, and stipulate that bedside ketone monitoring should be available.

Diabetic ketoacidosis necessitates close monitoring (vital signs, blood glucose, fluid balance, electrolytes and neurological state). Dehydration often causes hyperkalaemia (Higgins 2013), while osmotic diuresis can cause life-threatening hypokalaemia; hence the importance of monitoring potassium. However, polyuria can also cause significant loss of phosphate and magnesium (Keays 2014), which may necessitate replacement. See Chapter 36 for more on diabetic ketoacidosis.

Conclusion

Although plasma concentrations of all electrolytes, except sodium, are low, they have important (often vital) functions. Abnormalities can therefore cause significant and often life-threatening complications. Most electrolytes discussed in this chapter are measured in analysis of urea and electrolytes (U&Es). Staff caring for sicker patients should therefore to be able to interpret results in the context of their individual patients, identifying the likely causes of any abnormalities and what implications they may have for the individual patient. They should also recognise whether these abnormalities should be treated, and the most appropriate method of treating them.

References and further reading

Astle, S.M. (2005). Restoring electrolyte balance. *RN Journal.* **68** (5), 34–39.

Barrett, K.E., Barman, S.M., Boitano, S. & Brooks, H.L. (2010). *Ganong's Review of Medical Physiology.* 23rd edn. New York: McGraw Hill Lange.

Braun, C.A. & Anderson, C.M. (2011). *Pathophysiology: A Clinical Approach.* 2nd edn. Philadelphia: Lippincott, Williams and Wilkins.

Cely, C.M., Arora, P., Quartrin, A.A., Kett, D.H. & Schein, R.M.H. (2004). Relationship of baseline glucose homeostasis to hyperglycaemia during medical critical illness. *Chest.* **126** (3), 879–87.

Chapagain, A. & Ashman, N. (2012). Hyperkalaemia in the age of aldosterone antagonism. *QJM.* **105** (11), 1049–57.

Chalmers, C.A. (2008). 'Applied anatomy and physiology and the renal disease process' in N. Thomas (ed.) *Renal Nursing.* 3rd edn. Edinburgh: Baillière Tindall Elsevier, 27–72.

Cooper-DeHoff, R.M., Gong, Y., Handberg, E.M., Bavry, A.A., Denardo, S.J., Bakris, G.L. & Pepine CJ. (2010). Tight blood pressure control and cardiovascular outcomes among hypertensive patients with diabetes and coronary artery disease. *Journal of the American Medical Association.* **304** (1), 61–68.

Diabetes UK (2013). https://www.diabetes.org.uk/ (accessed 20 July 2015).

Drug Safety Update (April 2012). 5 (9). https://www.gov.uk/drug-safety-update (accessed 20 July 2015).

Fisher, L. & Macnaughton, P. (2006). Electrolyte and metabolic disturbances in the critically ill. *Anaesthesia and Intensive Care Medicine.* **7** (5), 151–54.

Higgins, C. (2013). *Understanding Laboratory Investigations.* 3rd edn. Oxford: Wiley-Blackwell.

Hillman, K. & Bishop, G. (2004). *Clinical Intensive Care.* 2nd edn. Cambridge: Cambridge University Press.

Isbister, J.P. (2014). 'Blood transfusion' in A.D. Bersten & N. Soni (eds) *Intensive Care Manual.* 7th edn. Edinburgh: Butterworth-Heinemann Elsevier, 973–86.

Jeschke, M.G., Klein, D. & Herndon, D.N. (2003). Insulin treatment improves the systemic inflammatory reaction to severe trauma. *Annals of Surgery.* **239** (4), 553–60.

Joint British Diabetes Societies (JBDS) for Inpatient Care Group http://www.diabetologists-abcd.org.uk/JBDS/JBDS.htm (accessed 20 July 2015).

Kaye, P. & O'Sullivan, I. (2002). The role of magnesium in the emergency department. *Emergency Medical Journal.* **19** (4), 288–91.

Keays, R. (2014). 'Diabetic emergencies' in A.D. Bersten & N. Soni (eds) *Intensive Care Manual.* 7th edn. Edinburgh: Butterworth-Heinemann, 629–36.

Mehanna, H.M., Moledina, J. & Travis, J. (2008). Refeeding syndrome: what it is, and how to prevent and treat it. *British Medical Journal.* **336** (7659), 1495–98.

National Institute for Health and Care Excellence (NICE) (2014). *Clinical Knowledge Summary (CKS) Hypercalcaemia.* http://cks.nice.org.uk/hypercalcaemia#!scenario:1 (accessed 3 September 2015).

National Patient Safety Agency (NPSA) (2002). *Patient Safety Alert. Ref PSA 01.* London: National Patient Safety Agency.

Ormerod, C., Farrer, K. & Lal, S. (2010). Refeeding syndrome: a clinical review. *British Journal of Hospital Medicine.* **71** (12), 686–90.

Overgaard-Steensen, C. (2010). Initial approach to the hyponatremic patient. *Acta Anaesthesiologica Scandinavica.* **55** (2), 139–148.

Parikh, M. & Webb, S.T. (2012). Cations: potassium, calcium, and magnesium. *Continuing Education in Anaesthesia, Critical Care & Pain.* **12** (4), 195–98.

Rang, H.P., Dale, M.M., Ritter, J.M., Flower, R.J. & Henderson, G. (2007). *Pharmacology.* 7th edn. Edinburgh: Elsevier Churchill Livingstone.

Renal Association (2014). *Emergency Treatment of Hyperkalaemia in Adults*
http://www.renal.org/guidelines/joint-guidelines/treatment-of-acute-hyperkalaemia-in-adults#sthash.K7ho15uc.dpbs (accessed 3 September 2015).

Resuscitation Council (UK). 2015. *Resuscitation Guidelines.* London. Resuscitation Council.

Reynolds, R.M., Padfield, P.L. & Seckl J.R. (2006). Disorders of sodium balance. *British Medical Journal.* **332** (7543), 702–705.

Sargent S. (2005). The aetiology, management and complications of alcoholic hepatitis. *British Journal of Nursing.* **14** (10), 556–62.

Taylor, B., Huey, W.Y., Buchman, T.G., Boyle, W.A. & Coopersmith, C.M. (2004). Treatment of hypophosphatemia using a protocol based on patient weight and serum phosphorus level in a surgical intensive care unit. *Journal of American College of Surgeons.* **198** (2), 198–204.

Van Den Berghe, G., Wouters, P., Weekers, F., Verwaest, C., Bruyninckx, F., Schetz, M., Vlasslelaers, D., Ferdinande, P., Lauwers, P. & Bouillon, R. (2001). Intensive insulin therapy in critically ill patients. *New England Journal of Medicine.* **345** (19), 1359–67.

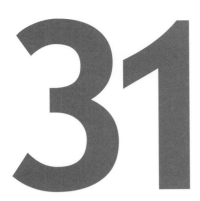

31 Renal failure

Russell Canavan and Michelle Webb

Renal failure is a common condition (Palevsky 2006) in which the excretory and metabolic function of the kidneys is insufficient to meet the body's requirements. The nephron is the functional unit of the kidney and has both passive and active functions in handling water and electrolytes. The kidney also has a role in blood pressure control, in stimulation of haemoglobin synthesis, and in bone metabolism.

By the end of this chapter, you should be able to identify patients at risk of renal impairment, and manage those patients in established renal failure.

Case scenario

A 43-year-old male lorry driver with a history of hypertension is admitted with shortness of breath. He has not been well for some time but has been reluctant to seek help from his GP. He is normally on lisinopril (10mg once daily) but he is away from home and has missed a couple of days of medication. On arrival, he is slightly agitated and confused.

A–Airway
He is maintaining his own airway.

B–Breathing
His respiratory rate is raised to 24 breaths per minute and his pulse oximeter reads 89% FiO$_2$ 0.21, increasing to 100% FiO$_2$ 0.85. Auscultation of his lungs reveals bi-basal crepitations.

C–Circulation
His pulses are all present but he has a blood pressure of 195/136 mmHg, which is repeated and still remains elevated.

D–Disability
He is alert on AVPU (see Box 2.1, p. 12) but is agitated and slightly confused. Pupils are normal.

E–Exposure and environment
There is nothing else to note.

Presentation of renal impairment

Renal impairment is often identified in the asymptomatic individual by the monitoring of urea and electrolytes (U&Es) or is noted as low urine output by the ward staff. These are both late signs in renal impairment. Renal impairment can be acute, chronic or acute on chronic. Both acute and chronic renal failure have some preventable underlying causes. Chronic renal impairment is managed by a nephrologist.

It is sometimes possible to anticipate which patients will develop renal impairment – for example, in a patient who has overdosed on paracetamol or a patient with prolonged hypotension, ischaemia or hypoxia. These patients should be adequately hydrated, and drugs that may compromise renal function avoided.

The Acute Kidney Injury Network (AKIN) classification of renal impairment is an attempt to classify renal impairment to deliver appropriate care (Table 31.1).

Table 31.1 The AKIN classification of renal impairment (based on AKIN 2015)

AKIN stages	Creatinine levels	Urine output
1	Serum creatinine increase ≥26.5µmol/litre (≥0.3mg/dl) or increase to 1.5–2.0-fold from baseline	<0.5ml/kg/h for 6 hours
2	Serum creatinine increase >2.0–3.0-fold from baseline	<0.5ml/kg/h for 12 hours
3	Serum creatinine increase >3.0-fold from baseline or serum creatinine ≥354µmol/litre (≥4.0mg/dl) with an acute increase of at least 44µmol/litre (0.5mg/dl) or need for RRT	

Firstly, check that there is no blockage or leak in the catheter; otherwise the patient may have renal impairment. Complete anuria is a blocked catheter until proved otherwise. Most commonly this is pre-renal (dehydration) but not always. A fluid challenge may be helpful in assessing whether the patient is dehydrated. Accurate fluid balance charts are crucial and good liaison with ward staff to ensure the quality of the charts is vital in early identification and monitoring of renal failure.

Creatinine

Creatinine (4–10µmol/litre in men; 6–10µmol/litre in women) is produced by the breakdown of creatinine in the body and is filtered by the glomerulus. It gives an estimated glomerular filtration rate but there are a number of confounding factors. As a breakdown product of muscle, creatinine can be artificially low in thin people. It also follows a logarithmic curve so that a change of 100 to 150 is vital but one of 400 to 450 is less so.

Recently the term eGFR has been introduced; eGFR is the estimated GFR calculated by the equation:

186.3 × (creatinine) – 1.154 × (age) – 0.203 × (0.742 if female) × (1.210 if black)

This is widely employed, but should be used with caution in the context of acute kidney injury.

Urea

This is a useful measurement to undertake in patients if it is relatively much higher than the creatinine would indicate. This implies the patient is dehydrated or has had a significant upper gastrointestinal bleed.

Potassium

This is a vital anion in cellular signalling. It is nearly all held intra-cellularly and low levels exist in the plasma. Small rises of plasma potassium can lead to life-threatening arrhythmias (see Chapter 30).

pH

pH is a logarithmic scale of hydrogen ions. Small changes outside the physiological pH lead to inactivation of cellular enzymes. There are a number of buffering systems in the body, which counteract small changes to maintain a stable pH. Consequently, acidaemia only occurs in extreme pathological states and is considered a poor prognostic factor in most disorders.

Sodium

Sodium is actively reabsorbed in the nephron. Damage to the nephron (e.g. acute tubular necrosis) results in a high loss of sodium in the urine (urinary sodium >40µmol/litre). In pre-renal failure, the urinary sodium will be low (<20µmol/litre) as the kidney tries to conserve water (see Chapter 30).

Urine osmolality

This is useful for establishing the cause of renal impairment (pre-renal versus renal). In pre-renal failure, the urine will be concentrated (>500mmol/litre). In intrinsic renal failure, the kidney loses its ability to concentrate urine and produces dilute urine (<350mmol/litre).

Causes of renal failure

Pre-renal causes

Renal failure is often due to dehydration or renal hypoperfusion but it can be due to renal artery stenosis or secondary to liver failure. Classically, small volumes of concentrated urine are produced.

Renal causes

This includes diseases of either the glomerulus or tubules. Acute kidney injury (Bonventre 2007) is most commonly seen on the ward. Other causes include drugs, glomerulonephritis, myeloma, haemolysis and rhabdomyolysis (see below for further explanation). In these conditions, the kidney loses its ability to concentrate urine and the patient often produces dilute urine. In many of the above causes, the urine dipstick will show at least significant proteinuria or haematuria.

Post-renal causes

Obstruction to the collecting system can be caused at any level and by renal stones or soft tissues (e.g. tumours, prostate or urethral strictures).

Acute tubular necrosis (ATN)

This is a common condition in the acutely ill patient. Either ischaemia or toxins damage the tubular cells. This leads to a reduction in the ability of the tubules to reabsorb water. The key to avoiding ATN is to avoid prolonged ischaemia or hypoxia and to ensure adequate filling.

Rhabdomyolysis

In acute muscle injury (whether through trauma or acute muscle disease), there can be a large amount of myoglobin in the serum. This is filtered into the urine and can cause damage to the renal tubules. It is characterised by dipstick positive haemoglobinuria (it is actually myoglobin) but negative urine microscopy for red cells, in the presence of a marked rise in serum creatinine kinase and renal impairment.

Emergency treatment

According to Thadhani et al. (1996) you should consider the following:

Precipitants

Avoid these. It is not uncommon to find the patient on hypotensive agents, ACE inhibitors, non-steroidal anti-inflammatories, etc. Even if these are not the cause of the renal failure, in the short term you should consider stopping them. Seek senior advice if the patient has cardiac problems before stopping the drugs.

Fluid balance

Early recognition is key. If you are unsure, a fluid challenge with 250ml of crystalloid is unlikely to cause much harm and, following reassessment, may tell you the patient's fluid status. The aid of a central venous line in managing fluid challenges is highly recommended. If the patient is overloaded, loop diuretics such as furosemide (Sumnall 2007) may help. A diuretic-sensitive patient may only need small doses of a loop diuretic to start with, but other people require large doses as a driver. Remember the action of furosemide lasts for 6 hours (hence Lasix™) and then the urine output will tail off again. Patients who are fluid-overloaded and resistant to diuretics may require removal of the fluid, using renal replacement therapy; referral to the intensive care team will be required.

Potassium

If potassium is greater than 6.0mmol/litre, treatment is usually recommended. The patient should have cardiac monitoring and their ECG should be assessed for signs of cardiac involvement. If treatment is indicated, it is generally accepted that 50ml of 50% glucose with 8 units of Actrapid™ insulin can be given as an infusion, and then check potassium.

If there is evidence of cardiac involvement, 10 ml 10% calcium gluconate is advised to stabilise the myocardium. If this fails, salbutamol, furosemide or exchange resins may all be useful. If they all fail, renal replacement may be called for.

pH

Acidaemia is not well tolerated. Sodium bicarbonate can normalise the extracellular pH but can worsen intracellular acidaemia. Appropriate fluid balance and oxygenation are often enough to correct acidaemia.

Renal replacement

The choice of therapy and when to start treatment depends on an overall assessment of the patient (Formica *et al.* 2007, Himmelfarb, 2007). Most commonly in the UK in the acute setting, the chosen therapy is haemofiltration. Generally, if the potassium, acidaemia and fluid overload fail to respond to medical therapy, renal replacement should be considered. There are essentially four main types of renal replacement:

1. **Dialysis:** This is used for chronic renal failure patients. Blood is run past a semipermeable membrane with fluid running on the other side of it. Toxins in the blood pass across the membrane by osmosis. Haemodialysis takes the blood out of the body through a line or fistula and runs it through an external membrane against a very pure water countercurrent with added solutes. Peritoneal dialysis uses the peritoneum as a dialysis membrane. Fluid is placed into the peritoneum via a peritoneal catheter and then washed out again. In both of the above, oncotic pressure is the predominant force. The amount of fluid removed can be determined by the concentration of the dialysate and the time given for fluid to diffuse across the membrane (see Box 31.2).

2. **Filtration:** This is used for acute renal failure patients who have failed to respond to medical therapy. It is a commonly available technique within the intensive care unit. Blood flows past a semipermeable membrane and hydrostatic pressure is used to extract waste products (e.g. water, potassium and hydrogen ions).

3. Transplant: When a patient is stable on long-term renal replacement, this may be an option. It is used in chronic renal failure and needs specialist referral to a transplant centre.

4. Haemodiafiltration: More recently, haemodiafiltration has been developed that is halfway between dialysis and haemofiltration. There is a theoretical benefit of being able to combine the advantages of both techniques. Some trials have been hopeful (Page *et al.* 2005) but more are needed.

Box 31.2 Managing patients on haemodialysis and continuous ambulatory peritoneal dialysis

It is preferable to manage **haemodialysis** patients in their base hospital, but occasionally patients are admitted to a hospital other than their own. Close liaison with the renal unit can help with managing drugs and fluid balance, as well as renal-related problems. With good communication, the only problem is logistical. Patients have to be off the ward having dialysis and therefore miss scans, for example, and often have longer stays in hospital.

Patients on **continuous ambulatory peritoneal dialysis** (CAPD) are seen less often by the renal unit and so are often managed in hospitals other than their home unit. Renal teams are still keen to help with their management. Patients are normally independent, normally exchanging one bag of fluid four times per day. Essentially, they have a catheter passing through the skin into the peritoneal cavity. The old dialysis solution is passed via the catheter into a waste product bag. The peritoneal cavity is then filled with a fresh bag of fluid for another 5 hours. The amount of fluid dialysed off can be altered by changing the osmolality of the dialysate solution. Solutions of varying strength are colour-coded and patients often mention their 'green' or 'yellow' bags. Again, fluid, drugs and diagnosis can be made much easier by liaising with the renal team.

Case scenario review

The case in the current scenario is likely to represent a hypertensive renal crisis. The diagnosis is confirmed by end-organ damage. The basal crackles represent pulmonary oedema (cardiac failure); the agitation and confusion represent leukoencephalopathy (brain failure); and the creatinine was elevated with a positive urine dipstick for protein (renal failure). Further examination by fundoscopy showed severe hypertensive retinopathy. The patient was oliguric. Following CT head (confirming leukoencephalopathy), an ultrasound Doppler of the renal arteries confirmed there was renal artery stenosis. This was angioplastied and within 24 hours the blood pressure was settled. Over the next few days, the creatinine fell and returned to almost normal. In the outpatient clinic, the patient was noted to have made a full recovery.

Conclusion

Acute renal failure (now called acute kidney injury) is a common problem in the acutely unwell patient and is often a result of the presenting illness. Early identification, fluid balance and consideration of the underlying problems can prevent deterioration of renal function. Existing renal patients can be managed away from their home unit with close cooperation with the renal team.

References and further reading

Acute Kidney Injury Network (AKIN) (2015). *Classification/staging system for acute kidney injury.* http://www.akinet.org/akinstudies.php (accessed 21 April 2015).

Bellomo, R., Kellum, J.A. & Ronco, C. (2007). Defining and classifying acute renal failure: from advocacy to consensus and validation of the RIFLE criteria. *Intensive Care Medicine.* **33** (3), 409–13.

Bonventre, J.V. (2007). Pathophysiology of acute kidney injury: roles of potential inhibitors of inflammation. *Contributions to Nephrology.* **156**, 39–46.

Formica, M., Inguaggiato, P., Bainotti, S., Gigliola G. & Canepari, G. (2007). Acute renal failure in critically ill patients: indications for and choice of extracorporeal treatment. *Journal of Nephrology.* **20** (1), 15–20.

Himmelfarb, J. (2007). Continuous renal replacement therapy in the treatment of acute renal failure: critical assessment is required. *Clinical Journal of the American Society of Nephrology.* **2**(2), 385–89.

National Institute of Health and Care Excellence (NICE) (2013). *Acute kidney injury Prevention, detection and management of acute kidney injury up to the point of renal replacement therapy. NICE clinical guideline 169.* https://www.nice.org.uk/guidance/cg169 (accessed 24 July 2015).

Page, B., Vieillard-Baron, A., Chergui K. *et al.* (2005). Early veno-venous haemodiafiltration for sepsis-related multiple organ failure. *Critical Care.* **9**, 755–63.

Palevsky, P.M. (2006). Epidemiology of acute renal failure: the tip of the iceberg. *Clinical Journal of the American Society of Nephrology.* **1**(1), 43–51.

Sumnall, R. (2007). Fluid management and diuretic therapy in acute renal failure. *Nursing in Critical Care.* **12**(1), 27–33.

Thadhani, R., Pascual, M. & Bonventre, J.V. (1996). Acute renal failure. *New England Journal of Medicine.* **334**, 1448–60.

Useful websites

Renal Association
http://www.renal.org (Accessed 24 July 2015)

NICE: Evidence Search

http://www.evidence.nhs.uk (Accessed 8 September 2015)

32

Emergency and massive blood transfusion

Alistair Challiner

Blood transfusion is not without risk. One of the most dangerous complications is incompatible transfusion, due to human error between sampling, documentation and giving the blood. To mitigate this risk, local policies on the transfusion process and related competencies should be followed by all staff involved.

When you have read this chapter, you will have an understanding of blood compatibility, transfusion triggers, blood components and the risks and benefits of massive transfusion.

Blood compatibility

There are numerous blood group considerations but the main ones for red cell transfusion are the blood group and antigens A, B, AB and O.

The frequency distributions within the population are (JPAC 2014):

- O – 47%
- A – 42%,
- B – 8%,
- AB – 3%

Group O is therefore the most common blood group and AB is the rarest.

Patients' plasma may have antibodies to other groups:

- Group O has anti-A and anti-B plasma
- Group B has anti-A plasma
- Group A has anti-B plasma
- Group AB has no antibodies.

Hence, in practical terms for red cell transfusions:

- Group AB can receive any blood group
- Group A can receive from A or O
- Group B can receive from B or O
- Group O can only receive from group O
- Group O is the universal donor and can donate to any group.

However, transfusion is more complex than just matching the blood group to reduce reactions and complications (such as Rhesus factors + or -, see below). In an emergency situation, O rhesus negative blood will normally be given.

HOT TIP

In an emergency situation, when there is no time to cross-match blood, O rhesus negative blood will normally be given. (This is particularly important for women of childbearing age.)

Platelet concentrates may contain red cells so they need to be grouped according to red cells to prevent adverse reactions.

Plasma concentrates, such as fresh frozen plasma (FFP), should be given according to the recipient's blood group. However, group AB is the universal donor, as it contains no antibodies compared to group O plasma, which has antibodies that would attack the recipient's red cells.

With regard to Rhesus (Group D) positive and negative, a rhesus negative person has no antibodies. If they receive rhesus positive blood, they will therefore form antibodies in the future, which may affect further transfusions or pregnancies (JPAC 2014). Approximately 30% of the population is rhesus negative.

The process of cross-matching involves sampling the patient's blood, grouping it and checking it for reactions with the donor blood bags. The process takes about half an hour in the laboratory but will detect incompatibilities, thus improving safety.

Transfusion triggers

Previously transfusions were commonly used to 'top up' haemoglobin (Hb) levels to normal limits. However, the evidence currently suggests that, in most patients, a restrictive policy with an Hb of 70g/litre (7g/dl) to 80g/litre (8g/dl) is adequate, even if they are critically ill. Hence transfusion would not improve outcome (Goodnough *et al* 2013).

This rationale is based on physiology, whereby the oxygen content of the normal blood is about four times higher than needed and the high viscosity of higher Hb levels may hinder delivery of oxygen in capillaries. Higher transfusion triggers of up to 90g/litre to 100g/litre may be indicated in symptomatic anaemia, myocardial ischaemia or a risk of continued bleeding.

In obvious bleeding, the Hb level is unreliable as it only measures the concentration of haemoglobin and doesn't compensate for the fluid lost. In an acute bleed with over a litre loss, the haemoglobin may not change, despite significant blood loss. However, following crystalloid or colloid infusions, the Hb may drop, due to dilution. The assessment of transfusion volumes in acute haemorrhage must also include haemodynamic signs of shock, the response to resuscitation measures and observed or estimated blood loss. Thus, Carson & Kleinman (2015) suggest transfusion should be guided by clinical signs, rather than Hb measurement alone.

Patients with iron deficiency anaemia may be effectively treated with direct iron infusions, rather than whole blood.

Blood component therapy

The main transfusion products available are:

Packed red cells

These are stored in a citrate-based solution to prevent clotting and they are concentrated to about twice the normal haematocrit of about 70%. This product replaces red cells as volume and oxygen-carrying capacity, and is stored for about 30 days at 4°Centigrade until required.

Fresh frozen plasma (FFP) and cryoprecipitate

These products are stored frozen to preserve shelf life and need to be thawed over about 20 minutes ready for use. They replace clotting factors. The prothrombin time (PT) and APTT tests are readily available to monitor the effectiveness of clotting.

Platelets

Platelets are stored at room temperature and are slowly agitated, with a shelf life of about 5 days. Platelets are essential, in conjunction with clotting factors, to form a clot.

The platelet count can guide platelet transfusions. The normal platelet count is between 150 and 450 billion (or 10^9) per litre of blood. A count of between 10×10^9/litre to 20×10^9/litre may be acceptable in non-injured patients with bone marrow disease. However, patients who are bleeding or who need to undergo surgical or vascular procedures should have a platelet count in the region of 100×10^9/litre.

Massive bleeding

Apart from major trauma, in the ward environment bleeding may occur in post-surgical patients, due to gastrointestinal bleeds from ulcers or oesophageal varices, and in obstetrics. Thus, patients' wounds and drains must be observed for excessive bleeding.

The initial management is based on **ABC** resuscitation, with volume replacement by intravenous fluids to treat shock (see Chapter 22 on hypovolaemic shock). In major blood loss, crystalloids and colloids do not carry oxygen, so red cells need to be transfused. In addition, clotting factors are consumed during bleeding. The ensuing dilutional coagulopathy will need to be treated by giving clotting factors and platelets.

In addition to transfusion, it is important to consider how to stop the bleeding using measures such as surgical intervention or inserting a Sengstaken-Blakemore tube (see Chapter 29 on oesophageal varices). The exact prescription will be decided by skilled senior clinicians, aided by the haematologist. However, a local massive transfusion protocol is advantageous in giving products together, as suggested by Pham and Shaz (2013):

- 6–10 units packed red cells
- 4 units fresh frozen plasma (FFP)
- 1–2 units platelets.

Continuous laboratory monitoring, with full blood count (FBC), clotting studies, calcium and potassium levels and blood gas analysis, is essential to guide further transfusion.

Other factors to consider

HOT TIP

Blood products are cold and may cause hypothermia, making coagulopathy worse. For this reason, massive and rapid transfusions should ideally be put through a warming device.

Group O negative blood is usually readily available for emergencies, but only in small quantities. A full cross-match may take about half an hour. Rapid and effective sampling documentation and transfer to the laboratory are therefore essential to save time.

Stored blood may contain a significant level of potassium from the red cells. The citrate anticoagulant works by absorbing calcium ions, which are an important clotting factor. Massive transfusion can therefore raise potassium levels and affect clotting ability.

HOT TIP

Remember that massive blood transfusion can raise potassium levels and affect clotting ability.

Blood transfusion should only be offered when the benefits outweigh the risks (JPAC 2014) and local or national guidance on transfusion should be followed. During transfusion it is vital to observe the patient for adverse effects and complications, and all products should be recorded in the patient's notes as per local policy. Significant complications can occur, including incompatibility reactions, anaphylaxis and fever. However, in massive transfusions it can be difficult to know if haemostasis is affected by the transfusion or by the patient's medical condition.

In the case of coagulopathy, expert help is required to advise on the appropriate regime. For severe coagulopathies, which do not respond to FFP and platelets, consider other clotting factors such as prothrombin concentrate, tranexamic acid or factor 7.

Tranexamic acid, given intravenously, has shown benefit in traumatic bleeding, with low cost and low side effects.

Conclusion

This chapter has given a brief overview of transfusion therapy but it is recommended that an expert (such as a haematologist) is consulted and local guidelines are followed. Even in an emergency, it is important to ensure that the right blood is given to the right patient (JPAC 2014), and the risk of errors naturally increases in any stressful situation.

Staff must also consider the issue of patient consent, as some clients refuse transfusion products for religious or cultural reasons. The JPAC (2014) offers guidance on the management of patients who do not accept transfusions.

Individual chapters throughout this book give detailed recommendations for blood transfusion related to particular conditions.

References and further reading

Carson, J.L. & Kleinman, S. (2015). *Indications and hemoglobin thresholds for red blood cell transfusion in the adult.* http://www.uptodate.com/contents/indications-and-hemoglobin-thresholds-for-red-blood-cell-transfusion-in-the-adult (accessed 6 April 2015).

Goodnough, L.T., Levy, J.H. & Murphy, M.F. (2013). Concepts of blood transfusion in adults. *The Lancet.* **381** (9880), 1845–54.

Joint United Kingdom (UK) Blood Transfusion and Tissue Transplantation Services Professional Advisory Committee (JPAC) (2014). *Transfusion Handbook.* 5th edn. http://www.transfusionguidelines.org/transfusion-handbook (accessed 6 April 2015).

Pham, H.P. & Shaz, B.H. (2013). Update on massive transfusion. *British Journal of Anaesthesia.* **111** (1), i71–i82. http://bja.oxfordjournals.org/content/111/suppl_1/i71.full (accessed 6 April 2015).

Useful website

Joint United Kingdom (UK) Blood Transfusion and Tissue Transplantation Services Professional Advisory Committee (JPAC) (2015). http://www.transfusionguidelines.org/ (Accessed 24 July 2015)

33 Pregnancy-related conditions

Diane Blake and Jo Cotton

This chapter aims to give general ward staff an overview of pregnancy-related issues that need consideration during an acute admission. Always inform the midwifery team (about a woman who is pregnant), at the point of hospital admission, for advice.

Pregnancy is the period from conception (when a female's egg is fertilised by a male sperm), to implantation in the uterus lining and the development of a placenta and embryo, until the birth of a foetus. This process usually takes 40 weeks, from the beginning of the woman's last menstrual period, and involves complex body changes in order to produce a well-developed baby. This chapter will provide an overview of the medical conditions that influence pregnancy. If you can recognise these conditions, you will be able to provide appropriate and timely referral and care.

However, you will need to undertake further reading to understand the normal physiology of pregnancy (Baston & Hall 2009, Stables & Rankin 2010, Johnson & Taylor 2010, Macdonald & Magill-Cuerden 2011, Coad & Dunstall 2011, Marshall & Raynor 2014). All systems in the female body are altered by hormonal changes during pregnancy, which is a natural biological event. These hormonal changes should be understood above and beyond this introductory chapter, particularly if you have regular contact with this service user group.

Physiological considerations

The normal physiology of pregnancy involves three trimesters (see Table 33.1) and there are numerous adverse conditions that can cause complications at any stage, such as vaginal bleeding, abdominal pain, sexually transmitted diseases, thrush or other vaginal or systematic infections, thrombosis, haemorrhage and hypertension. In addition, pregnancy has an impact on major body systems such as the individual's cerebral and psychological state, cardiovascular circulation, and their respiratory, renal, reproductive and gastrointestinal systems (Macdonald & Magill-Cuerden 2011, Robson & Waugh 2013, Marshall & Raynor 2014).

Table 33.1 The three trimesters

Trimester	Weeks
First	1–12
Second	13–28
Third	29–40

Conditions commonly associated with the first trimester include nausea and vomiting, early vaginal bleeding or implantation bleed, sexually transmitted diseases and vaginal or systemic infections such as thrush and cystitis. Issues in the second trimester can include abdominal pain, constipation and heartburn, while the third trimester can involve thrombosis, haemorrhage and hypertension. Given that each trimester is marked by specific embryo/foetal developments, these conditions may well be significant and could potentially have an adverse effect on the pregnancy.

Assessment

Observations of maternal well-being during pregnancy require careful interpretation and ought to be carried out using the appropriate Modified Early Obstetric Warning Score (MEOWS) charts (RCOG 2008). The MEOWS charts (Healthcare Quality Improvement Partnership 2007) have specific parameters that clearly outline sources of negative influence on pregnancy, meaning that liaison with obstetricians, midwives and other specialist staff is required (NMC 2015, Midwifery 2020 UK Programme 2010, CMACE 2011). Ward staff must therefore ensure that they identify adverse signs and symptoms, providing referrals to midwives and obstetricians to ensure the provision of collaborative and expert care early in the patient's admission (NMC 2015, CMACE 2011, NMC 2012).

Furthermore, having an awareness of difference in blood tests (see Table 33.2) and an understanding of the commonly used medications during pregnancy (see Table 33.3) requires an interprofessional approach (RCP & RCN 2012, RCM 2011). Allied health professionals, such as pharmacists, may also need to be involved to ensure that other medications are not contraindicated during pregnancy.

Table 33.2 Most common blood tests taken in pregnancy
(based on Cunningham 2010)

Blood test	Non-pregnant	Pregnant
Haemoglobin	12–16g/dl	9–11.5g/dl
White blood cell (WBC)	4–10.6mm$_3$	6–20mm$_3$
Platelets	165–415^9/litre	150–430^9/litre
Mean corpuscular volume (MCV)	79–93μm$_3$	81–99μm$_3$
Alanine aminotransferase (ALT)	7–41U/litre	2–30U/litre
Aspartate aminotransferase (AST)	12–38U/litre	4–32U/litre
Alkaline phosphatase (ALP)	33–96U/litre	38–229U/litre

Creatinine	0.5–0.9mg/dl	0.4–0.9mg/dl
Sodium (Na)	136–146mEq/litre	130–148mEq/litre
Potassium (K)	3.5–5mEq/litre	3.3–5.1mEq/litre
Urea	7–20mg/dl	3–11mg/dl
Uric acid	2.5–5.6mg/dl	3.1–6.3mg/dl

Table 33.3
Some examples of medications that are safe to take in pregnancy

Medication	Safe dose
Folic acid	400µg
Paracetamol	500mg–1g
Codydramol	500mg–1g
Ranitidine	150mg
Maxalon	10mg
Gaviscon	10–15ml
Peppermint water	10ml
Magnesium hydroxide	10ml
Sodium citrate	10ml
Labetalol	100–200mg
Nifedipine	10–20mg

NB: This list is not exhaustive. Please refer to the British National Formulary for further information on dosage and side effects.

The health and well-being of the foetus or neonate must also be a major consideration but this assessment must only be carried out by a midwife and/or obstetrician (NMC 2012, RCOG 2009). Midwives have a duty of care to women accessing maternity services. There is a statutory requirement that safeguards women and their babies, ensuring that they receive care and advice from a midwife who holds a functioning midwifery qualification (NMC 2012). It is therefore vital to inform midwifery services of any pregnant women admitted to acute services promptly.

Systems overview
The following section gives an overview of important areas to consider for a pregnant woman within the acute ward setting. These relate to issues that may be due to the pregnancy, or issues that may complicate other conditions that the woman has presented with. They will need further investigation and consideration to ensure maternal wellbeing.

Reproductive system

Early vaginal bleeding in the first trimester could be the result of placental implantation, vaginal erosions or polyps, coitus and miscarriage or, in some cases, unknown (Stables & Rankin 2010, Johnson & Taylor 2010, Coad & Dunstall 2011). Rest and reassurance may be the only treatment that can be prescribed during this time. Sensitive care is extremely important during this trimester, as the developing embryo is not recognised as a foetus until 12 weeks and the pregnancy is not considered viable until 24 weeks (Holt 2004, Coad & Dunstall 2011). During this early stage, there is some overlap of care provision. Pregnant women are generally managed by the gynaecology team but the midwife can also provide guidance and support.

This means that ward staff need to be aware of additional symptoms such as abdominal pain and increasing vaginal blood loss. Ward staff must observe and also ask about the amount of vaginal bleeding and carefully record and monitor blood pressure, pulse and oxygen saturations in order to pre-empt and avoid maternal shock, especially if there is significant blood loss. A full blood count, group and save and Kleihauer (if the mother is rhesus negative) blood assessment will also be required to exclude anaemia and determine if a blood transfusion and Anti D (gamma globulin given to rhesus negative women to prevent them making antibodies against their rhesus positive foetus) are required.

However, low blood pressure in early pregnancy is a normal physiological event and therefore may not indicate signs of deviation: a 24–48 hours in-patient assessment would be the recommended course of action in this case (Hutcherson 2011). Complaints of abdominal pain or cramps, as described by women during the first trimester, may suggest uterine contractions (accumulation of bleeding in the uterine cavity will stimulate contractions), which may lead to a miscarriage or premature labour (Hossain *et al.* 2007).

Causes of vaginal bleeding that occur in the first trimester, and which are mentioned above, may also arise in the second or third trimester. In all cases, immediate referral to the obstetric team is fundamental to manage foetal wellbeing as well as maternal health (Hutcherson 2011). Substantial blood loss during the second or third trimester is considered an antepartum haemorrhage and may be due to placental abruption (premature separation of the placenta from the uterine wall) or placenta praevia (when the placenta is situated in the lower segment of the uterus, either completely, partially or close to the internal os), which is life-threatening for both the woman and her baby (CMACE 2011). The importance of monitoring blood loss by ward staff is therefore an integral part of care. Staff also need to record notable changes in vital signs such as blood pressure and pulse, as these will assist in detecting any deterioration (NICE 2011).

Gastrointestinal system

Many pregnant women experience nausea and vomiting during the first trimester due to the release of hormones that aid pregnancy (Isbir & Mete 2010). Other symptoms, such as heartburn and constipation (progesterone causing the motility of the gut to become sluggish), pica (cravings for unusual foods) and changes in the tastebuds (food tastes bland), are hormone-induced but these are minor ailments and will usually be resolved by the end of the first trimester.

However, some of these symptoms may continue throughout the pregnancy into the second and third trimester. In this case, practical methods of treatment (such as small regular meals, increased fluid intake, gentle exercise or laxatives and antacids) may help to manage these conditions and reassure the woman. Ward staff may consider referral to the General Practitioner for additional support and guidance, once the woman has been discharged from hospital.

Continued nausea and vomiting during the first three months may lead to dehydration and affect the woman's electrolyte balance, which in turn could be toxic for the foetus (Wegrzyniak, Repke &

Ural 2012). In this case, a diagnosis of hyperemesis may need to be considered. This condition requires immediate hospitalisation to hydrate the woman intravenously. Referral to the gynaecology team should also be undertaken by the ward nurse. Blood tests should be carried out to monitor electrolyte balance, in addition to the monitoring of temperature, blood pressure and pulse. Assessment of foetal wellbeing may be prescribed via an ultrasound scan if vomiting persists into the second trimester. Hyperemesis rarely affects the foetus but in severe cases it can result in low birth weight and skeletal malformations (Doughty & Waugh 2013).

Renal system

Biological changes in the renal system during pregnancy are usually incidental. For example, by the third trimester the growth of the uterus applies pressure on the bladder, causing more frequent micturition. The action of progesterone on the kidneys affects the renal pelvis, causing it to dilate, and on the walls of the ureters to develop curves which may collect urine (Shortland 2009, Gibson & Rosene-Montella 2008). As a result, the maturation of micro-organisms occurs, predisposing the woman to develop bacterial infections within the urinary tract. These infections may occur in any of the three trimesters (Kenny 2011, Porth 2011). Good renal function is important throughout pregnancy, hence the importance of undertaking urinalysis during any admission and during every antenatal appointment to exclude micro-organisms, which may lead to conditions such as urethritis, cystitis or less commonly pyelonephritis (Health Protection Agency 2012).

Child-bearing women are at risk of urinary tract infections (UTIs) so urinalysis must be undertaken and a mid-stream urine specimen should be assessed in the laboratory to see if micro-organisms are present. The usual maternal observations of blood pressure, pulse, respiration (and more specifically temperature to monitor for fever), should be taken and recorded. Other than a positive urine specimen, if other vital signs are asymptomatic, the woman may be treated with antibiotics and should attend a follow-up appointment with her community midwife. However, assessment of foetal wellbeing and uterine activity must be considered and undertaken by a midwife, since a UTI can increase the risk of uterine contractions, which may develop into miscarriage or premature labour (Kean 2011). The inflammation produced by the infection will cause the hormones known as prostaglandins to be released, which will trigger uterine contractions (Bewley 2011). Referral to a midwife to auscultate the foetal heart and palpate the uterus is an important part of the examination, particularly in the second and third trimester.

Glycosuria and/or proteinuria (two pluses or more on urinalysis) may suggest other complex conditions such as gestational diabetes or pre-eclampsia (Webster, Dodd & Waugh 2013, Gregory & Todd 2013) and will require further clinical assessment and additional investigations, as well as immediate referral to the obstetric team.

Cardiovascular circulation

The physiological changes that occur during pregnancy affect the cardiac and circulatory system, including blood volume, cardiac output and blood viscosity. For example, the demands of pregnancy cause cardiac output to surge by 35–50%, heart rate to rise by 10–20%, and blood volume to increase by 30–50%. There is also an increase in blood plasma, leading to haemodilution (Hassall 2014). Mean cell volume (MCV) must therefore be taken into consideration to ensure that the woman has not become anaemic (Baston 2014).

Existing hypertension, smoking, obesity or other risk factors may also complicate pregnancy and induce conditions such as myocardial infarction, ischaemic heart disease, thrombosis and other complications related to the cardiac and circulatory systems. The CMACE (2011) has identified 17–38 cerebral vascular accidents, deep vein thrombosis, hypertension and other major conditions that require collaboration and intervention by an obstetric and cardiology team. While these conditions are usually associated with the third trimester, they can occur at any stage. Fortunately, these disorders are rare in maternity care but do require careful assessment and prompt referral if suspected.

Signs and symptoms may vary and blood tests will be utilised, which can then be interpreted by an appropriate specialist. Regarding the above conditions, nurses should undertake the monitoring of blood pressure, pulse, temperature, respiration and oxygen saturation. The parameters of normal vital signs for a pregnant woman are better understood by a midwife and obstetrician – so referral and careful interpretation will be necessary. It is crucial to record the maternal observations on a MEOWS chart (which provides the parameters for pregnancy vital signs) and seek advice from a senior midwife to clarify the results (RCOG 2008).

Conditions such as cerebral vascular accidents, deep vein thrombosis, pulmonary embolism and hypertension may present as headaches with visual disturbances, redness and pain in the calf, shortness of breath, cyanoses and pain in the chest (Tucker 2013). These symptoms are not dissimilar to those of a non-pregnant patient presenting with the same disorders. The nurse must therefore follow the appropriate plan of care. However, the effects of these conditions on the pregnant woman will also have an impact on the foetus. A team of specialists must therefore diagnose and prescribe the most appropriate care, interventions and medication.

In the intervening period, healthcare staff must be aware of how to resuscitate the pregnant woman effectively. While the basic principles remain the same as for any collapsed adult, resuscitation of a pregnant woman requires careful positioning. The woman must be placed in a supine position, with her left side elevated, using a pillow under her back, to allow successful resuscitation for both maternal and foetal circulation (Resuscitation Council UK 2015). The correct maternal position is vital, as this will prevent aortocaval compression due to the weight of the enlarged uterus. It is essential to understand the significance of maternal resuscitation during pregnancy so that this technique can be applied correctly (Resuscitation Council UK 2015).

Respiratory system

The blood flow to the respiratory system during pregnancy is augmented because of increased cardiac output. This can result in oedema and hyperaemia in the upper respiratory mucosa, which may cause epistaxis, a minor ailment of pregnancy (Hassall 2014). As the pregnancy advances and the growing uterus expands to accommodate the developing foetus, the rib cage is displaced upwards and the diaphragm is elevated up to 4cm (Hassall 2014). Lung capacity is reduced by 5%, meaning that breathing becomes testing for the woman with a gravid uterus from about 30–33 weeks into the pregnancy (McNabb 2011).

Women experiencing breathlessness on exertion, in the absence of any other adverse conditions, may not be presenting with anything significant but nurses must ensure that this observation is supported by assessing maternal vital signs, in particular temperature and respiration, using the MEOWS scoring chart. Changes in these signs may signify an infection or embolic disorder, which require further investigations such as blood tests and x-rays. Recognising the signs and symptoms of a pulmonary embolism will demand collaborative work with the appropriate senior team.

Cerebral disorders

Although cerebral thrombosis or haemorrhage is a rare condition in pregnancy, ward staff must be vigilant and watch for signs of raised blood pressure and falling pulse that may manifest as headaches, visual disturbances, nausea or vomiting, and tingling and/or numbness in the limbs. These symptoms must be reported immediately to the medical and obstetric team. The CMACE (2011) reported two deaths because of cerebral vein thrombosis between 2006 and 2008. While this figure is extremely low and offers the reassurance of improvement in care, any maternal death is one too many. Considering the cerebral changes during pregnancy (such as the effect of the hormone progesterone on cerebral vessels, which swell and soften due to increased blood flow), it is not uncommon for pregnant women to experience headaches (Coad & Dunstall 2011). Such headaches may not be significant and may only warrant medication with a mild analgesia (such as paracetamol) and rest, along with simple remedies such as maintaining hydration, drinking up to 3 litres of fluid daily and eating balanced nutritious meals.

Again, it is expected that maternal vital signs of temperature, pulse, blood pressure, respirations and oxygen saturation will be taken and reviewed, to ensure that they are within normal pregnancy parameters. However, it is essential that adverse signs and symptoms are not missed. Headaches accompanied by visual disturbances and hypertension may be indicative of pre-eclampsia and this condition requires prompt referral to the obstetric team (NICE 2011). Additional medication could be considered to treat any hypertension but medical staff must refer to the Joint Formulary Committee, BNF (2014), to ensure the appropriate use of medication and seek advice on potential side effects. Some hypertensive medication such as methyldopa, can cause harm to the foetus; therefore a careful choice of the most appropriate medication is essential.

Psychological disorders

During pregnancy, a woman's emotions are very labile; women need support and reassurance to ensure that the management and treatment of their condition is in their best interests and those of their baby (NICE 2007). It should be routinely ensured that the woman has one or two daily visits from a midwife while on the ward to auscultate or monitor the foetal heart rate. Additional advice on avoiding anxiety and stress during admission is essential to allay unnecessary concerns. If women understand the care they will receive from the medical staff and feel confident that appropriate treatment will be provided, they will feel empowered and will have fewer apprehensions. Mental health concerns will also need careful monitoring, especially for those women with a history of mental illness. Specialist advice and liaison from the mental health team and community midwives are essential for immediate and follow-up care.

Conclusion

It is important to understand that pregnancy is a normal physiological event in which hormonal changes affect all systems in the female body, and these changes are vital to sustain foetal development. Pregnancy is a very large, complex topic; the present chapter should therefore only be considered as a brief introduction. You will need to read additional midwifery and obstetric texts to gain a full understanding of the pathological and adverse conditions that may occur during pregnancy.

It is hoped that practitioners will find this chapter valuable, and that it will help them recognise various adverse medical conditions, and provide the appropriate care for pregnant women. However it is crucial for ward nurses to make referrals to specialist staff, once deviations are recognised. Ultimately, collaborative practice must be undertaken to ensure that pregnant women and their babies receive effective care.

References and further reading

Baston, H. & Hall. J. (2009). *Midwifery Essentials: Antenatal Volume 2.* London: Churchill Livingstone Elsevier.

Baston, H. (2014). 'Antenatal Care' in J. Marshall & M. Raynor (eds) *Myles Textbook for Midwives.* 16th edn. London: Churchill Livingstone Elsevier. pp. 179–203.

Bewley, C.A. (2011). 'Medical disorders of pregnancy' in S. Macdonald & J. Magill-Cuerden (eds). *Mayes Midwifery.* 14th edn. London: Churchill Livingstone Elsevier. pp. 771–87.

Centre for Maternal and Child Enquiries (CMACE) (2011). Saving Mother's Lives: Reviewing Maternal Deaths to Make Motherhood Safer: 2006–2008. The Eighth Report on Confidential Enquiries into Maternal Deaths in the United Kingdom. *BJOG: An International Journal of Obstetrics and Gynaecology.* **118** (1).

Coad, J. & Dunstall, M. (2011). *Anatomy and Physiology for Midwives.* 3rd edn. London: Churchill Livingstone Elsevier.

Cunningham, G.F. (2010). 'Laboratory Values in Normal Pregnancy' in J.T. Queenan, J.C. Hobbins & C.Y. Spong (eds) *Protocols for High-Risk Pregnancies: An Evidence-Based Approach.* 5th edn. Dallas: Blackwell Science Ltd. pp. 587–95.

Doughty, R. & Waugh, J. (2013). 'Metabolic Disorders' in S.E. Robson & J. Waugh (eds). *Medical Disorders in Pregnancy: A Manual for Midwives.* 2nd edn. Oxford: Wiley-Blackwell. pp. 241–55.

Gibson, P. & Rosene-Montella, K. (2008). *Medical Care of the Pregnant Patient.* 2nd edn. Philadelphia: ACP Press.

Gregory, R. & Todd D. (2013). 'Endocrine Disorders' in S.E. Robson & J. Waugh (eds) *Medical Disorders in Pregnancy: A Manual for Midwives.* 2nd edn. Oxford: Wiley and Blackwell. pp. 105–25.

Hassall, J. (2014). 'Change and adaptation in pregnancy' in J. Marshall & M. Raynor (eds) *Myles Textbook for Midwives.* 16th edn. London: Churchill Livingstone Elsevier. pp. 143–79.

Health Protection Agency (2012). *UK standards for microbiology investigations: Investigation of urine.* Wales: The Standards Unit, HPA.

Healthcare Quality Improvement Partnership (2007). *Example of Obstetric Early Warning Score Chart* http://www.hqip.org.uk/assets/NCAPOP-Library/CMACE-Reports/27.-2007-Saving-Mothers-Lives-Early-Obstetric-Warning-Chart.pdf. (accessed 25 July 2015).

Holt, J. (2004). 'Screening and the perfect baby' in L. Frith & H. Draper (eds) *Ethics and Midwifery.* 2nd edn. London: Churchill Livingstone Elsevier. pp. 143–61.

Hossain, R., Harris, T., Lohsoonthorn, V. & Williams, M.A. (2007). Risk of preterm delivery in relation to vaginal bleeding in early pregnancy. *European Journal of Obstetrics, Gynecology and Reproductive Biology.* **135** (2), 158–63.

Hutcherson, A., (2011). 'Bleeding in Pregnancy' in S. Macdonald & J. Magill-Cuerden (eds) *Mayes Midwifery.* 14th edn. London: Churchill Livingstone Elsevier. pp. 753–71.

Isbir, G.G. & Mete, S. (2010). Nursing care of nausea and vomiting in pregnancy: Roy Adaptation Model. *Nursing Science Quarterly.* **23** (2), 148–55.

Johnson, R. & Taylor, W. (2010). *Skills for Midwifery Practice.* 3rd edn. London: Churchill Livingstone Elsevier.

Joint Formulary Committee (2014). *British National Formulary (BNF).* London: BMJ Publishing Group Ltd and the Royal Pharmaceutical Society.

Kean, L. (2011). 'Obstetric history taking and examination' in P.N. Baker & L.C. Kenny (eds) *Obstetrics by Ten Teachers.* 19th edn. London: Hodder and Stoughton Ltd. pp. 1–13.

Kenny, L.C. (2011). 'Antenatal obstetric complications' in P.N. Baker & L.C. Kenny (eds) *Obstetrics by Ten Teachers.* 19th edn. London: Hodder and Stoughton Ltd. pp. 27–43.

Macdonald, S. & Magill-Cuerden, J. (eds) (2011). *Mayes Midwifery.* 14th edn. London: Churchill Livingstone Elsevier.

Marshall, J. & Raynor, M. (eds) (2014). *Myles Textbook for Midwives.* 16th edn. London: Churchill Livingstone Elsevier.

McNabb, M. (2011). 'Maternal and fetal responses to pregnancy' in S. Macdonald & J. Magill-Cuerden (eds) *Mayes Midwifery.* 14th edn. London: Churchill Livingstone Elsevier. pp. 397–411.

Midwifery 2020 UK Programme (2010). *Midwifery 2020: Delivering Expectations.* Cambridge: Midwifery 2020 Programme.

National Institute for Health and Care Excellence (NICE) (2007). *Guidelines on Antenatal and Postnatal Mental Health.* London: NICE.

National Institute for Health and Care Excellence (NICE) (2011). *Hypertension in pregnancy: The management of hypertensive disorders during pregnancy.* Manchester: NICE.

Nursing and Midwifery Council NMC (2015) *The Code.* Available at: http://www.nmc.org.uk/standards/code/ (accessed 29.11.2015)

Nursing and Midwifery Council (NMC) (2012). *Midwives Rules and Standards.* London: NMC.

Porth, C.M. (2011). *Essentials of Pathophysiology: Concepts of Altered Health States.* Philadelphia: Wolters Kluwer Health and Lippincott Williams and Wilkins.

Queenan, J.T., Hobbins, J.C. & Spong, C.Y. (eds). (2010). *Protocols for High-Risk Pregnancies: An Evidence-Based Approach.* 5th edn. Dallas: Blackwell Science Ltd. pp. 587–95

Resuscitation Council UK (2015). *Resuscitation Guidelines: Advanced Life Support.* The NICE Accreditation Scheme.

Robson, S.E. & Waugh, J. (2013). *Medical Disorders in Pregnancy: A Manual for Midwives.* 2nd edn. Oxford: Wiley-Blackwell.

Royal College of Midwives (RCM) (2011). *The Royal College of Midwives Research and Development Action Plan.* London: RCM.

Royal College of Obstetricians and Gynaecologists (RCOG) (2008). *Standards for Maternity Care: Report of a working party.* London: RCOG.

Royal College of Obstetricians and Gynaecologists (ROCG) (2009). *Green-Top Guideline No. 37, Reducing the risk of thrombosis and embolism during pregnancy and the puerperium.* London: RCOG.

Royal College of Physicians (RCP) and Royal College of Nursing (RCN) (2012). *Ward Rounds in Redicine: Principles for Best Practice.* London: RCP.

Shortland, J.R. (2009). *General and Systemic Pathology.* 5th edn. London: Elsevier Limited.

Stables, D. & Rankin, J. (2010). *Physiology in Childbearing: With Anatomy and Related Biosciences.* 3rd edn. London: Bailliere Tindall Elsevier.

Tucker, S. (2013). *Maternal, Fetal and Neonatal Physiology: A Clinical Perspective.* 4th edn. USA: Elsevier.

Webster, S., Dodd, C. & Waugh, J. (2013). 'Hypertensive Disorders in Medical Disorders' in S.E. Robson & J. Waugh J. (eds) *Pregnancy.* 2nd edn. Chichester: Wiley Blackwell Publishing. pp. 27–43.

Wegrzyniak, L.J., Repke, J.T. & Ural S.H. (2012). Treatment of Hyperemesis Gravidarum. *Obstetrics and Gynecology.* **5** (2), 78–84.

Useful websites

British National Formulary
http://www.bnf.org/bnf/index.htm (Accessed 25 July 2015)
Royal College of Midwives
https://www.rcm.org.uk/ (Accessed 27 July 2015)
Royal College of Obstetricians and Gynaecologists
https://www.rcog.org.uk/en/ (Accessed 27 July 2015)

· A B C D E ·

Disability

34 Assessing and managing aspects of consciousness and disability

Ann M. Price

By the end of this chapter, you should be able to explain the basic pathophysiology of the key 'D' disability aspects, define 'normal' consciousness and gain an overview of assessment methods (particularly those related to consciousness, pain and blood glucose levels). You should also be able to recognise a deterioration in level of consciousness and other 'D' aspects, and understand the initial interventions required to prevent further deterioration.

This chapter will focus on aspects of the 'D' for disability section of the assessment of the acutely ill adult. Often the focus is on the neurological status of the patient (Tait *et al.* 2012) but pain and blood glucose assessment are also key areas to consider (Mulryan 2011). These are all huge, complex subjects and this chapter will therefore only outline the key aspects that should be considered to ensure that the acutely ill patient is assessed fully. Thus, it will include some common assessment methods and major initial patient management interventions. The chapter starts with a brief overview of pathophysiology.

Pathophysiology overview

The A, B, C assessment is undertaken before 'D' because issues within these first three categories can affect the 'D' area and need to be excluded first. Jevon (2010) notes that monitoring conscious level plays an essential part in detecting critical illness. For example, hypoxia or hypotension will lead to inadequate cerebral perfusion and could result in confusion or reduced consciousness (Braun & Anderson 2011).

Pain is a complex mechanism that includes objective and subjective aspects. In acute illness, it has a protective focus that helps to prevent further damage (Braun & Anderson 2011). Thus, although it is vital to monitor pain in order to manage the patient's condition effectively, other signs are generally more suggestive as early indicators of a life-threatening condition. However, increasing pain may indicate changing status and should not be ignored. Equally, the stress response is initiated during an acute illness episode, which means that blood glucose would normally be raised (Braun & Anderson 2011), so blood glucose measurement is normally left until later. Having said all this, in the clinical setting many of these aspects will be performed simultaneously or may be prioritised, depending on the patient's presentation and history.

Consciousness — characteristics and definitions

Consciousness is a mental state in which we are aware of our surroundings and able to interact with the environment (Waterhouse 2005, Boss & Huether 2012). Altered consciousness is usually caused by an event that affects the reticular activating system (RAS) within the brain. The RAS is normally involved in the wake/sleep cycle and adverse events can cause disruption of this system (Tortora & Nielsen 2009). Disturbance of conscious level is usually manifest by difficulty in arousing the patient and possibly coma (unrousable).

Confusion, which can be caused by injury to various parts of the brain cortex, is when a person becomes disorientated in relation to their surroundings. Confusion can vary in severity and can affect specific aspects of consciousness. For instance, an individual may be disorientated in current time but still remember past events clearly (Boss & Huether 2012). Confusion and altered consciousness can be sudden or slow in onset, depending on whether the disease process is an acute event or a degenerative process. See Table 34.1 for descriptions of different types of altered consciousness.

Table 34.1
Description and characteristics of altered states of consciousness

Description	Characteristics
Normal consciousness	Easily aroused, wakeful, aware of environment (Haymore 2004)
Lethargy, obtunded, stupor	These are poorly defined terms and should be avoided; specific information about the patient's response to verbal and tactile stimuli is more useful (Haymore 2004)
Confusion	Unable to think rapidly, diminished judgement and decision-making ability, loss of rationality (Boss & Huether 2012)
Coma	Boss & Huether (2012) say 'light' coma is associated with purposeful movement; 'coma' with non-purposeful movement; and 'deep' coma with no response (all with stimulus being applied)
Brainstem death (see Chapter 43 on organ donation)	Irreversible loss of entire brain function, including brainstem, cerebellum and cortical functions (Boss & Huether 2012)
Cerebral death or irreversible coma	The cerebral hemisphere dies but brainstem and cerebellum functions remain. Haemostasis is maintained but cognitive function, awareness and movement are significantly impaired. Related terms include 'persistent vegetative state (PVS)', 'minimally conscious state (MCS)' and 'locked-in syndrome' (Boss & Huether 2012).
Related areas	
Dementia	Progressive failure of many cerebral functions, often resulting in disorientation, decline in memory and decision-making, and altered behaviour (Boss & Huether 2012)
Acute confusional states (ACS), delirium	Transient changes in awareness, often secondary to illness, drugs or withdrawal from substances; delirium is a term that is often used for ACS (Boss & Huether 2012)

Delirium (or acute confusional state) is a term that is frequently used for critically ill patients. This means that the patient has an acute cerebral dysfunction, which may include inattention, change in mental status, disorganised thinking or decreased consciousness (Karnatovskaia *et al.* 2015) which is often associated with an acute illness episode.

There are *primary* neurological causes of altered consciousness such as head injury, brain tumour, meningitis, electrolyte imbalances, metabolic disturbances (e.g. diabetic ketoacidosis) and cerebrovascular accident (CVA or stroke), that result from a disease process (Haymore 2004). There are also *secondary* causes of neurological dysfunction such as drugs, pain, alcohol, dementia and psychological causes. These can be termed delirium or psychosis and often need to be dealt with differently from primary causes (Haymore 2004).

Please refer to separate chapters on neurological compromise secondary to electrolyte imbalance (Chapter 35), diabetic ketoacidosis (Chapter 36), and NICE (2008) Stroke Clinical Guideline 68 for more detail on these conditions.

Pathophysiology/aetiology and mechanism of condition and therapy

The reticular activating system (RAS) is an area of specialised cells situated in the brainstem (Tortora & Nielsen 2009). The RAS has to interact with the brain (cerebral) hemispheres to produce consciousness. Consciousness is described as involving three elements: arousal, awareness and activity (Barlow 2012). Damage to the RAS, or parts of the cerebral hemispheres, can lead to altered conscious level and (in severe cases) unconsciousness (Geraghty 2005). The type and severity of neurological dysfunction depends on the size of injury, cause of dysfunction and the area of brain affected. Initial signs that may be significant include headache, vomiting, amnesia, drowsiness, being 'knocked out' and seizures, which may escalate to unconsciousness (NICE 2014).

Intracranial pressure (ICP) is the result of pressure in the skull from the components of brain tissue (the major component), blood and cerebral spinal fluid (CSF) (approximately 300ml) (Woodrow 2012). In normal people, the ICP will rise transiently (for example, when coughing); but in head-injured patients the brain swells, leading to increasing ICP and reducing blood flow to the brain, so leading to further brain ischaemia (often termed secondary injury). A normal ICP is 0–15mmHg (Woodrow 2012) although this can only be measured when the patient is being cared for in an intensive care setting. Many nerves emanating from the brain cross to the opposite side at the level of the brainstem, before travelling down the spinal cord to the body. Thus, if an injury occurs on the left side of the brain then the right side of the body's limbs will be affected.

Neurological assessment

A full neurological assessment requires consideration of mental, motor, pupillary, cranial nerve function, reflexes and sensation, as well as vital signs (Hilton 2013). However, there are two main tools that are used for the initial neurological assessment of acutely ill patients:

- AVPU – Alert, Verbal, Pain, Unresponsive
- Glasgow Coma Score (GCS).

Pupillary assessment is also a vital element – in addition to the above tools (Jevon 2010). Both these tools require regular refresher training and experienced practitioners to ensure accuracy of assessment is maintained (Chan *et al.* 2013).

The AVPU is used when a quick assessment of consciousness is required as part of a general assessment (Resuscitation Council UK 2005). It is a good way to measure a patient's deterioration, as many illnesses and complications can lead to changes in level of consciousness. A normal person should be 'alert', and any changes may indicate a worsening condition.

The GCS is used to assess the level of consciousness in more detail (Cree 2003, Waterhouse 2005, Barlow 2012). A normal GCS is 15. A GCS of 3–8 is considered to be severe neurological impairment (coma); 9–12 moderate impairment; and 13 mild impairment (Woodrow 2012). Any sudden change of 13 and under needs further investigation (NICE 2014). Sustained changes in GCS of 2 points or more for over 30 minutes are considered significant and require prompt referral (NICE 2014). Specific limb response and pupil reactions give additional information on the nature of the neurological dysfunction. In severe neurological insults, or injury that affects the brainstem, vital functions (such as respiration and pulse) can be affected.

The GCS is used as an indicator of morbidity and mortality (Barlow 2012) but it has limitations in consistency between different practitioners. NICE (2014) recommends that patients admitted who require GCS should have recordings every half-hour for 2 hours, then every hour for 4 hours and then every 2 hours. If there is any deterioration in the readings, the assessment should increase back to half-hourly. See Table 34.2 for further details of how to take a Glasgow Coma Score.

Remember that there are tools designed to assess specific conditions, such as the FAST tool (**F**acial weakness, **A**rm weakness, **S**peech problems, **T**est all of these) used for suspected stroke (NICE 2008). A full discussion of these is beyond the scope of this chapter.

Table 34.2
How to undertake a Glasgow Coma Score (GCS) properly

THERE ARE 3 SECTIONS TO COMPLETE TO OBTAIN A GCS SCORE. Add the 3 scores together to produce Glasgow Coma Score – and record the E, V and M scores separately.

A score below 9 is considered a coma, and a deterioration of 2 or more points is considered significant. The lowest score possible is 3 (completely unresponsive) and the highest is 15 (normal).

Section 1 Open Eyes (E)	Score	Tips
Approach patient. Patient opens eyes spontaneously.	Score 4	Normal response – eyes open without speech or touch.
If no response to approach, try speaking to patient – and score if they open their eyes.	Score 3	Take care not to approach, speak and touch all at the same time, as you won't know which caused the response. Consider hearing problems.
If no response to speech, try painful stimuli – and score if they open their eyes.	Score 2	Try touch or gentle shaking before using painful stimuli. Use a minimal level to elicit a response (maximum of 30 seconds), slowly increasing intensity of pain. Severe pain can make the patient shut their eyes! (See 'Painful stimuli' below.)

No response to pain. Patient deeply unconscious.	Score 1	Consider drug-induced unconsciousness.
If eyes are closed, this could be due to injury or swelling.	Score C	Inability to open eyes (e.g. due to trauma or swelling) scores C.
Section 2 Best Verbal Response (V)	**Score**	**Tips**
Orientated – patient knows where they are, who they are, why they are there, talks in sentences, and recognises people.	Score 5	Consider that patients lose track of time and date during hospital stay but should know month and year. More difficult to assess in children.
Confused – muddled information, not sure of where and who they are; patient talks in sentences.	Score 4	Some patients seem to be talking sense and then make strange incorrect statements. Remember that some patients may not be able to express themselves but may be able to understand you.
Inappropriate words – patient uses recognisable words but odd or incomplete sentences.	Score 3	Words may be swear words or odd and out of context.
Patient makes incomprehensible sounds – no words, only grunts, moans and groans.	Score 2	Check that the sounds are not signs of airway obstruction (e.g. gurgling).
No response.	Score 1	Consider injuries that may limit speech such as jaw fracture or tracheostomy/ET tube.
Tracheostomy or endotracheal (ET) tube.	Score T	Don't assume that a tracheostomy patient can speak – record T on chart.
Section 3 Best Motor Response (M)	**Score**	**Tips** **Remember to record 'best' response as limbs may differ**
Patient obeys commands – even if their limbs are weak.	Score 6	Don't ask the patient to 'squeeze your hand' as this is a reflex response to touching the palm. Ask them to lift their left arm or leg, stick out their tongue, etc. Be specific!
Patient localises to pain – moves an arm or leg purposefully away from pain.	Score 5	The peripheral pain method is usually more useful, as the central method gives a more generalised response. Patients are localising if they try and pull at lines, endotracheal or nasogastric tubes, or try and push you away.

Withdrawal from pain – patient moves an arm or leg away from pain but *not* in a purposeful way.	Score 4	This differs from purposeful removal from pain, as the patient may move all limbs away because they can't distinguish where the pain is originating.
Flexion to pain – if the patient demonstrates 'decorticate posturing'.	Score 3	The arms will bend at the elbow and the wrists flex. This response is slower than withdrawal from pain.
Extension to pain – if the patient demonstrates 'decerebrate posturing'.	Score 2	The arms and legs straighten, and there is internal rotation of the shoulder and wrist. This is a very abnormal response.
No response at all.	Score 1	Consider drug-induced problems (such as paralysing agents) or spinal injury.

Painful stimuli (based on Woodrow 2012)

Central pain

- Sub-orbital pressure: Place your thumb on the patient's eyebrow ridge and apply pressure.
- Jaw pressure: Apply pressure to the angle of the jaw. This is unsuitable for patients with possible facial injuries or those with severe bruising.
- Trapezium pinch: Squeeze the patient's trapezium muscle (on the top of the shoulder at the base of the neck) between your fingers and thumb. This has few side effects.
- Sternal rub: Rub the centre of the chest on the sternum. This causes bruising if excessive pressure is used or there is a clotting disorder (not recommended).

Peripheral pain

This includes pain on the side of a fingernail – *not* on the nailbed, as this damages the nail. It is useful for assessing limb strength in deeply unconscious patients. It is *not* suitable for assessing GCS, as it only elicits a local reflex response (Cree 2003).

Management of the unconscious patient

The National Institute for Care and Health Excellence now emphasises the need for early diagnostic testing and intervention for a number of neurological conditions, such as head injuries (NICE 2014) and stroke (NICE 2008). The aim of nursing care and medical treatment is to reduce the damage from the physical injury and control intracranial pressure. It is therefore vital to refer patients to appropriate specialist services for medical intervention, such as the hospital Stroke Team, and follow the NICE (2008) stroke guideline. Table 34.3 outlines the key areas to consider when an acutely ill patient presents with a reduced level of consciousness.

Any brain injury can lead to long-term disability that has an impact on the patient and their family. Early recognition and management of the disease can reduce the initial damage and improve the long-term outcome for many patients. It takes a lot of time to meet the needs of the unconscious patient and reduce potential risks (Geraghty 2005). This is often a traumatic period for relatives and friends, who will require assistance and information. Rehabilitation and social support are needed to ensure that the patient is enabled to achieve the best possible recovery.

Table 34.3 Key considerations for the patient with reduced level of consciousness

Issue	Management	Rationale
Airway	• Consider using recovery position; use airway adjuncts (e.g. oropharyngeal airway), watch for signs of obstruction such as gurgling, stridor. • Inability to cough. • If patient has GCS <9, refer to anaesthetist.	• To ensure there is no airway obstruction, which would limit oxygen supply to brain and increase ischaemic injury (Resuscitation Council UK 2005). • If patient cannot cough, they do not clear their airway and may need an endotracheal tube (Hartshorn & Gauthier 2001). • A GCS of 8 or less means that the patient cannot maintain their airway effectively and should be considered for intubation.
Respiration	• Monitor respiration rate, depth, rhythm and pattern for abnormalities. • Give oxygen therapy as prescribed. • Monitor oxygen saturations.	• Report changes in pattern and low/high rates, which can indicate deterioration in neurological condition. • Giving oxygen reduces risk of further hypoxic brain damage (Geraghty 2005).
Cardiovascular	• Monitor pulse and blood pressure, as patient may need treatment for hypotension or hypertension, tachycardia or bradycardia. • Monitor temperature.	• The brain needs an adequate supply of blood to maintain function so a low blood pressure is as bad as a high one (Cree 2003). • High temperature is a rare complication of severe head injury when the hypothalamus is affected. However, it has been suggested that elevated temperature has a negative impact on mortality (Greer *et al.* 2008).
Level of consciousness	• If patient is stable, assess GCS half-hourly for 2 hours; then reduce to hourly for 4 hours, and 2-hourly after this. • Remember to include pupillary reaction and size and report differences/changes (NICE 2014). • Follow local guidelines and consider patient's condition after this.	• After the initial injury, there is a risk of extension of damage; early recognition and treatment can improve outcome. • Conscious level should slowly improve (for most patients) after the initial insult.

Fluid and nutritional intake	• Give intravenous fluids or nasogastric feeding until patient is able to eat and drink. • The patient should be assessed to check swallowing ability if there is any concern (e.g. coughing when drinking). • The hospital policy for swallow tests should be adhered to.	• Depressed conscious level means that the patient will not be able to drink adequate fluids and is at risk of dehydration. • Aspiration of fluids into the lungs needs to be avoided, as it complicates recovery (and can be fatal) (Cree 2003). • Around 50% of stroke patients have swallowing impairment and so a swallow test is vital before freely giving fluids and food orally (The Stroke Association 2008). • A nasogastric tube may be needed for feeding or to prevent aspiration if vomiting but can also increase the risk of respiratory infection (Brogan *et al.* 2015).
Bed rest	• Assess for signs of deep vein thrombosis (DVT), e.g. swollen and warm calves. Anti-embolism stockings and prophylactic anticoagulation may be ordered (Geraghty 2005). • Encourage limb movements (if able) and physiotherapy; encourage deep breathing. • Sit up at 30 degrees or follow local policy.	• Bed rest is common in the first few days after a neurological event to promote recovery. However, complications of bed rest can delay recovery through DVT and pneumonia. • Sitting the patient up reduces the risk of aspiration and aids intracranial pressure (Cree 2003). • Note: anticoagulation therapy may not always be used in some types of head injury if there is concern about further brain bleeding, and the use of anti-embolism stockings is controversial (NICE 2010).
Pressure ulcers	• Assess Waterlow Score (or other pressure risk score). • Use pressure-relieving devices where appropriate. • Promote side lying and position changes. • Assess the patient's ability to move themselves.	• Reduced conscious level often means that the patient cannot or does not move themselves. For example, one-sided weakness in cerebrovascular accident (CVA) patients can make it difficult for them to adjust their own position.

Mobility and risk of falls	• Assess the patient's understanding of commands. • Assess their movement and strength in their limbs. • Use appropriate moving and handling aids (e.g. a hoist). • Assess whether there is a need for cot sides. Establish a physiotherapy regime if needed.	• Altered conscious level and confusion can affect mobility and put the patient at risk of falling. Independence and mobility should be promoted but this needs to be done carefully to ensure the safety of the patient and others (Geraghty 2005). • Some neurological conditions lead to poor balance and spatial awareness. • Cot sides should be used with patient consent or according to local policy.
Incontinence	• Assess bladder and bowel control. • Patient may need urinary catheter or bowel management regime. • If there is a risk of constipation, consider laxatives.	• Bladder and bowel control can be affected in head injury and is a particular problem in stroke patients. • Incontinence adds to pressure ulcer risk so measures to limit soiling are needed. • Constipation often results from prolonged immobility (Geraghty 2005).
Unable to maintain hygiene	• Assess the patient's ability to carry out skin care and mouth and eye care.	• Hygiene needs will be individually adjusted to meet the patient's needs and promote independence where possible (Geraghty 2005).
Psychological	• Assess for fear, anxiety, agitation, aggression, mood swings and depression. • Antidepressants may be used in some patients or they may need to be reviewed by a psychologist. • Assess for difficulty with communicating.	• Any brain injury can create huge anxiety and fear for patients about the long-term effects. • Stroke patients are particularly at risk of difficulties as they try to cope with changes in mood, physical function and difficulties in mental processing (Stroke Association 2008). • Observe non-verbal signs as well as verbal interaction to aid communication (Geraghty 2005).

Pain

Pain is defined as 'An unpleasant sensation occurring in varying degrees of severity as a consequence of injury, disease, or emotional disorder' (*The Free Dictionary* 2014). However, pain in the acutely ill patient can give an indication of the severity of, or a deterioration in, the patient's condition. Pain can manifest in a variety of ways in the acutely ill adult, including fear, anxiety, restlessness, immobility and sleep disturbances (Jevon 2012). The sensation of pain may be verbalised or may be evident through the patient's behaviours or physiological signs. Healthcare workers therefore need to be observant in order to pick up non-verbal and verbal cues suggesting pain.

In the acutely ill patient, pain can be seen as a secondary issue, with the priority being to stabilise the condition (Jevon 2012). However, pain is a significant factor in triggering the stress response and sympathetic nervous system, leading to further physiological instability (Middleton 2003). The effects of untreated pain can affect both short- and long-term recovery and may also lead to psychological disturbances (Jevon 2012). Thus, pain needs to be recognised and addressed adequately, and as quickly as possible, in the acute illness phase.

There are numerous pain scoring tools available, which are adjusted according to the clinical area and the patient's ability to understand (as for elderly people and children). However, in acutely ill adult patients, a tool that is quick and simple to use is preferable and a numerical rating scale is commonly utilised (Jevon 2012). Numerical rating scales allow patients to score their pain from 0 to 10 (some areas use a 0–3 scale), where 0 is no pain and 10 is the worst pain imaginable. This is an easy scale for most patients to understand and requires no special tools.

Pain assessment in the acutely ill patient should include pain score, location, intensity, type and anything that affects the pain; all this information should be documented and any changes reported. Healthcare professionals have a vital role in assessing pain and ensuring that appropriate analgesia is prescribed and administered (Jevon 2012). Obviously the type of analgesia and delivery method will vary, depending on the patient's condition and local policy. However, the response to analgesia should be recorded and any specific observations (as for epidural analgesia) should be adhered to. Difficulty in controlling pain, or increasing analgesia requirements, may mean that the underlying condition is worsening; this should be investigated further to exclude complications. Pain assessment and pain management are discussed in detail in Chapter 38.

Blood glucose

Monitoring of blood glucose levels is routinely undertaken as part of the assessment of the acutely ill adult patient and the normal range is 4.0–5.9mmol/litre (Diabetes.co.uk 2014). Readings below 3mmol/litre should be treated immediately (Resuscitation Council UK 2005).

The stress response is triggered, as previously mentioned, in the acutely ill patient and this normally leads to hyperglycaemia. A stress response hyperglycaemia is defined as a random glucose >11·1 mmol/litre without evidence of previous diabetes (Dungan et al. 2009). This has been viewed as the body's way of enabling energy to be available for the cells to utilise, although evidence shows that mortality increases in critically ill patients whose blood glucose remains high (Corathers & Falciglia 2011). However, most of the studies into hyperglycaemia in the critically ill have been undertaken in intensive care patients and caution should be applied in transferring this finding to general ward settings.

Hypoglycaemia is more unusual in acutely ill patients but is a poor prognostic sign, particularly for those without diabetes (Glynn et al. 2014). Patients particularly at risk of hypoglycaemia are diabetic patients, those with poor nutritional intake, some metabolic disorders and low body glucose reserves. These patients may not utilise nutrition appropriately (either they metabolise too quickly or there is insufficient uptake of glucose to cells) and so their glucose levels drop.

Alternatively, there may have been inappropriate administration of hypoglycaemic agents, causing glucose levels to drop. Patients with diabetes mellitus are particularly at risk when they are acutely ill, as they may not eat properly but continue to take medication. These patients often need careful management to maintain their glucose intake, whilst enabling their bodies to process this effectively through insulin metabolism.

Monitoring blood glucose levels is clearly vital and should be undertaken as part of the initial assessment and continued according to the local policy. Continued monitoring and management of acutely ill patients with blood sugar abnormalities is needed, and specialist advice should be sought to address individual needs.

Conclusion

This chapter has given an overview of areas related to the 'D' aspect of assessment. This type of assessment is essential in order to detect deterioration and consider wider issues that may affect the critically ill adult patient.

References and further reading

Barlow, P. (2012). A practical review of the Glasgow Coma Scale and Score. *The Surgeon.* **10** (2), 114–19.

Brogan, E., Langdon, C., Brookes, K., Budgeon, C. & Blacker, D. (2015). Can't swallow, can't transfer, can't toilet: Factors predicting infections in the first week post stroke. *Journal of Clinical Neuroscience.* **22** (1), 92–97. DOI: 10.1016/j.jocn.2014.05.035

Boss, B.J. & Huether, W.E. (2012). 'Alterations in cognitive systems,cerebral hemodynamics, and motor function' in S.E. Huether & K.L. McCance (eds) *Understanding Pathophysiology.* 5th edition. Missouri: Mosby Inc, 347–76.

Braun, C.A. & Anderson, A.M. (2011). *Pathophysiology: A Clinical Approach.* 2nd edn. Philadelphia: Lippincott, Williams & Wilkins.

Chan, M.F., Mattar, I. & Taylor, B.J. (2013). Investigating factors that have an impact on nurses' performance of patients' conscious level assessment: a systematic review. *Journal of Nursing Management.* **21** (1), 31–46.

Corathers, S.D. & Falciglia, M. (2011). The role of hyperglycaemia in acute illness: supporting evidence and its limitations. *Nutrition.* **27** (3), 276–81.

Cree, C. (2003). Acquired brain injury: acute management. *Nursing Standard.* **18** (11), 45–56.

Diabetes.co.uk (2014). *Blood Sugar Level Ranges.* http://www.diabetes.co.uk/diabetes_care/blood-sugar-level-ranges.html (accessed 26 June 2014).

Dungan, K.K., Braithwaite, S.S. & Preiser, J. (2009). Stress hyperglycaemia. *The Lancet.* **373** (9677), 1798–1807.

Geraghty, M. (2005). Nursing the unconscious patient. *Nursing Standard.* **20** (1), 54–64.

Glynn, N., Owens, L., Bennett, K., Healy, M.L. & Silke, B. (2014). Glucose as a risk predictor in acute medical emergency admissions. *Diabetes Research and Clinical Practice.* 103 (1), 119–26.

Greer, D.M., Funk, S.E., Reaven, N.L., Ouzounelli, M. & Uman, G.C. (2008). Impact of fever on outcome in patients with stroke and neurologic injury: a comprehensive meta-analysis. *Stroke.* **39**, 3029–35.

Hartshorn, J.C. & Gauthier, D.M. (2001). 'Nervous system alterations' in M.L. Sole, M.L. Lamborn & J.C. Hartshorn (eds). *Introduction to Critical Care Nursing.* 3rd edn. London: W.B. Saunders.

Haymore, J. (2004). A neuron in a haystack: advanced neurological assessment. *AACN Clinical Issues.* **15** (4), 568–81.

Hilton, G. (2013). 'Patient Assessment: Nervous System' in P.G. Morton & D.K. Fontaine (eds). *Critical Care Nursing: a holistic approach.* 10th edn. Philadelphia: Lippincott, Williams & Wilkins, 723–43.

Jevon, P. (2010). How to ensure patient observations lead to effective management of altered consciousness. *Nursing Times.* **106** (6), 17–18.

Jevon, P. (2012). *Monitoring the Critically Ill Patient.* 3rd edn. Oxford: Wiley-Blackwell.

Karnatovskaia, L.V., Johnson, M.M., Benzo, R.P. & Gajic, O. (2015). The spectrum of psychocognitive morbidity in the critically ill: A review of the literature and call for improvement. *Journal of Crtical Care.* **30** (1), 130–37. DOI: 10.1016/j.jcrc.2014.09.024.

Middleton, C. (2003). Understanding the physiological effects of unrelieved pain'. *Nursing Times.* **99** (37), 28. http://www.nursingtimes.net/nursing-practice/clinical-zones/pain-management/understanding-the-physiological-effects-of-unrelieved-pain/205262.article (accessed 13 February 2014).

Mulryan, C. (2011). *Acute Illness Management.* London: Sage.

National Institute for Health and Care Excellence (NICE) (2008). *Stroke Clinical Guidance 68.* http://www.nice.org.uk/nicemedia/live/12018/41331/41331.pdf (accessed 7 February 2014).

National Institute for Health and Care Excellence (NICE) (2010). *Venous thromboembolism: reducing the risk: reducing the risk of venous thromboembolism (deep vein thrombosis and pulmonary embolism) in patients admitted to hospital. Clinical Guideline CG92.* https://www.nice.org.uk/guidance/cg92 (accessed 15 April 2015).

National Institute for Health and Care Excellence (NICE) (2014). *Head Injury Clinical Guideline 176.* http://www.nice.org.uk/guidance/cg176 (accessed 12 August 2015).

Resuscitation Council UK (2005). *A Systematic Approach to the Acutely Ill Patient.* https://www.resus.org.uk/resuscitation-guidelines/a-systematic-approach-to-the-acutely-ill-patient-abcde/#disab (accessed 12 August 2015).

Tait, D., Barton, D., James, J. & Williams, C. (2012). *Acute and Critical Care in Adult Nursing*. London: Learning Matters.

Tortora, G.J. & Nielsen, M.T. (2009). *Principles of Human Anatomy*. 11th edn. Chichester: John Wiley & Sons.

The Free Dictionary (2014). *Definition of pain*. http://www.thefreedictionary.com/pain (Accessed 13 February 2014).

Waterhouse, C. (2005). The Glasgow Coma Score and other neurological observations. *Nursing Standard*. **19** (33), 56–64.

Woodrow, P. (2012). *Intensive Care Nursing: A Framework for Practice*. 3rd edn. London: Routledge.

Useful websites

Headway: the Brain Injury Association
https://www.headway.org.uk
(Accessed 12 August 2015)

Stroke Association
https://www.stroke.org.uk/
(Accessed 12 August 2015)

Neurological compromise secondary to electrolyte imbalance

Amanda Sudan and Sally A. Smith

This chapter discusses a case of rapid correction of low sodium levels (hyponatraemia), resulting in neurological compromise (osmotic demyelination syndrome) in a previously fit and well 45-year-old man. It should be read in conjunction with Chapter 30 (on electrolytes) and also the other 'Disability' chapters (34 and 36–40).

Hyponatraemia is an electrolyte imbalance that is commonly found in the hospital setting. It occurs from sodium loss, water gain or inadequate sodium intake. Common causes include loss of electrolytes from the gut through diarrhoea and vomiting, and water excess from over-infusion of 5% dextrose or over-use of diuretics. Medical conditions resulting in hyponatraemia include renal disease, severe cardiac failure and cirrhosis of the liver (Kumar & Clark 2012).

Osmotic demyelination syndrome (ODS) or central pontine myelinolysis (as it was previously known) is a recognised complication resulting from the overly rapid correction of hyponatraemia (Pearce 2009). It is a condition that does not occur spontaneously; rather it is a complication of treatment for pre-existing medical conditions (Norenberg 2010). The morbidity and mortality of central/extrapontine myelinolysis have been reduced through recognition of predisposing conditions, early diagnosis, modern neuro-imaging and cautious intensive treatment (Kumar *et al.* 2006). It is therefore imperative that nursing and medical staff are able to recognise, assess and prevent its onset. This requires them to be competent in neurological assessment and fluid management care for their patients. This chapter covers the management of a patient with hyponatraemia and suggests appropriate correction methods.

By the end of this chapter, you should have an understanding of the aetiology and management of low sodium levels; have sufficient knowledge to assess, monitor and manage a patient with ODS; be able to recognise potentially life-threatening complications.

Background and definitions

Normal serum sodium level is 135–145mmol/litre (Longmore *et al.* 2014); therefore hyponatraemia is defined as a sodium level below 135mmol/litre (Mattson-Porth 2006). The clinical context in which hyponatraemia develops may be useful in differentiating acute from chronic hyponatraemia, which is relevant to its treatment (Decaux & Soupart 2003). The functions of sodium in the body are explained in Chapter 30 (on electrolytes).

Case scenario

A 45-year-old man was admitted to a medical ward with a history of diarrhoea and vomiting. On admission all physical examination findings were unremarkable, but his blood sodium concentration was 109mmol/litre. He was admitted for rehydration and correction of hyponatraemia with intravenous fluids (mainly normal saline).

The following day, he suffered several *grand mal* seizures. Arterial blood gases taken at the time showed: pH 7.0, pCO_2 3.7kPa, HCO_3 6.8mmol/litre, base deficit −24.8 (severe metabolic acidosis) and a serum sodium that had increased to 132mmol/litre. Over the next day, he received a large amount of normal saline rapidly and 150ml 8.4% sodium bicarbonate to correct his acidosis. An intravenous phenytoin infusion was commenced.

The next day, his condition remained stable and medical management was oral fluid restriction, continuation of intravenous fluids, and measurement of electrolytes. He then suffered two further seizures with a diagnosis of seizures secondary to rapid sodium correction and a severe metabolic acidosis of unknown cause. The critical care outreach team was called to review the patient, due to his decreased level of consciousness. Intensive care intervention was requested and a diagnosis of osmotic demyelination syndrome was assumed.

The previous day, this patient's blood test results were:

	At 23:15	At 00:05	At 01:55
pH	7.0	7.05	7.38
pCO_2	3.7	2.5	4.05
HCO_3	6.8	5.1	17.6
Base excess	24.8	25.7	5.9
Sodium		132	130
Lactate			1.8

Physiology of osmotic demyelination syndrome

ODS is a demyelinating condition often affecting the brainstem (pons). The name was changed from central pontine myelinolysis because demyelination can be more diffuse, affecting areas beyond the pons (Sahay & Sahay 2014). The destruction of the myelin sheath, which coats the nerves, inhibits impulse conduction within the cells, thus decreasing their ability to communicate with other cells.

ODS is most commonly caused by a rapid correction of sodium levels in a person with chronic hyponatraemia, of at least several days' duration (Pearce 2009, Norenberg 2010). Clinically, this may present as a biphasic course: the patient demonstrates complications of hyponatraemia (seizures and encephalopathy), then recovers rapidly after correction of serum sodium, only to deteriorate several days later.

The clinical manifestations of myelinolysis vary considerably, depending on the degree of pontine involvement and the presence of extrapontine lesions (Kiley *et al.* 1999). Dysarthria and dysphagia (corticobulbar tract involvement) appear initially before the patient progresses from flaccid quadriparesis (corticospinal tract) to spastic quadriparesis (basis pontis). Further progression to the tegmentum may present with pupillary and occulomotor dysfunction. 'Locked-in syndrome' may also result (Alleman 2007).

ODS usually presents with spastic tetraparesis (complete or partial loss of all movement and/or sensation from the neck downward) and pseudobulbar palsy. Examination may indicate involvement of all four extremities or weakness of the face, arms and legs (upper motor neuron syndrome). Reflexes may be abnormal, and eye examination may show loss of control of the eye muscles, particularly cranial nerve VI paralysis. Symptoms include weakness and muscle spasm, reduced and/or double vision, reduced alertness and poor enunciation. Psychiatric manifestations (such as confusion and delirium) have been reported in the literature, along with behavioural changes including personality changes and disinhibition. Florid signs of brainstem and pyramidal tract dysfunction usually overshadow neuropsychiatric symptoms.

Although not fully understood, the mechanisms for this condition are becoming more evident with continuing research. One of the leading factors in the pathogenesis of ODS is osmotic stress. Rapid correction of hyponatraemia can cause osmotic stress, which is associated with the disruption of the blood brain barrier (Chang *et al.* 2014). This endothelial injury and opening of the blood brain barrier results in the release of myelinotoxic or oligodendroglial destructive factors (Norenberg 2010).

ODS is an emergency disorder with no known cure. Treatment is focused on relieving symptoms, with the prognosis involving persistence of serious chronic disability (Afsari & Posin 2002). However there are some reversible causes with acute oedema that subsides and there are reports of remyelination occurring (Tosaka & Kogha 1998). An MRI scan, which in the early stages may be normal, is the primary diagnostic study. Serum sodium levels are also imperative.

Assessment

On examination, the patient in the case scenario was lying on his back with a nasopharyngeal airway in situ and he appeared comatose. He opened his eyes briefly to his name but no other response could be elicited. He was monitored but had no oxygen in situ and he was clammy and sweating.

Immediate care

Airway management is the priority in a patient who has disordered conscious level. The man in this case scenario had his airway maintained with a nasopharyngeal airway. However, because of the initial finding of a Glasgow Coma Score of 5/15, he was placed for his own safety in the left lateral position to ensure absolute protection of his airway, despite the nasopharyngeal airway and before any further assessment was carried out. The results of the physical assessment can be found in Box 35.1.

Discussion and implications for practice

The diagnosis of ODS for this man was a grave one. He had received large amounts of supplementary intravenous sodium to correct his hyponatraemia. He was clearly exhibiting adverse signs and symptoms, with great risk to his airway and prognosis. The knowledge and skills of the nursing and medical staff were critical to managing this patient and preventing the condition. A patient such as this requires thorough neurological assessment at regular intervals, and timely reporting of any trends and changes. The nursing care of these patients includes a comprehensive assessment of airway, breathing, circulation and disability (neurological status). Nursing staff will routinely undertake vital sign observations, including assessment of conscious level, such as **AVPU** (**A**lert, responds to **V**erbal stimulation or command, responds to **P**ainful stimuli, **U**nresponsive) (NICE 2007).

In this particular patient, formal neurological observations were not recorded. It was therefore difficult to ascertain a trend with regard to his deterioration. An important aspect of managing acutely ill patients is reviewing their response to any treatment and interventions instigated (NICE 2007). This includes reviewing results and tests and also any trends, not only with respect to vital signs but also fluid management. Correcting this patient's hyponatraemia too rapidly may have caused a deterioration in his conscious level with the onset of ODS.

With chronic hyponatraemia, the brain undergoes adaptation and generally needs gradual correction. There is a high risk of ODS if serum sodium is 120meq/litre or less, or if comorbidities such as alcoholism, liver disease, malnutrition or severe hypokalaemia are present (Sahay & Sahay 2014). These authors suggest that an increase of 4–6 mmol/litre is sufficient, with a maximum of 8mmol/litre in a 24-hour period, using 3% NaCl (1ml/kg of 3% NaCl is estimated to raise the serum Na by 1meq/litre). If chronic hyponatraemia is symptomatic (with seizures or confusion) or severe (serum sodium concentration below 125meq/litre), aggressive therapy is indicated, using 3% NaCl, with or without vasopressin receptor antagonists. Patients with mild symptoms (such as dizziness, forgetfulness or gait disturbance) should be treated with less aggressive therapy. Expert help should be sought in these situations, and referral to the intensive care unit will be needed if a patient's conscious level and airway are compromised.

Monitoring includes continuous cardiac and oxygen saturation monitoring. Frequency of vital sign recording needs to be assessed at the time, according to the patient's condition. For the case scenario patient, neurological observations should have been undertaken every 15 minutes, and reduced to 30 minutes when he was stabilised. Fluid input and output should also have been accurately recorded. In this case, a diagnosis of ODS was suspected – and supported by a specialist neurological unit, who were contacted for advice. As a result of supportive management, the patient continued to improve and made a recovery to his previous level of health. An MRI scan performed several days later confirmed the diagnosis of ODS.

Box 35.1 Physical assessment of patient in case scenario

Respiratory system

Inspection:

- Patent airway maintained, equal chest expansion
- No peripheral or central cyanosis
- Respiratory rate 24 breaths per minute; deep breathing
- No use of accessory muscles
- Oxygen saturations 98% on air.

Palpation:

- Trachea central with symmetrical expansion.

Percussion:

- Both lung fields resonant.

Auscultation:

- Bilateral vesicular breath sounds, quiet to bases
- No added sounds.

Cardiovascular system

- Heart rate monitored in sinus tachycardia rate 104 per minute
- Blood pressure 140/70mmHg
- Temperature 36.5°C
- Patient sweating and clammy
- Peripherally warm with capillary refill of 1–2 seconds.

Neurological system

- Glasgow Coma Scale 5/15 (eyes 3, verbal 1, motor response 1)
- Nasopharyngeal airway tolerated
- Pupils size 3 and both reactive to light
- Phenytoin infusion in progress to control seizures.

Summary of remaining relevant assessment

- 10ml dilute urine in 3 hours
- Urine positive for ketones, blood protein and glucose
- No intravenous fluids running
- Positive balance of 3 litres from previous day
- No oral intake for last 12 hours, due to reduced level of consciousness
- Blood glucose 10.9mmol/litre
- Abdomen soft.

Conclusion

The man in this case scenario was clearly exhibiting adverse signs and symptoms with great risk to his airway and prognosis. The knowledge and skill base of the nursing and medical staff were key to his management and to prevent any worsening of his condition. Thorough neurological assessments at regular intervals were required, as well as timely reporting of any trends and changes. ODS usually has a poor prognosis. While it is not commonly seen in general wards, drowsiness due to low serum sodium is a common condition and is often overlooked as healthcare professionals search elsewhere for a cause. This chapter has described a severe case of hyponatraemia that required urgent intervention by critical care, close monitoring and management of fluid status, electrolytes, neurological care and airway management.

References and further reading

Afsari, K. & Posin, J.P. (2002). Central pontine myelinolysis. *Annals of Internal Medicine.* **137** (6), 553.

Alleman, A.M. (2007). Osmotic demyelination syndromes: Central and extra pontine myelinolysis. *Journal of Clinical Neuroscience.* **14**, 684–88.

Chang, K. Y., Lee, I., Kim, G. J., Cho, K., Park, Hoon S. & Kim, H.W. (2014). Plasma exchange successfully treats central pontine myelinolysis after acute hypernatremia from intravenous sodium bicarbonate therapy. *BMC Nephrology.* **15**, 56.

Decaux, G. & Soupart, A. (2003). Treatment of symptomatic hyponatraemia. *The American Journal of Medical Sciences.* July, 25–30.

Kiley, M.A., King, M. & Burns, R.J. (1999). Central pontine myelinolysis. *Journal of Clinical Neuroscience.* **6** (2), 155–57.

Kumar, P. & Clark, M. (2012). *Clinical Medicine.* 8th edn. London: W.B. Saunders.

Kumar, S., Fowler, M., Gonzalez-Toledo, E. & Jaffe, S.L. (2006). Central pontine myelinolysis, an update. *Neurological Research.* **28**, 360–66.

Longmore, M., Wilkinson, I. Baldwin, A. & Wallin, E. (2014). *Oxford Handbook of Clinical Medicine.* 5th edn. Oxford: Oxford University Press.

Mattson-Porth, C. (2006). *Essentials of Pathophysiology. Concepts of Altered Health States.* London: Lippincott, Williams and Wilkins.

National Institute for Health and Care Excellence (2007). *NICE Guidelines 50: Acutely ill patients in hospital: Recognition and response to acute illness in adults in hospital.* London: NICE.

Norenberg, M.D. (2010). Central pontine myelinolysis: historical and mechanistic considerations. *Metabolic Brain Disease.* **25** (1), 97–106.

Pearce, J.M.S. (2009). Central pontine myelinolysis. *European Neurology.* **61** (1), 59–62.

Sahay, M. & Sahay, R. (2014). Hyponatraemia: A practical approach. *Indian Journal of Endocrinology and Metabolism.* **18** (6), 760–71.

Tosaka, M. & Kogha, H. (1998). Extrapontine myelinolysis and behavioural change after transsphenoidal pituitary surgery: Case Report. *Neurosurgery.* **43** (4), 993–96.

36 Diabetic ketoacidosis

Ann M. Price and Russell Canavan

Diabetic ketoacidosis (DKA) occurs when there is a deficiency of insulin and extreme hyperglycaemia, leading to metabolic acidosis and osmotic diuresis (Braun & Anderson 2011). DKA is a true medical emergency that, if managed well, can be rewarding to treat. Early appropriate diagnosis and treatment can result in the patient's rapid recovery. This chapter cannot replace your Trust guidelines, but it can give you an insight into the principles of managing such a patient.

By the end of this chapter, you should understand the principles of diabetic ketoacidosis management. You should also understand how to diagnose and treat patients with diabetic ketoacidosis.

Background and definitions

Insulin is a hormone that is produced from the Islets of Langerhans in the pancreas (Braun & Anderson 2011). There is cleavage of pre-insulin to insulin and C peptide, which is then released into the portal circulation to regulate carbohydrate, protein and fat metabolism and maintain a stable blood sugar level via insulin receptors in the systemic circulation (Pessin & Saltiel 2000). Diabetes mellitus comprises a number of conditions related to insulin that lead to a state of chronic hyperglycaemia and subsequent organ damage. The main types of diabetes are known as type 1 and type 2.

Type 1 diabetes

Type 1 diabetes is an autoimmune condition characterised by destruction of the insulin-secreting pancreatic cells. It is multifactorial but often occurs at an early age. As the pancreatic cells are destroyed, the systemic levels of insulin fall and glucose levels rise (Braun & Anderson 2011). Insulin drives movement of glucose from the serum into the cell so the systemic circulation may have high glucose levels while the cell has low levels due to lack of insulin transport.

Extreme low intracellular glucose stimulates production of glucose via lipolysis, in which fats are broken down, producing ketones and fatty acids. This leads to a high glucose level (hyperglycaemia) with severe insulin deficiency. The presence of high levels of ketones leads to metabolic acidosis and the high glucose promotes diuresis and excessive water loss via the kidneys. Thirst, high urine output, fatigue and weight loss are classic symptoms when diagnosing type 1 diabetes. Left untreated, it becomes diabetic ketoacidosis.

It is important to note that only a small amount of insulin is needed to avoid ketoacidosis but, in type 1 diabetics, the lack of insulin means that blood sugars rise quickly and the patient deteriorates relatively rapidly (over a few days).

Type 2 diabetes

Type 2 diabetes is characterised by insulin resistance where there is inadequate insulin production and/ or reduced tissue sensitivity to insulin (Braun & Anderson 2011). The pancreas may be stimulated to produce very high circulating levels of insulin but the insensitive tissues mean that glucose levels are not controlled adequately. After many years, the pancreas starts to fail and levels of insulin reduce. As there is still circulating insulin, ketoacidosis does not occur. Diagnosis is often delayed, as symptoms are subtle. Therefore, glucose levels can rise much higher over a prolonged period of time and exceed the renal threshold. Glucose in the urine acts as an osmotic diuretic and the patient becomes dehydrated. This continues until the patient becomes hyperosmolar. This is known as hyperosmolar non-ketosis (HONK) or hyperglycaemic hyperosmolar nonketotic syndrome (HHNK) (Braun & Anderson 2011).

Diabetic ketoacidosis

Diabetic ketoacidosis is a catastrophic metabolic condition, in which no physiologically significant circulating insulin is present. It results in a metabolic acidosis (pH <7.3 or bicarbonate <15 mmol/litre), ketonuria and often hyperglycaemia (although this is not a necessary criterion). Approximately half of patients with DKA have an underlying source of infection (Noble-Bell & Cox 2014).

Case scenario

A 17-year-old girl with known type 1 diabetes has a long history of non-attendance at clinic and is admitted via the emergency department with abdominal pain and vomiting. You are asked to review her, as she is clearly unwell.

A–Airway
She is maintaining her own airway.

B–Breathing
Her respiratory rate is 30 per minute with saturation of 100% on air. Her chest is clear.

C–Circulation
She is cold and clammy to touch but all pulses are present. She has a blood pressure of 95/50mmHg.

D–Disability
She is drowsy and groaning but responsive to voice. Her capillary blood glucose is noted to be raised, at 14mmol/litre.

E–Exposure and environment
She is covered in vomit.

Physical examination reveals:

- Inspection: As above.
- Palpation: She is guarding over her abdomen.
- Percussion: Her abdomen is tympanic.
- Auscultation: She has a succussion splash (see Box 36.1).

Box 36.1 Succussion splash

To test for a succussion splash, explain to the patient what you are about to do. Place your stethoscope over their stomach and gently rock the abdomen. If there is a large gastric residual (in this case secondary to gastroparesis/gastric stasis), a 'splash' will be heard.

Diagnosing diabetic ketoacidosis

Unless this is a first presentation, the patient will be a known diabetic. They may have had a preceding illness, or they may have missed their insulin. The patient can have a wide variety of symptoms such as abdominal pain and vomiting. They are likely to have polyuria (excessive urine output) and polydipsia (excessive thirst).

On examination, patients vary from acutely unwell to unconscious and peri-arrest. The patient's condition is related to the speed of onset of the illness and the severity of the metabolic disturbance. You may smell acetone (pear drops) on their breath. (See Box 36.2 for criteria for the diagnosis of DKA.)

Box 36.2 Criteria for the diagnosis of diabetic ketoacidosis (JBDS 2013)

1 Hyperglycaemia
Serum glucose of >11 mmol/litre (normal 3.5–7.8mmol/litre) or known diabetes.

2 Ketonaemia
>3.0mmol/litre (normal <0.6mmol/litre) or significant ketonuria
(more than 2+ on standard urine sticks)

May be smelt on the breath as pear drops (acetone).

3 Acidaemia
A pH of <7.3 (normal 7.35–7.45) or serum bicarbonate of <15 mmol/litre (normal 22–26mmol/litre).

A high respiratory rate with normal saturations could be a sign of acidosis. Not all diabetic ketoacidotic patients have a particularly raised blood glucose.
Some people cannot smell pear drop breath.

Pathophysiology, aetiology and mechanism of condition and therapy

Diabetes care and support have improved in recent years but some patients find it difficult to accept their condition and comply with their treatment. These issues often complicate their care so it is important to contact the diabetic team for information (Noble-Bell & Cox 2014). Engaging some patients can be challenging, and it is essential to take a non-critical approach.

The patient in the case scenario has lost contact with her diabetes service and is likely to be neglecting glycaemic control. It is still possible that she has another underlying medical condition that has precipitated her deterioration. Hyperglycaemia itself causes gastroparesis, vomiting and abdominal pain so this may be a manifestation of DKA, rather than the primary pathology.

Despite having hyperglycaemic serum, her intracellular glucose is low, and insulin signalling is essential for transmembrane glucose transport. Soon the intracellular glucose is used up and the body switches to fat metabolism. The metabolism of fat leads to the production of ketones and acidaemia (Braun & Anderson 2011).

Patients with hyperglycaemia often pass glucose into their urine and this acts as an osmotic diuretic, causing excessive loss of water and electrolytes. The patients often feel very thirsty but, if they are unable to drink, they will get dehydrated very quickly. Patients can be grossly dehydrated (by up to 10 litres or more) – in both intracellular and extracellular compartments – due to the fluid shifts that occur during DKA.

Assessment, monitoring and management

Every unit should have its own DKA guidelines, which should be followed meticulously. Early discussion with a diabetologist or diabetic nurse specialist should be sought for every patient in DKA. Often, these staff members will know the patient well or will have been looking after them for many years. Early aggressive treatment can give satisfying results but it is not uncommon for a patient to decline or fail to improve if not carefully monitored. A venous line occlusion or insulin pump failure can be left alarming for a few minutes, leading to a decline in the patient's clinical condition. Meticulous monitoring of infusions and serum biochemistry can have the patient well by the next day.

A-Airway

In this case scenario, the patient is maintaining their airway. If there is any change in conscious level then airway protection is vital. Patients with DKA have a high incidence of vomiting and are at high risk of aspiration.

B-Breathing

Patients may seem to have abnormally deep and laboured respirations as a way of hyperventilating to combat acidosis. This is known as Kussmaul's breathing (Noble-Bell & Cox 2014). The treatment described below will reduce the metabolic acidosis and improve respiratory pattern.

If the oxygen saturation level falls, an arterial blood gas and chest X-ray are indicated (JBDS 2013).

C-Circulation

Vital signs should be monitored according to local guidelines (usually a minimum of half-hourly in the acute phase), including accurate fluid balance. Tachycardia and hypotension may be seen, due to dehydration (Noble-Bell & Cox 2014) and there is a risk of cardiac arrhythmias, due to hypokalaemia.

Key investigations are (JBDS 2013, p. 18):

- Blood ketones (recommended hourly)
- Capillary blood glucose
- Venous plasma glucose
- Urea and electrolytes
- Venous blood gases

- Full blood count
- Blood cultures
- ECG
- Chest radiograph if clinically indicated
- Urinalysis and culture
- Continuous cardiac monitoring.

Restoring fluid volume, establishing glycaemic control and maintaining electrolyte balance are key to successful management.

Fluid management

Fluids (0.9% saline) need to be commenced before initiating the insulin regime. Establishing venous access is a priority. If blood pressure (BP) is <90mmHg, a fluid challenge of 500ml 0.9% saline over 10–15 minutes is recommended (JBDS 2013). This can be repeated if the patient's BP does not improve.

In the case scenario, the patient's BP is >90mmHg and the JBDS (2013, p. 18) recommend the following:

1. 1 litre 0.9% saline over first hour
2. 1 litre 0.9% saline with potassium chloride over the next 2 hours
3. 1 litre 0.9% saline with potassium chloride over the next 2 hours
4. 1 litre 0.9% saline with potassium chloride over the next 4 hours
5. 1 litre 0.9% saline with potassium chloride over the next 4 hours
6. 1 litre 0.9% saline with potassium chloride over the next 6 hours.

Remember that some patients may require 0.5% dextrose solution, to maintain blood glucose and prevent hypoglycaemia, as they respond to the treatment regime.

Insulin

The JBDS (2013) recommend a fixed rate intravenous insulin infusion (FRIII) of 0.1 units/kg/hour in DKA (or follow local hospital guidelines) because this takes into account the individual patient's requirements. Only a small amount of insulin is needed to switch off fatty acid metabolism. Intravenous human soluble insulin (such as Actrapid™) has a half-life of 4–7 minutes; and a regime of 50 units insulin in 50ml of 0.9% saline is suggested. It is important that the infusion is not interrupted (for instance, by bending of the arm, occlusion of the infusion, or if the pump stops), as the patient can deteriorate very quickly.

The aim of treatment is (JBDS 2013, p. 19) to:

- Reduce blood ketones by 0.5mmol/litre/hr
- In the absence of ketone measurements, aim to increase bicarbonate by 3mmol per hour and decrease blood glucose by 3mmol per hour
- Avoid hypoglycaemia.

If these targets are not achieved, the insulin regime may be increased by 1 unit/hour (JBDS 2013). Continue the FRIII until the ketone measurement is less than 0.6mmol/litre, venous pH over 7.3 and/or venous bicarbonate over 18mmol/litre (JBDS 2013, p. 20).

Once the DKA has resolved and the patient can eat and drink, a subcutaneous dose of insulin can be given (usually before a meal) and the insulin infusion discontinued one hour later (see JBDS 2013 guidelines for more details). Newly diagnosed diabetics should be commenced on a human NPH insulin (such as Lantus® or Levemir®) to prevent rebound ketosis.

An easy to remember sliding scale infusion is set up as 50 units of short-acting insulin (e.g. human Actrapid™), made up to 50ml with 0.9% saline and infused in conjunction with fluid replacement. In patients with DKA, a fixed rate intravenous insulin infusion (FRIII) of 0.1 units/kg/hour is recommended (JBDS 2013).

HOT TIP

A type 1 diabetic *must* always have a small dose of insulin in progress, even if their blood sugar is low or normal. This is because the short half-life of intravenous insulin means that, within an hour, the capillary blood glucose will rise and the patient will be ketotic again.

Potassium

The patient is initially acidaemic, dehydrated and insulin depleted; this leads to hyperkalaemia as potassium leaks from intracellular to extracellular spaces. As the insulin regime is established, the biochemistry corrects and potassium re-enters the cell. It is not uncommon to see a dramatic drop in the serum potassium (Noble-Bell & Cox 2014), which can lead to life-threatening complications (such as arrhythmias). Serum potassium should therefore be closely monitored (at least every 4 hours initially).

JBDS (2013, p. 19) recommend:

- No potassium replacement required if blood level is >5.5mmol/litre
- 40mmol/litre potassium replacement if blood level is 3.5–5.5mmol/litre
- If blood level <3.5mmol/litre, urgent senior advice should be sought.

Remember that potassium chloride cannot normally be administered in concentrations greater than 40mmol/litre in the ward setting – check your local policies.

Disability

The patient may require a urinary catheter to be inserted, to monitor fluid balance. A nasogastric tube may also be required, to drain gastric contents and prevent aspiration, especially if the patient has a decreased level of consciousness.

Blood samples (particularly pH, bicarbonate and U&Es) will be required at regular intervals – usually at 2 hours, 6 hours and 12 hours.

Exposure

The patient needs to be examined for possible sites of infection or injuries that may have led to the DKA. Women of child-bearing age should have a pregnancy test (JBDS 2013).

Aftercare

An episode of DKA should never be assumed to be a 'one-off'. There are a number of treatment options available to the diabetes team, following an episode of DKA. They may know the patient well and be able to offer physical, social and psychological support, in conjunction with community services. To prevent long-term problems, reduce the chance of readmission, and provide continuity of care, patients should be seen by the diabetes team prior to discharge.

Hyperglycaemic hyperosmolar nonketotic syndrome (HHNK)

HHNK is less common than DKA in current western practice. Patients with HHNK are usually older, have multiple comorbidities, have a very high glucose, and have a high mortality. The deterioration is often triggered by sepsis. As the patient is not ketotic, they can progress to more marked hyperglycaemia until their blood becomes thicker and more viscous (hyperosmolar). This leads to the patient being more at high risk of ischaemic or thrombotic events (Scott 2006).

If the serum sodium is high in a hyperglycaemic patient, this should raise the suspicion of HHNK. Sending a serum osmolality as well as a glucose on these patients will confirm the diagnosis. (See Box 36.3 for more on diagnosing HHNK.)

Box 36.3 Diagnosis of hyperglycaemic hyperosmolar nonketotic syndrome (HHNK)

Signs indicating HHNK:

- Blood glucose >35mmol/litre
- Serum osmolality >320mmol/litre
- Dehydration
- No ketosis
- Reduced conscious level.

Patients with HHNK have a high mortality and care needs to be taken not to fluid-overload the patient or correct the biochemistry too fast. The full management of HHNK is beyond the scope of this book but most hospitals have treatment guidelines that can be followed.

Conclusion

DKA is a time-consuming medical emergency that requires attention to detail. Careful maintenance of insulin and fluid infusions, close biochemical monitoring and airway protection to prevent aspiration are all required. It is quite rewarding to see both the patient and their biochemistry gradually improve as a direct result of your care.

References and further reading

Braun, C.A. & Anderson, C.M. (2011). *Pathophysiology: A Clinical Approach.* 2nd edn. Philadelphia: Lippincott, Williams & Wilkins.

De Beer, K., Michael, S., Thacker, M. *et al.* (2008). Diabetic ketoacidosis and hyperglycaemic hyperosmolar syndrome – Clinical guidelines. *Nursing in Critical Care.* **13**(1), 5–11.

Joint British Diabetics Societies (JBDS) (2013). *The management of diabetic ketoacidosis in adults.* http://www.diabetologists-abcd.org.uk/JBDS/JBDS_IP_DKA_Adults_Revised.pdf (Accessed 5 April 2015).

Noble-Bell, G. & Cox, A. (2014). Management of diabetic ketoacidosis in adults. *Nursing Times.* **10** (10), 14–17.

Pessin, E. & Saltiel, A. (2000). Signaling pathways in insulin action: molecular targets of insulin resistance. *Journal of Clinical Investigation.* **106** (2), 165–69.

Scott, A. (2006). Hyperosmolar hyperglycaemic syndrome. *Diabetic Medicine.* **23** (3), 22–41.

Useful websites

Association of British Clinical Diabetologists
http://www.diabetologists-abcd.org.uk/home.htm
(Accessed 13 August 2015)

Diabetes UK
https://www.diabetes.org.uk/
(Accessed 13 August 2015)

National Institute for Health and Care Excellence
http://www.nice.org.uk/
(Accessed 13 August 2015)

37 Neurogenic shock

Ann M. Price

Neurogenic shock is most commonly associated with spinal cord injuries. However, the incidence of neurogenic shock is lower than expected. Guly *et al.* (2008) noted that neurogenic shock was a complication in 19% of cervical spinal injury cases, in 7% of thoracic spinal injury cases and only 3% of lumbar spinal injuries in the initial emergency phase. Gawor *et al.* (2012) note that spinal injuries can also be due to falls, violence and sports injuries and the average patient age is increasing, meaning that more elderly patients are affected. Whatever the cause, neurogenic shock is a life-threatening complication of spinal cord injury that needs to be recognised and treated promptly.

The National Institute for Health and Care Excellence (NICE) is due to publish guidelines on the assessment of spinal injuries, related to trauma, in 2016. Neurogenic shock is usually described as hypotension in the presence of a spinal injury when other possible causes have been excluded (Summers *et al.* 2012). By the end of this chapter, you should understand how to diagnose, treat and manage patients with neurogenic shock.

Definitions, signs and symptoms

The terms neurogenic shock and spinal shock are often used interchangeably (Fox 2014) but there are some important differences.

Neurogenic shock (Summers *et al.* 2012)

This usually occurs in spinal injuries. It is characterised by hypotension, bradycardia, reduced cardiac output and hypothermia due to disruption to sympathetic nerve impulses. It is more usually associated with lesions at T6 and above.

Spinal shock (Fox 2014)

This is a transient depression of cord reflexes below the level of injury. There is a loss of all sensorimotor functions and catecholamine release causes an initial increase in blood pressure followed by hypotension. The symptoms, including flaccid paralysis and bowel and bladder dysfunction, last from hours to weeks until the reflex arcs below the injury level start to function.

Autonomic dysreflexia (AD)

This is a syndrome that occurs in spinal cord injury patients where massive reflex sympathetic discharge leads to hypertension, bradycardia, profuse sweating and flushed appearance (Stephenson & Berliner 2015). The syndrome usually occurs in patients where the injury is above the splanchnic sympathetic outflow (T5–T6). Usually AD results when reflexes return after a period of spinal shock.

> ### Case scenario
>
> A 23-year-old man was involved in a motorcycle accident earlier today. He has suffered a spinal injury at C5 level and is being cared for on an orthopaedic ward until a specialist opinion is sought. He says he is feeling unwell and observations note hypotension at 80mmHg systolic blood pressure, a pulse of 60 beats per minute and a temperature of 35°C.

Box 37.1 Indicative signs of neurogenic shock (Summers *et al.* 2012)

- Hypotension
- Bradycardia
- Reduced cardiac output
- Hypothermia.

Pathophysiology

The autonomic nervous system contains both sympathetic and parasympathetic motor fibres. These fibres are important for the function of smooth muscle, including cardiac muscle. The sympathetic pathways are mainly transported via the spinal cord, whereas the parasympathetic pathways are mainly transported via the vagal nerve (tenth cranial nerve) (Ciechanowski *et al.* 2005). This difference in nerve impulses explains why, in spinal injuries, the sympathetic pathways are suppressed and the parasympathetic dominate.

Thus, patients with high spinal cord injuries lack sympathetic stimulation and are prone to bradycardia, hypotension secondary to vascular dilation (Fox 2014) and hypothermia due to dilation and heat loss. Summers *et al.* (2012) note that hypotension under 100mmHg and bradycardia below 80 beats per minute are considered significant signs of neurogenic shock. Other functions that are affected due to the loss of sympathetic input include bowel and bladder function.

Monitoring and management

Any patient with a spinal injury will initially need close and frequent monitoring to identify neurogenic shock. This includes temperature, blood pressure, respirations and continuous cardiac monitoring via an ECG machine. Patients will require large-bore cannulae (Fox 2014) and may require invasive monitoring such as arterial and central venous lines for fluid management.

In multiple trauma situations, the condition is complicated by the possibility of hypovolaemic shock from bleeding, and the masking of injuries by an absence of pain below the spinal lesion. These cases will require critical care and trauma centre referral.

Treatment of hypotension is initially with fluid challenges. The patient may require large volumes of fluid to compensate for the vasodilation and venous pooling of blood that occurs, although care must be taken to avoid fluid overload (Fox 2014). Patients who are unresponsive to fluids should be considered for vasopressor drugs (Fox 2014), such as norepinephrine via a central line, to induce vascoconstriction. Bradycardia can be limited by the use of atropine, although Bilello *et al.* (2003) note that a number of patients will require cardiac pacing to treat the bradycardia associated with neurogenic shock. Patients should be kept warm using blankets and other aids but this can induce further hypotension, which should be corrected quickly.

Patients who develop neurogenic shock should ideally be managed within a critical care setting until they have stabilised and no longer require intensive treatment.

Box 37.2 Management of neurogenic shock

- Initially fluid challenges for hypotension
- If hypotension is not resolved by fluid, administer vasopressor drugs
- Atropine or pacing for bradycardia
- Use warming aids but this may reduce blood pressure further
- Manage in a critical care unit with continuous ECG monitoring
- Referral and advice from a spinal injuries centre is vital.

Conclusion

Several syndromes are associated with spinal injuries, with varying time frames for onset. Neurogenic shock is an early and life-threatening complication of spinal injury that needs swift fluid resuscitation and management of bradycardia to compensate for vascular dilation and hypotension.

References and further reading

Bilello, J.F., Davis, J.W., Cunningham, M.A., Groom, T.F., Lemaster, D. & Sue, L.P. (Oct 2003). Cervical spinal cord injury and the need for cardiovascular intervention. *Archives of Surgery.* **138** (10), 1127–29.

Ciechanowski, M., Mower-Wade, D., McLeskey, S.W. & Stout, L. (2006). 'Anatomy and physiology of the nervous system' in P.G. Morton, D.K. Fontaine, C.M. Hudak & B.M. Gallo (eds) (2006) in *Critical Care Nursing: a Holistic Approach.* 8th edn. Philadelphia: Lippincott, Williams & Wilkins.

Fox, A. (Nov 2014). Assessment and treatment of spinal cord injuries and neurogenic shock. *Journal of Emergency Medical Services.* http://www.jems.com/article/patient-care/assessment-and-treatment-spinal-cord-inj (Accessed 18 December 2014).

Gawor, G., Biese, K. & Platts-Mills, T.F. (2012). Delay in spinal cord injury due to sedation; a case report. *The Journal of Emergency Medicine.* **43** (6), e413–e418.

Guly, H.R., Bouramra, O. & Lecky, F.E. (2008). The incidence of neurogenic shock in patients with isolated spinal cord injury in the emergency department (on behalf of Trauma Audit and Research Network). *Resuscitation.* **6** (1), 57–62.

Stephenson, R.O. & Berliner, J. (2015). *Autonomic Dysreflexia in Spinal Cord Injury.* http://emedicine.medscape.com/article/322809-overview (accessed 13 September 2015).

Summers, R.L., Stephen, O., Baker, D., Sterling, S.A., Porter, J.M. & Jones, A.E. (2012). Characterization of the spectrum of hemodynamic profiles in trauma patients with acute neurogenic shock. *Journal of Critical Care.* **28** (4), 531.e1–531.e5.

Useful websites

US National Library of Medicine

http://www.nlm.nih.gov/medlineplus/spinalcordinjuries.html

(Accessed 17 August 2015)

Hub Pages

http://medicalmd.hubpages.com/hub/Neurogenic-Shock-Definition-Symptoms-Causes-Treatment

(Accessed 17 August 2015)

38 Severe acute pain

Jane Donn

For a number of reasons, the relief of acute pain is often poorly managed. A general lack of understanding of the pharmacology and pharmacokinetics of analgesia, compounded with inappropriate attitudes and organisational barriers, has left the acutely ill patient exposed to the harmful side effects of unresolved pain.

By the end of this chapter you will be able to identify the patient in acute pain; have a working knowledge of the harmful effects of unresolved acute pain; and be able to direct logical prescribing of the most commonly used analgesics. You will also have an awareness of potential barriers to effective pain management; and understand the role of patient-controlled and epidural analgesia in the acutely unwell patient.

Understanding pain

The International Association for the Study of Pain describes pain as 'an unpleasant sensory and emotional experience associated with actual or potential tissue damage, or described in terms of such damage' (Merskey & Bogduk 1994). Acute pain is defined as 'pain of recent onset and probable limited duration. It usually has an identifiable temporal and causal relationship to injury or disease' (Ready & Edwards 1992).

The ability to detect noxious and potentially tissue-damaging stimuli is an important protective mechanism that involves both central and peripheral mechanisms. Pain may be classified by inferred physiology into two major types: *nociceptive pain*, in which stimuli arise from somatic and visceral structures; and *neuropathic pain* (Braun & Anderson 2011), in which stimuli are abnormally processed by the nervous system. Nociceptive pain is the type most often encountered in the acute setting.

The four basic processes of pain transmission (Braun & Anderson 2011) are:

- Transduction: This process occurs in the periphery when a noxious stimulus causes tissue damage. The damaged cell releases sensitising substances that cause an action potential.

- Transmission: The action potential is transmitted from the site of the damage to the spinal cord and on to the higher centres.

- Perception of pain: This is the conscious experience of pain.
- Modulation: The neurons originating in the brainstem descend to the spinal cord and release endogenous opioids, serotonin and norepinepherine, which inhibit the transmission of nociceptive impulses (Pasero *et al.* 1999).

In addition, the perception and experience of pain is overlaid with psychological, cultural and environmental factors (Linton 2005, Pavlin *et al.* 2005).

Harmful effects of unresolved pain

The presence of trauma, surgical insult or the pain of disease triggers a number of physiological responses. This is called the 'stress response' and its purpose is to activate the sympathetic nervous system and alert the body to impending or existing harm. If left unmanaged, this response can lead to a number of harmful effects (Desborough 2000), as outlined in Table 38.1.

In addition to these potentially life-threatening physiological effects, there is a basic humanitarian imperative to prevent suffering in a fellow human being. This philosophy is supported by Liebskind and Melzack, cited by Harmer (2007), who believe that by any standard, freedom from pain should be a basic human right. Its limitations should only be our current evidence and knowledge regarding treatment.

Table 38.1 The effects of pain on the body (adapted from Pasero *et al.* 1999)

System	Physiological changes	Effect on the body
Endocrine	• Increased ACTH, cortisol, ADH, epinephrine, glucagon, renin, angiotensin II, catecholamines • Decreased insulin, testosterone	• Excess production of hormones
Metabolic	• Hyperglycaemia • Insulin resistance • Muscle protein catabolism	• Raised blood sugar
Cardiovascular	• Increased heart rate, myocardial oxygen consumption, SVR • Hyper coagulation	• Hypertension, DVT • Myocardial ischaemia • Tachycardia
Respiratory	• Decrease tidal volume, cough • Splinting • Increased respiratory rate	• Sputum retention • Chest infection • Hypoxaemia
Genitourinary	• Increased release of hormones regulating urinary output	• Urinary output down • Urinary retention • Hypokalaemia • Fluid overload
Gastrointestinal	• Decreased gastric and bowel activity	• Delay in return to function

Musculoskeletal	• Fatigue • Immobility	• Pressure damage • DVT • Chest infection
Immune	• Depression of immune system	• Pneumonia • Wound infection • Sepsis

ACTH, adrenocorticotrophic hormone; ADH, antidiuretic hormone; DVT, deep vein thrombosis; SVR, systemic vascular resistance.

Case scenario

A 29-year-old man attends A&E with a history of upper abdominal pain. He describes it as severe, deep and gnawing. It travels from left of the midline through to his back. He rates the severity as 10 out of 10. The pain is reduced when he leans forward. He is sweaty and distressed.

He has been vomiting, complains of breathlessness and has a fever. His vital signs are BP 102/56mmHg, temperature 38.2°C, heart rate 119 beats per minute, and oxygen saturation is 92% on air. He has decreased breath sounds. Bowel sounds are sluggish.

Blood tests show an amylase of 938 U/L, white blood cell count of 11.2 x 10^9/L, sodium 141mmol/litre, potassium 3.1mmol/litre, creatinine 117μmol/litre, and blood glucose 10.3mmol/litre.

He gives a history of attending a stag weekend in Scotland and becoming unwell on the journey home. He admits to drinking large quantities of alcohol over two days. He has no allergies.

On catheterisation, his urine is dark and concentrated and there is a residual volume of 110ml.

Assessing pain

The starting point of any successful pain management plan must be assessment. Because pain is a subjective experience, the gold standard is the patient's self-report of pain (McCaffery & Pasero 1999). This approach may cause concern for those who fear being duped, but it should be remembered that malingerers are rare. Although accepting every patient report of pain may result in being fooled by the few, the alternative is to doubt every patient and risking 'under-analgesing' the vast majority. If a patient is successful in duping a healthcare professional, the responsibility rests with that patient.

Different types of validated pain assessment tool are available to the clinician and it is important to choose the right tool for the specific clinical situation (Bird 2003). For the unwell patient in acute pain, there are two main elements of the initial assessment – how *much* does it hurt and *where* does it hurt?

How much does it hurt?

The unwell patient does not want to be bothered with charts and diagrams – they just want to quickly get over to you how bad things are. To this end, the most useful tool is a numerical pain scale. The most commonly used scale is a 0–10 scale, where 0 is no pain on movement and 10 is the worst pain imaginable, but others can be used. The important factor is that the same scale is used throughout the patient's journey to ensure consistency. The patient in this case scenario rated his pain as 10.

Once the pain is better under control and the patient's condition has been stabilised, a more detailed pain history can be taken. While nociceptive pain is more frequently seen in the acute setting, misdiagnosing neuropathic pain may lead to delay in appropriate treatment. Features that may suggest neuropathic pain include (Hogan-Quigley *et al.* 2012):

- Pain described as burning, shooting or stabbing
- Hyperalgesia (a heightened response to normally painful stimulus)
- Allodynia (abnormal response to a stimuli that does not normally cause pain such as light stroking)
- Abnormal or unpleasant sensations such as crawling, numbness or tingling (Stacey 2005).

While neuropathic pain may be partially responsive to opioids, the ongoing management can be complex and the clinician is advised to obtain advice from the hospital pain team, or the team responsible for the patient's pain management.

Where does it hurt?

As well as ascertaining how bad the pain is, it is important to regularly check *where* the pain is. Patients do not always think to mention that the pain is now in their chest or other leg, and changes in their clinical condition may therefore be missed. This is particularly important to remember if the patient is administering their own analgesia. Any acute change in the severity or nature of the pain in a patient whose pain has previously been well managed must result in a full reassessment.

An inability to communicate does not mean that the patient is not experiencing pain. In the absence of a patient self-report, a commonsense approach should be adopted. If a broken leg would reasonably give you pain, then it will be giving your patient pain too. In addition, behavioural responses (such as a particular facial expression or a reluctance to use a limb) or physiological responses (such as a tachycardia or raised blood pressure) can indicate that your patient is in pain (Davies *et al.* 2004). Patients with special needs or communication difficulties may need additional help to express their pain. A carer, close relative or friend may be familiar with how the patient is responding and know how to help the staff caring for them elicit a pain assessment.

The pain management plan

Once a pain management plan has been formulated, pain assessment needs to be ongoing to enable evaluation of the plan. Further uncontrolled pain should trigger a reassessment of the diagnosis or alert healthcare staff to developing complications.

Having identified that the patient is in pain, action needs to be swift, especially if the patient is also unwell. The healthcare professional has access to effective analgesics but they are often not used effectively. Keeping things simple, and using these analgesics well, will improve pain management for 99% of patients.

Step 1

Exclude any medications that the patient is allergic to, or that are contraindicated (such as non-steroidal anti-inflammatory drugs in poor renal function, clotting abnormality and gastric ulceration). Ensure that the patient is reporting an allergy and not a side effect that can be managed (such as nausea with opioids). Also consider what analgesics have already been tried and how the pain responded to them.

Caution is required if using opioids in patients with major organ failure. In this case, start with less than the usual recommended dose and titrate gradually upward. All opioids are metabolised to some extent by the liver, and in patients with liver disease adverse effects may be seen from higher than expected plasma concentrations. The metabolism of morphine and methadone is not significantly altered in liver disease, so these drugs are well tolerated (Portenoy 1996). However, methadone should only be used for pain management under the supervision of a pain specialist.

Caution and close monitoring are recommended when using morphine in a patient with renal insufficiency. Synthetic opioids, such as hydromorphone or oxycodone, may be better tolerated (Portenoy 1996). In moderate to severe renal insufficiency, opioids that are not renally excreted (such as buprenorphine or fentanyl) may be required.

There is no rationale for delaying the appropriate administration of an opioid to a patient presenting with an acute abdomen. There is good evidence that opioids can be safely given before assessment and diagnosis without increasing the risk of errors in diagnosis or treatment (National Institute for Clinical Studies 2008).

For the patient in the case scenario, non-steroidal anti-inflammatory analgesics are contraindicated, due to poor renal function.

Step 2

After allergies and contraindications have been taken into account, the next step is to choose an analgesic of the appropriate efficacy. This can be easier said than done. There are many myths and misconceptions about the relative efficacy of analgesics amongst healthcare professionals. This has led to mass under-dosing of patients and inappropriate preparations being used.

Thankfully, researchers have developed league tables that can enable logical progression of prescribing. Analgesics at different strengths, and by different routes, are allocated a 'number needed to treat' (NNT). The NNT is calculated from the proportion of patients with at least 50% pain relief over 4–6 hours, compared with placebo (in randomised, double-blind, single dose studies in patients with moderate to severe pain). The lower the NNT, the more effective that drug or dose is likely to be. Although the NNT may vary between individual patients, it is a good place to start. The NNT table is available from the Oxford Pain Research Unit site (2008). Remember that relative strength may be dose related.

In the current case scenario, the patient requires an easily titratable analgesic that is suitable for severe pain. Opioids are the analgesic group of choice. Non-steroidal anti-inflammatory analgesics can be very effective for severe pain, but were contraindicated in this case. (see Box 38.1 for Overview of available analgesics)

HOT TIP

The 'Electronic Medicines Compendium (eMC)' lists numerous drugs and gives full information about uses, dosage, cautions and contraindications at: https://www.medicines.org.uk/emc/

Step 3

Having decided what you are *not* going to give your patient and which analgesics are likely to be effective, the available routes of administration need to be considered (see Box 38.2). Does the patient have intravenous access? Is the oral route appropriate? Can the rectal route be utilised?

Step 4

Another and sometimes unsatisfactory consideration is when the patient asks 'what is available to me?' Different institutions have different formularies and this may unfortunately play a part in your decision-making. Short-acting preparations are the most appropriate for quick titration of analgesia.

Box 38.1 Overview of available analgesics

Paracetamol: This is an important, but sometimes overlooked, drug when planning an effective analgesic regime. Its mechanism of action is not clearly understood but it is primarily thought to be a cyclooxygenase inhibitor, acting through the central nervous system. It is well absorbed from the gastrointestinal tract, whereas rectal administration is unpredictable and erratic. The intravenous preparation is undoubtedly being more commonly used in the acute setting. Intravenous dosing must be carefully based on the patient's weight. Studies have shown that, when taken at recommended doses, paracetamol can be used safely in patients with liver disease (Benson *et al.* 2005).

Non-steroidal anti-inflammatory drugs (NSAIDs): These can be very effective for many patients but are often the most troublesome, in terms of side effects and contraindications, for the acutely unwell patient. NSAIDs work by reducing prostaglandin and other mediator synthesis chemicals, causing pain and inflammation. However, prostaglandins and other mediators have beneficial effects on platelet function, renal blood flow and bronchodilation. NSAIDs should therefore be avoided in any patient with:

- Renal impairment
- Active bleeding (or high likelihood of bleeding)
- An active or past history of gastric ulceration
- Heart failure
- Severe asthma.

NSAIDs also increase the risk of cardiovascular events. Diclofenac is associated with higher cardiovascular risks than the other non-selective NSAIDs, and similar cardiovascular risks to the COX-2 inhibitors. Naproxen and low-dose ibuprofen are still considered to have the most favourable cardiovascular safety profiles of all non-selective NSAIDs. For all patients, NSAIDs should be prescribed at the lowest effective dose and for the shortest time necessary (NICE 2013).

Some analgesics are limited in use due to a maximum safe daily dose, e.g. paracetamol.

Opioids: At doses that are not causing over-sedation or respiratory depression, opioids do not have a maximum daily dose. They are therefore important in the management of severe acute pain.

Morphine should be considered the first-line strong opioid. Oxycodone is an alternative, should the patient experience intolerable side effects from morphine.

Codeine alone has limited use in the management of severe pain. Once absorbed, codeine is metabolised in the liver to morphine, its active form (Reisine & Pasternak 1996). However, up to 8% of Caucasians cannot metabolise codeine (Kroemer & Eichelbaum 1995).

Pethidine is arguably the most inappropriately used opioid for moderate to severe acute pain and therefore not recommended. Pethidine is very short acting and therefore the patient is likely to be exposed to periods of unmanaged pain. In addition, and probably more significantly, pethidine has a toxic metabolite, norpethidine. When allowed to accumulate, norpethidine acts on the central nervous system, ultimately causing convulsions, especially (but not exclusively) in patients with renal dysfunction. There is no rationale for choosing pethidine over morphine in patients with biliary colic, as has previously been suggested (Nagle & McQuay 1990).

Adjuvants: In some cases, where pain control is complicated by pre-existing high opioid use, drugs such as ketamine and clonidine may be required. These should only be prescribed by experienced practitioners and following local protocols. Antineuropathics may also be beneficial, depending on the underlying cause of the pain.

In acutely unwell patients, remember:

- The intravenous route is the preferred choice
- The intramuscular route of administration is not recommended
- Transdermal preparations play no part in acute pain management.

Step 5

The next step is to ensure that your ongoing analgesic regime is balanced. Reliance on a single analgesic may necessitate its use at high doses and is therefore likely to be more troublesome. As a general rule, choose one analgesic from each group and use them together (e.g. paracetamol and diclofenac and morphine) but not two from the same group.

Table 38.2 shows the main analgesic groups. The patient in our case scenario should be administered up to 10mg morphine intravenously and 1g paracetamol intravenously. He should be assessed for effect after 5 and 15 minutes. The initial dose of morphine is the start dose only. Be prepared to adjust. There is no correlation between weight and analgesic requirements. Age, on the other hand, is a valid consideration (Gnjidic *et al.* 2008) and doses should be adjusted for people at the extremes of age (Macintyre & Jarvis 1996, Braun & Anderson 2011).

Box 38.2 Routes of administration

For the relief of severe acute pain, speed is of the essence and the intravenous route is therefore the preferred choice. Fine titration of dose is achievable with this route.

Although commonly used, the intramuscular route of administration is *not* recommended. This route has numerous disadvantages, the key one being unreliable absorption with a 30–60-minute delay to peak effect (Austin *et al.* 1980).

Transdermal preparations play no part in acute pain management.

The route of choice for the case scenario patient is the intravenous route. This allows rapid onset of effect and careful titration of dose.

Barriers to effective pain management

Acute pain management continues to be poorly understood and the effects of unresolved pain discounted. It is important for the healthcare professional to examine their own practice and deal with any education deficits or attitude issues that they have (Clarke *et al.* 1996). The challenge for educational institutions is to ensure that pain management education is high on their list of priorities (Twycross 2000).

It is worth noting that patients attending hospitals with 'self-inflicted' illnesses are often exposed to high levels of prejudice and negative attitude. Healthcare professionals have the same duty of care to these patients and should indeed take the opportunity to exert a positive influence. While nurses and doctors are often keen to promote smoking cessation advice, discussions about alcohol and illicit drug taking are often avoided. When the patient in the current scenario has recovered from this acute episode, the opportunity to provide health education should be taken.

Patients themselves present barriers to successful pain management. Many people are frightened to use opioids because of the risk of addiction, and healthcare professionals often do nothing to correct this misunderstanding. Large studies have estimated an iatrogenic addiction rate of less than 1% (Porter & Jick 1980). The elderly, who are also the most vulnerable, do not like to trouble nursing or medical staff and will suffer in silence. A cultural disposition may also encourage the 'stiff upper lip' approach (Davidhizar & Giger 2004).

Hospital staff encourage the patient to endure mismanaged pain by being positive towards patients who do not request analgesia and negative towards those who do (Carr & Thomas 1997). The correct approach is to actively encourage the patient to report pain (Hogan-Quigley *et al.* 2012) and to simply prescribe analgesia regularly and not on an 'as and when' basis.

Organisational barriers to effective pain management also exist (Schafheutle *et al.* 2001, Mann & Redwood 2000). For example, it is not a legal requirement to double-check controlled drugs but in some institutions it remains a local policy. Double-checking has not prevented error or diversion of drugs but it has been found to cause delay in analgesia administration. These risks need to be weighed up within a culture of patient safety and patient need.

Table 38.2 Analgesic groups, with examples

NSAIDs	Ibuprofen Diclofenac Aspirin Ketorolac Celecoxib
Others	Paracetamol
Opioids (weak)	Codeine Dihydrocodeine Tramadol
Opioids (strong)	Morphine Oxycodone Fentanyl Diamorphine
Adjuvants	Amitriptyline Gabapentin Diazepam
Anaesthetics	Entonox Local anaesthetics

Maintaining analgesia

Once severe escalating pain has been brought under control, a plan for ongoing management is required. There are several options for this. Sticking to the principle of keeping things simple, the oral route is the preferred route. However, this may not be available for the acutely unwell patient – for example, if they are 'nil by mouth' or drowsy. The rectal route is an underused route in the UK. Regular (as opposed to 'as and when') prescribing is likely to be most effective. Long-acting opioid preparations are available, but when dealing with acute escalating pain, short-acting preparations that can be rapidly titrated are required.

Patient-controlled analgesia

The concept of patient-controlled analgesia (PCA) allows very small doses of analgesia to be administered frequently, from a syringe pump with a timing device, on the patient's demand. Thus the patient can titrate their own analgesic dose within certain limits. PCA may be considered but is not suitable for use until pain is under control. It should be used as a 'top-up' rather than a 'catch up'. Patients report positively on its use (Hudcova *et al.* 2005) but it does have disadvantages. It has been effectively used in patients with severe pain from pancreatitis (Di Vadi *et al.* 1999).

Some patients report that nursing staff spend less time with them. Also sleep can be difficult, as pain wakes the patient and it may take some time before enough doses can be taken from the machine to get it back under control. One study using subcutaneous diamorphine for PCA has shown better results for night-time pain relief (Dawson *et al.* 1999).

Continuous infusions of opioids are an alternative but if patients are not suitably observed they may cause more over-sedation because the infusion will continue even if the patient does not require analgesia at that time.

Epidural analgesia

Epidural analgesia is an effective technique for post-operative or trauma pain. The infusion of local anaesthetics and opioids into the epidural space causes blockade of afferent impulses to the brain. It has the potential to provide complete analgesia while the infusion is running. It has one major advantage over other techniques in that it can attenuate the stress response to trauma and surgery, as discussed at the beginning of this chapter (Kehlet & Holte 2001, Fotiadis *et al.* 2004). This is a valuable effect to remember.

The Royal College of Anaethsetists (2010) have produced a Best Practice Guide for using epidural analgesia in hospital. The use of epidural analgesia is contraindicated in patients:

- Who refuse the technique
- Who have local infection around the potential insertion site
- Who have systemic infection or sepsis
- Who have raised intracranial pressure
- Who have some allergy or sensitivity to local anaesthetics
- Who have uncontrolled coagulation disorders.

There are several benefits of epidural analgesia:

- By limiting systemic opioid use and by blocking nociceptive and sympathetic reflexes, duration of post-operative ileus is reduced, which can allow for earlier enteral feeding.
- There is a reduction in the incidence of atelectasis and chest infection.
- There is a reduction in the incidence of myocardial infarction.
- The hypercoagulable response to surgery is attenuated.

Many institutions run a ward-based epidural service and if staff are adequately trained and supervised it is a very safe technique to employ in the general ward area.

Conclusion

This chapter has aimed to present a logical and systematic approach to developing an effective pain management plan for the acutely unwell patient. The benefits of adequate pain management have been outlined, and considerations when assessing and deciding on pain relief have been discussed. The case scenario has shown, in a practical sense, how pain in an acutely unwell person may be managed.

References and further reading

Austin, K., Stapleton, J. & Mather, L. (1980). Multiple intramuscular injections: a major source of variability in analgesic response to Meperidine. *Pain.* **8**, 47–62.

Benson, G.D., Koff, R.S. & Tolman, K.G. (2005). Therapeutic use of acetaminophen in patients with liver disease. *American Journal of Therapeutics.* **12** (2), 133–41.

Bird, J. (2003). Selection of pain measurement tools. *Nursing Standard.* **18** (13), 33–39.

Braun, C.A. & Anderson, C.M. (2011) *Pathophysiology: a clinical approach.* 2nd edition. Philadelphia: Lippincott, Williams & Wilkins

Carr, E.C. & Thomas V.J. (1997). Anticipating and experiencing post-operative pain: the patients' perspective. *Journal of Clinical Nursing.* **6** (3), 191–201.

Clarke, E., French, B., Bilodeau, M., Capasso, V. & Edwards, A. (1996). Pain management knowledge, attitudes and clinical practice: The impact of nurses' characteristics and education. *Journal of Pain and Symptom Management.* **11** (1), 18–31.

Davies, E., Male, M., Reimer, V. & Turner, M. (2004). Pain assessment and cognitive impairment; Part 2. *Nursing Standard.* **19**, (13) 33–40.

Davidhizar, R. & Giger, J. (2004). A review of the literature on care of clients in pain who are culturally diverse. *International Nursing Review.* **51**(1), 47–55.

Dawson, L., Brockbank, K., Carr, E. & Barrett, F. (1999). Improving patients' postoperative sleep: a randomised control study comparing subcutaneous with intravenous patient controlled analgesia. *Journal of Advanced Nursing.* **30** (4), 875–81.

Desborough, J.P. (2000). The stress response to trauma and surgery. *British Journal of Anaesthesia.* **85** (1), 109–17.

Di Vadi, P., Schnepel, B., Bunton, T., Luffingham, N., Condon, D. & Lanigan, C. (1999). The use of patient-controlled analgesia in acute and chronic relapsing pancreatitis. *The Pain Clinic.* **11** (4), 345–48.

Fotiadis, R., Badvie, S., Weston, M. & Allen-Mersh, T. (2004). Epidural analgesia in gastrointestinal surgery. *British Journal of Surgery.* **91**(7), 828–41.

Gnjidic, D., Murnion, B. & Hilmer, S. (2008). Age and opioid analgesia in an acute hospital population. *Age and Aging.* **37**(6), 699–702.

Harmer, M. (2007). Postoperative pain relief – time to take our heads out of the sand? *Anaesthesia.* **46** (3), 167–68.

Hogan-Quigley, B., Palm, M.L. & Bickley, L. (2012). *Bates' Nursing Guide to Physical Examination and History Taking.* London: Lippincott, Williams & Wilkins.

Hudcova, J., McNicol, E., Quah, C., Lau, J. & Carr, D. (2005). Patient controlled intravenous opioid analgesia versus conventional opioid analgesia for postoperative pain control: A quantitative systematic review. *Acute Pain.* **7**, 115–32.

Kehlet, H. & Holte, K. (2001). Effect of postoperative analgesia on surgical outcome. *British Journal of Anaesthesia.* **87** (1), 62–72.

Kroemer, H.K. & Eichelbaum, H.K. (1995). It's the genes stupid; the molecular bases and clinical consequences of genetic cystochrome P450 2D6. *Polymorphism, Life Sciences.* **46** (26), 2285–98.

Linton, S.J. (2000). A review of psychological risk factors in back and neck pain. *Spine.* **25**, 1148–56.

Macintyre, P.E. & Jarvis, D.A. (1996). Age is the best predictor of postoperative morphine requirements. *Pain.* **64**, 357–64.

Mann, E. & Redwood, S. (2000). Improving pain management: breaking down the invisible barrier. *British Journal of Nursing.* **9** (19), 2067–72.

McCaffery, M. & Pasero, C. (1999). 'Assessment. Underlying complexities, misconceptions and practical tools' in M. McCaffery & C. Pasero (eds) *Pain: Clinical Manual.* 2nd ed. St Louis: Mosby.

Merskey, H. & Bogduk, N. (1994). *Pain terms: a current list with definitions and notes on usage. Classification of Chronic Pain.* 2nd edn. Seattle: IASP Publications.

Nagle, K. & McQuay, H. (1990). Opioid receptors: Their role in effect and side-effect. *Current Anaesthesia and Critical Care.* **1**, 247–52.

National Institute for Clinical Studies (2008). *Pain Medication for Acute Abdominal Pain. A summary of best available evidence and information on current clinical practice.* Canberra: National Health and Medical Research Council.

National Institute for Health and Care Excellence (2013). *Non-steroidal anti-inflammatory drugs* http://www.nice.org.uk/guidance/ktt13/chapter/Evidence-context (accessed 19 August 2015).

Oxford Pain Research Unit (2008). *The Oxford League Table of Analgesic Efficacy.* http://www.medicine.ox.ac.uk/bandolier/booth/painpag/acutrev/analgesics/lftab.html (accessed 19 August 2015).

Pasero, C., Paice, J.A. & McCaffery, M. (1999). 'Basic mechanisms underlying the causes and effects of pain' in M. McCaffery & C. Pasero (eds) *Pain: Clinical Manual.* 2nd ed. St Louis: Mosby.

Pavlin, J. D., Sullivan, M. J. L., Freund, P. & Roesen, K. (2005). Catastrophizing; a risk factor for post-surgical pain. *Clinical Journal of Pain.* **21**, 83–90.

Portenoy, R.K. (1996). 'Opioid analgesics', in R. Portenoy & R. Kanner (eds), *Pain Management Theory and Practice.* Philadelphia:

F.A. Davis. 249–76.

Porter, J. & Jick, H. (1980). Addiction rare in patients treated with narcotics. *New England Journal of Medicine.* **302**, 123.

Ready, L.B. & Edwards, W.T. (1992). *Management of Acute Pain; A practical guide. Taskforce on Acute Pain.* Seattle: IASP Publications.

Reisine, T. &Pasternak, G. (1996). Opioid analgesics and antagonists. *The Pharmacological Basis of Therapeutics.* **9**, 521–55.

Royal College of Anaesthetists (2010). *Best Practice in the Management of Epidural Analgesia in the Hospital Setting.* http://www.rcoa.ac.uk/system/files/FPM-EpAnalg2010_1.pdf (accessed 25 September 2015).

Schafheutle, E., Cantrill, J. & Noyce, P. (2001). Why is pain management suboptimal on surgical wards? *Journal of Advanced Nursing.* **33** (6), 728–37.

Stacey, B.R. (2005). Management of peripheral neuropathic pain. *American Journal of Physical Medicine and Rehabilitation.* **84**, S4–S16.

Twycross, A. (2000). Education about pain; a neglected area. *Nurse Education Today.* **20**, 244–53.

39 Nutrition in the acutely unwell patient

Wendy-Ling Relph

The importance of nutrition in the critically ill patient cannot be overstated. It is vital to aid healing, hasten recovery and improve prognosis. In the acute situation, a patient's nutritional state is often not considered part of the priority assessment or treatment. Yet a poor nutritional state may have contributed to the patient's deterioration and is likely to be a consequence of the illness.

By the end of this chapter you will be able to assess the acute patient's nutritional requirements, improve their nutritional intake, and take steps to avoid the risks of malnutrition and refeeding syndrome.

Background and definitions

When someone is acutely unwell, they need to eat the right foods, in the right amounts, at the right time (Royal College of Nursing (RCN) 2008). However, there are some significant concerns relating to patient malnutrition in the UK:

- Malnutrition is estimated to affect 1 in 7 patients over 65 years of age (British Association for Parenteral and Enteral Nutrition (BAPEN) 2012b).
- Between 30% and 40% of people admitted to hospitals, care homes or mental health units are at risk of malnutrition (BAPEN 2008).
- 1 in 3 adults admitted to hospital or care homes are malnourished on admission (Best 2011) suggesting poor nutritional status in the community.
- Malnutrition is estimated to cost the UK more than £ 13 billion a year (BAPEN 2011).
- Malnourished patients stay in hospital longer, are more likely to develop complications during surgery, and have a higher mortality rate (BAPEN 2011 & 2012a).

Patients with a critical illness may be unable to eat, have restricted diets, poor appetites or be 'nil by mouth' (Moore & Woodrow 2004). Patients with symptoms such as pyrexia, increased respiratory rate and tachycardia will have increased metabolic rates because increased energy is required to maintain this state and to recover from this acute stage of illness. If the supply of energy from nutrition is not sufficient, catabolism begins to occur. This is when the body starts to break down muscle in order to use the protein molecules to provide energy. This leads to muscle weakness, resulting in increased risk of the patient falling over. In severe cases, it can start to break down the heart muscle and eventually lead to death.

Most acute patients will need increased opportunities to eat food that is high in calories and protein. They may need additional supplements or they may need to be artificially fed. A nutritional care plan (based on screening and assessment of the patient's nutritional status) should be instigated as soon as possible after the onset of critical illness and ideally within the first 24–48 hours.

Malnutrition

Malnutrition (or undernutrition) is when the body is receiving insufficient nutrients to maintain its normal functions. Nutrition support should be considered in people who are malnourished, as defined by any of the following:

- A body mass index (BMI) of less than 18.5kg/m²
- Unintentional weight loss greater than 10% within the last 3–6 months
- A BMI of less than 20kg/m² and unintentional weight loss greater than 5% within the last 3–6 months.

Those at risk of malnutrition should also be considered for nutrition support if they have (NICE 2006):

- Eaten little or nothing for more than 5 days and/or are likely to eat little or nothing for 5 days or longer
- A poor absorptive capacity and/or high nutrient losses and/or increased nutritional needs from causes such as catabolism.

Assessing patients' nutritional requirements

The first step in identifying patients who are malnourished or are at risk of becoming malnourished is to use a screening tool. There are many tools available but the one that is used most widely for the general adult patient in hospitals across the UK is the Malnutrition Universal Screening Tool (MUST). This was developed by BAPEN (2003). Other screening tools are used for specific patient groups such as paediatric or renal patients. The locally agreed screening tool should be used to ensure consistency. Screened patients who are at risk of malnutrition should be referred to the dietician and nutrition support teams, depending on local policies, for specialist assessment and further nutritional care. A key point to remember for critically ill patients is that fluid shifts and oedema can cause them to look more overweight than they actually are. (See Figure 39.1.)

Meeting patients' nutritional requirements

Once the risk of malnutrition has been identified, it is important to implement strategies to improve nutritional intake. Many patients who are acutely unwell are unable to eat large amounts of food at designated mealtimes. It is important to ensure that they are given the opportunity to eat small amounts regularly, throughout the day, to ensure that they are able to take in optimum calories and nutrients. This could be in the form of small, regular meals, snacks in between meals and milk-based drinks. Consider:

- Using red food trays or red mats to identify those patients who need monitoring or assistance
- Filling in food and fluid daily record charts to monitor their intake
- Having 'protected mealtimes', to ensure that patients are uninterrupted and have time to eat their meals in a conducive environment.

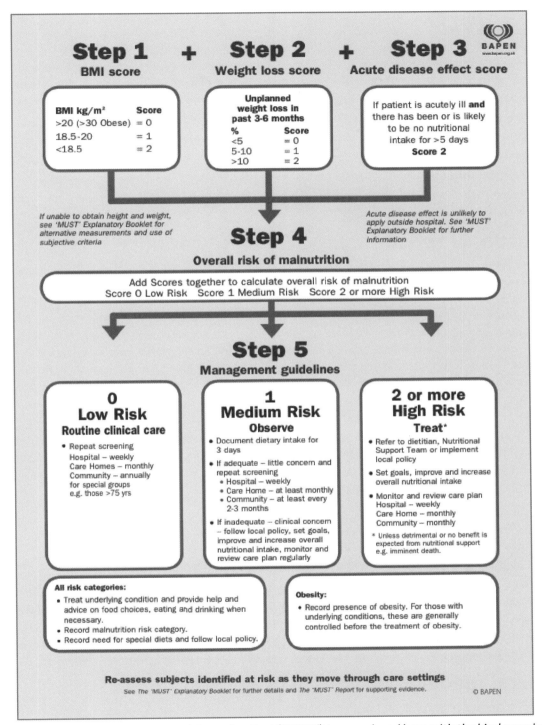

Figure 39.1 *The Malnutrition Universal Screening Tool ('MUST') is reproduced here with the kind permission of the British Association for Parenteral and Enteral Nutrition (BAPEN). Copyright © BAPEN 2012. For further information on 'MUST', see www.bapen.org.uk*

Treatment should always be tailored to the needs of the individual, but in general, if a person is able to eat, then the first step would be to encourage this with a 'Food first' approach. This may be in the form of advice on meals, snacks, nourishing drinks and food fortification. Patients and carers should be involved in these treatment plans, which should include setting goals for treatment and a plan for monitoring to ensure that these goals are met. If simple measures are not working or the patient has a reduced appetite, then dietetic assessment may recommend oral nutritional supplements (BAPEN 2012b).

Nutrition support methods are used to improve or maintain nutritional intake. These include:

- Oral nutrition support – for example, fortified food, additional snacks and/or supplements
- Enteral tube feeding – the delivery of a nutritionally complete feed directly into the gut via a tube
- Parenteral nutrition – the intravenous delivery of nutrition.

All patients who need nutrition support should receive this in a co-ordinated way from the multidisciplinary team.

Nutritional requirements for obese patients

Obese patients are at risk of not being given enough food when acutely ill in hospital. There is a general sense among patients themselves, members of the public and healthcare professionals that obese patients who are acutely ill could use this opportunity to lose weight. However, these patients will have higher than average calorie and nutrient requirements to maintain their bodily functions when healthy. They will therefore need more calories than average to help them recover during their acute phase of illness.

These patients are easily overlooked nutritionally and can slip into a catabolic state if they are not closely monitored. Once these patients are well and over the acute phase of their illness, then discussions can begin about eating more healthily.

Dysphagia

Patients who have had acute or chronic neurological problems, or those who have had treatment to the upper gastrointestinal tract, are at high risk of developing dysphagia (swallowing problems). Some of the more obvious symptoms of dysphagia are:

- Difficulty controlling food or liquid in the mouth
- Drooling
- Speaking with a hoarse or 'wet' voice
- Slow or painful chewing and swallowing
- Coughing or choking during or after swallowing.

Healthcare professionals with relevant skills and training in the diagnosis, assessment and management of swallowing disorders, such as speech and language therapists, should regularly monitor and reassess people with dysphagia. If patients are able to continue to take oral food and drinks, there are some options that may help prevent them aspirating food into their lungs. These include thickening their drinks and puréeing their food. If this is not possible, then enteral feeding may be required.

Enteral feeding

Patients who are critically ill and not able to eat enough to meet their requirements, should receive enteral nutrition (ESPEN 2006). The easiest and most commonly used type of enteral tube feeding in hospital is via the nasogastric (NG) route, which is a tube that is passed through the nose and down into the stomach. This is usually for short-term feeding of less than 4 weeks.

If the patient has delayed gastric emptying, there will be high gastric aspirates and poor absorption rates. To help counteract this, a gut motility agent may be prescribed, such as metoclopramide. For longer-term feeding into the stomach, a tube is usually placed through the abdomen directly into the stomach. This is usually done via endoscopy and known as a percutaneous endoscopic gastrostomy (PEG) or via radiology and known as a radiologically inserted gastrostomy (RIG).

Occasionally it is not possible to use the stomach, due to impaired gastric function or increased vomiting. In this case, one option is to place the feeding tube into the jejunum. For the first 4 weeks, a nasojejunal tube can be used, but for longer-term feeding a jejunostomy tube can be placed directly through the abdominal wall.

The types of enteral feed and the amount of micro-nutrients required should be assessed and monitored by healthcare professionals and dieticians with specialist knowledge. Careful documentation of fluid balance and the amount of feed administered is required to maintain optimum homeostasis (Bloomfield 2012).

Parenteral nutrition

Patients who are malnourished, or at risk of malnutrition, and have a non-functioning, inaccessible or perforated (leaking) gut should be assessed by the multidisciplinary team for parenteral nutrition (PN). PN should be introduced progressively and closely monitored, usually starting at no more than 50% of the patient's estimated needs for the first 24–48 hours. PN can be withdrawn once adequate oral or enteral nutrition is tolerated and nutritional status is stable. Withdrawal should be planned, with a daily review of the patient's progress.

PN is a sterile feed, which can be given directly into the bloodstream via a dedicated centrally placed central venous catheter or a dedicated peripherally inserted central catheter. A free dedicated lumen in a multi-lumen centrally placed catheter may also be used. However, administration of PN via a peripheral venous catheter may be considered for patients who are likely to need short-term PN (less than 14 days) and who have no need for central access for other reasons.

Care should be taken with catheter choice, and in attention to pH, tonicity and long-term compatibility of the PN formulations in order to avoid administration or stability problems. Intravenous catheters should be monitored and managed safely by competent healthcare professionals.

Refeeding syndrome

Nutrition support should be cautiously introduced in seriously ill or injured patients, or those who have eaten little or nothing for more than 5 days. It should be started at no more than 50% of the estimated target energy and protein needs. It should then be built up to meet full needs over the first 24–48 hours, according to metabolic and gastrointestinal tolerance.

If this is not adhered to, refeeding syndrome could result. This is when, due to an episode of starvation, the sudden reintroduction of micro-nutrients can trigger a hormone and electrolyte shift within the body. The main reason for this is that when the high glucose content of feeds is introduced to a previously starved body, excess insulin is produced in order to maintain blood glucose levels. This results in increased cellular uptake of glucose and electrolytes, leading to sudden shifts of fluid (Yantis & Velander 2009).

In these circumstances, it is crucial to closely monitor clinical status and biochemical blood levels. Of particular interest are the phosphorus, potassium and magnesium levels. Healthcare professionals who are competent in monitoring serum levels should be involved in order to rapidly identify whether refeeding syndrome is present, before increasing feed rates to meet full clinical requirements (Mehanna *et al.* 2008).

If refeeding syndrome occurs, symptoms may include abnormal heart rhythm due to potassium imbalance, fluid overload and therefore breathlessness, hypotension and oedema. In severe cases, the patient can suffer from confusion, seizures and eventually death. Close monitoring of serum blood levels and subsequent titration of feeds will help prevent refeeding syndrome. Treatment involves electrolyte replacement, fluid review and symptom control. Refeeding syndrome is rare, but it can have catastrophic effects on patients so those at risk must be monitored closely.

Case scenario

Anne, a 75-year-old woman, is admitted with a fractured neck of femur, following a history of falling over at home. She wears dentures, which fall out when she speaks. She is a widow, who lives alone, and her wedding ring moves easily on her finger. Anne says she eats OK but feels lonely so she often doesn't bother too much if it is just herself eating. She hasn't weighed herself for years and doesn't know if she's lost weight recently. Due to the pain in her hip, you are unable to weigh her. As per BAPEN guidance (2011), you use her mid upper arm circumference to estimate her weight and then work out her 'MUST' score. She has a score of 1, meaning that she is medium risk.

Case scenario considerations

Anne doesn't need immediate referral to dietetics. However, you have noted that her dentures fall out easily and that her wedding ring is loose. These are both indicators suggesting that she has lost weight. She has also admitted to being lonely and possibly not eating as much as she used to.

In order to fully assess her, you should commence a food record chart to understand how much she eats. She should have a red mat or red tray to identify her as needing monitoring of her eating. To help her to eat as much as possible, she should have her likes and dislikes documented and be provided with the meals and snacks that she prefers. She admits to feeling lonely, so a mealtime companion would be useful. This could be a volunteer, other patients eating nearby or a member of the healthcare team. Foods and snacks that are high in calories and full-fat milky drinks will help too.

If her food chart shows that she is eating inadequate amounts after 3 days (despite these amendments to care), she may benefit from being referred to a dietician for specialist assessment and review.

Conclusion

This chapter has outlined the nutritional requirements of an acutely ill patient. It has explained how to assess these requirements and the particular considerations that healthcare professionals need to take into account.

References and further reading

BAPEN (2008). *Nutrition Screening Survey in the UK in 2007: Nutrition Screening Survey and Audit of Adults on Admission to Hospitals, Care Homes and Mental Health Units.*
http://www.bapen.org.uk/pdfs/nsw/nsw07_report.pdf (accessed 21 August 2015).

BAPEN (2011). *The MUST Explanatory Booklet: A guide to the 'Malnutrition Universal Screening Tool (MUST) for adults.* Revised version. Redditch: BAPEN. http://www.bapen.org.uk/pdfs/must/must_explan.pdf (accessed 21 August 2015).

BAPEN (2012a). *The Cost of Disease Related Malnutrition in the UK.* http://www.bapen.org.uk/professionals/publications-and-resources/bapen-reports/the-cost-of-disease-related-malnutrition-in-the-uk (accessed 15 September 2015).

BAPEN (2012b). *The 'MUST' report Executive Summary.*
http://www.bapen.org.uk/screening-for-malnutrition/must/must-report/the-must-report-executive-summary
(accessed 21 August 2015).

Best, C. (2011) 'Malnutrition needs identifying in the community. *Nursing Times.* **107** (22), 16–17.

Bloomfield (2012). Improving nutrition and hydration in hospital: The nurse's responsibility. *Nursing Standard.* **26** (34), 52–56.

Elia, M., Stratton, R.J., Russell, C., Green, C. & Pang, F. (2005). *The cost of disease related malnutrition in the UK and economic considerations for the use of oral nutritional supplements (ONS) in adults.* Redditch: BAPEN.

ESPEN (2006). Guidelines on Enteral Nutrition: Intensive Care. *Clinical Nutrition.* **25**, 210–23.

Mehanna, H., Moledina, J. & Travis, J. (June 2008). Refeeding Syndrome: What it is and how to prevent and treat it. *British Medical Journal.* **336**, 1495–98.

Moore, T. & Woodrow, P., (2004). *High Dependency Nursing Care.* London: Routledge.

National Institute for Health and Care Excellence (NICE) (2006). *Nutrition support in adults: Oral nutrition support, enteral tube feeding and parenteral nutrition. Clinical Guideline 32.* London: NICE.

Royal College of Nursing (RCN) (2008). *Nutrition Now: Enhancing Nutritional Care.* London: RCN.

Stratton, R.J., King, C.L., Stroud, M.A., Jackson, A.A. & Elia, M. (2006). 'Malnutrition Universal Screening Tool' ('MUST') predicts mortality and length of hospital stay in acutely ill elderly. *British Journal of Nutrition.* **95**, 325–30.

Yantis, M. & Velander, R. (2009). How to recognise and respond to refeeding. *Nursing Critical Care.* **4** (3), 14–20.

Useful websites

British Association of Parental and Enteral Nutrition
http://www.bapen.org.uk/
(Accessed 21 August 2015)

National Nurses Nutrition Group
http:/www.nnng.org.uk
(Accessed 21 August 2015)

40 Placement of a nasogastric tube

Ian Setchfield

A nasogastric (NG) tube is a flexible tube that can be inserted transnasally into the stomach. They are commonly used in surgical patients to allow aspiration and drainage of gastric secretions. They are also used to provide enteral nutrition in acutely ill patients. It is essential for the nutritional needs of patients within the acute care setting to be met, in order to promote healing, decrease mortality rates and facilitate a safe discharge (Alberda *et al.* 2009). If patients are unable to swallow effectively, they are at risk of developing aspiration pneumonia, which is associated with an increased risk in mortality (Lanspa *et al.* 2013).

The National Patient Safety Agency (NPSA) classifies the misplacement of a nasogastric tube, which is not detected prior to use, as a never event (NPSA 2005). Appropriate training should be provided for staff prior to insertion of NG tubes. They must also be aware of NG tube contraindications.

By the end of this chapter you will be understand the indications and contraindications for use of NG tubes. You will also know how to assess patients for NG tubes and how to carry out the insertion procedure.

Types of nasogastric tube

A nasogastric tube can have a wide-bore (Ryle's) tube, which is used for drainage or gastric aspiration. Alternatively, it can have a fine-bore tube for short or medium-term feeding (NICE 2006). Short-term use NG tubes can be made from polyvinyl chloride (PVC), such as Ryle's tubes. Fine-bore NG tubes, which can be kept in for much longer periods of time as recommended by the manufacturers, are usually made of polyurethane.

Indications for NG tubes

One of the most common indications is for gastric drainage after an operation. NG tubes are also used for nutritional support and hydration in patients who:

- Have a functioning gastrointestinal (GI) tract
- Require short-term tube feeding (up to 4–6 weeks)

- Are unable to fulfil their nutritional requirements with normal or modified diet nutritional supplements
- Have increased nutritional requirements due to sepsis, trauma, post-operative stress or burns.

Contraindications for NG tubes

One important contraindication is basal skull fracture, as the tube may enter the brain if incorrectly positioned (orogastric positioning may be appropriate in this case). Other contraindications include obstructive pathology (such as stricture, tumour or pharyngeal pouch) in the oropharynx or oesophagus, which may prevent passage of the tube.

Possible complications related to NG tubes

These include:

- Epistaxis
- Oesophageal gastric and duodenal perforation
- Pneumothorax
- Nasal and mucosal ulceration
- Pulmonary intubation.

Assessment for a nasogastric tube

Patients must be assessed prior to insertion of an NG tube to ascertain if it is appropriate, and the decision must be recorded in the patient's medical notes. Informed consent must be obtained (as per Trust policy) and recorded in the patient's medical notes. If the patient lacks the capacity to give consent, the decision to treat must be made within the patient's best interests.

NG tube insertion procedure

Staff must have had the appropriate training and be deemed competent by their organisation to insert NG tubes. The procedure must be undertaken according to *The Code: Professional standards of practice and behaviour for nurses and midwives* (NMC 2015):

1. Prepare the patient. If the patient can communicate, it is important to agree upon a 'stop signal' that they can give if they wish to stop the procedure, should they feel any discomfort or pain.

2. Put the patient in a semi-upright position in the bed or chair, if clinically appropriate. Support the patient's head with pillows.

3. The NEX measurement is used to mark the distance the tube has to be passed by measuring the distance from the bridge of the patient's nose to their earlobe and then to the bottom of the xiphisternum (NPSA 2011).

4. Check that the patient's nostrils are patent by asking the patient to sniff with one nostril closed.

5. Wash hands and put on non-sterile gloves and an apron.

6. Lubricate the NG tube and insert the proximal end into the patient's clear nostril, along the floor of the nose into the nasopharynx. If an obstruction is felt, withdraw the tube, re-insert at a different angle or try the other nostril.

7. If the patient is able to drink, small sips of water may be given at this stage to aid the passage of the NG tube.

8. If at any time the patient starts to gag, appears to be in respiratory distress or develops cyanosis, the procedure should be stopped and the NG tube removed. This indicates that the NG tube may have been inserted into the trachea.

9. Reposition the patient, reassure them and attempt to insert the NG tube again.

10. Advance the NG tube down the patient's oesophagus until the appropriate depth is reached (NEX measurement).

11. Check the position of the NG tube (see Box 40.1). If a **fine-bore NG feeding tube** is inserted, the metal stylet should be withdrawn before attempting to obtain a gastric aspirate.

Box 40.1 Confirming the NG tube position

- Do not flush the tube until gastric confirmation has been obtained, as this may alter the pH of the aspirate (NPSA 2012).
- The pH testing of the gastric aspirate must be Merck CE certified – a 0.5 gradients pH testing indicator strip is the **first line** test method. Indicator strips distinguish between gastric (pH <5.5) and bronchial secretions (pH >6), confirming the NG tube is in the correct position (NPSA 2011).
- If the pH is greater than 5.5 or you are unable to obtain gastric aspirate, an x-ray must be requested as a **second line** test method. The x-ray must be reported by an appropriately competent person, as per individual organisation policy.
- If a patient is on a proton pump inhibitor (PPI), the gastric pH can be raised. If this is the case, and an electromagnetic bedside placement device is not being used, the patient should be x-rayed. It is not usually in the patient's best interest to have daily x-rays. Therefore, if there is no reason to suspect displacement, external observation of the tube (including its length and fixation of the tape) and usage must be documented as per organisational policy.

Note: Auscultation of the NG tube by injecting air into it (the 'whoosh test') or using litmus paper *must not* be used as a means of confirming placement.

Interpreting absence of respiratory distress as an indicator of correct positioning is ineffective, as is monitoring bubbling at the end of the tube (NPSA 2005).

Once the NG tube position has been correctly confirmed:

- Secure the NG tube, using appropriate tape or a fixation device
- Dispose of all waste according to your local Trust policy
- Wash or clean your hands, as per Trust policy.

Finally, the procedure must be documented, including:

- Type and size of NG tube
- Who inserted it
- Which nostril was used for the NG tube
- The cm measurement on the NG tube at the exit point of the nostril
- The method used to confirm the position of the NG tube.

Positioning the patient's chin on their chest, or rotating the tip of the tube upwards, positions the tube in line with the nasopharyngeal wall and may assist in the successful insertion of the NG tube.

When to check confirmation of placement

After initial NG tube insertion, placement should be checked:

- At least once per shift if continuous feeds are in progress
- If the measurement marking the tube's exit from the nose has changed
- Before each bolus feed, fluid or drug administration
- If the patient suddenly shows signs of respiratory distress, such as breathlessness or cyanosis.

Orogastric tubes

At times the patient's clinical condition will require them to have an orogastric tube. In this case, the tube is passed through the mouth and into the stomach, rather than through the nostrils. The guidance for checking whether the tube is positioned in the stomach will be the same as for nasogastric tubes.

Fine-bore nasogastric tubes

Fine-bore NG tubes are commonly size 8–10Fr and have a stylet, which aids the insertion of the fine-bore NG tube. Due to the narrow lumen of the fine-bore NG tube, there is an increased risk that the tube may enter the bronchus, resulting in a lung placement. It may also be difficult to obtain gastric aspirate. The NPSA (2011) acknowledge that bedside electromagnetic devices (see Figure 40.1) are increasingly being used as a second-line testing method (Windle *et al.* 2010), but if you do not obtain aspirate or aspirate with a pH <5.5, a chest X-Ray must be the definitive second-line test, not the electromagnetic device trace.

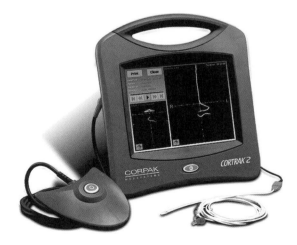

*Figure 40.1. **Example of an electromagnetic place device.** (Photograph used with permission of Corpak Medsytems.)*

Electromagnetic devices can visualise the position of the stylet in real-time during insertion. This provides a number of key benefits, when compared with standard methods of fine-bore feeding tube placement confirmation. Using an electromagnetic device:

- Minimises the risk of tube misplacement into the lungs
- Minimises the time needed to confirm tube placement and reduces the delay before feeding can begin
- Virtually eliminates the need to confirm tube placement with an x-ray, resulting in decreased patient exposure to potentially harmful radiation (Ackerman & Mick 2006).

In addition, the record, playback and printing functions allow for later review of the procedure, which can be useful for teaching purposes.

Conclusion

This chapter has explained the purpose of NG tubes, how to assess patients for NG tubes, how to position them and how to monitor their use. They are a vital tool in the management of critically ill patients but should be removed, as soon as practicable, to prevent complications.

References and further reading

Ackerman, M.H. & Mick, D.J. (2006). Technologic approaches to determining proper placement of enteral feeding tubes. *AACN Advanced Critical Care.* **17** (3), 246–49.

Alberda, C., Gramlich, L., Jones, N. *et al.* (2009). The relationship between nutritional intake and clinical outcomes in critically ill patients: results of an international multicentre observational study. *Intensive Care Medicine.* **35**, 1728-37.

Lanspa, M.J., Jones, B., Brown, S.M. *et al.* (2013). Mortality, morbidity, and disease severity of patients with aspiration pneumonia. *Journal of Hospital Medicine.* **8** (2), 83–90.

National Institute for Health and Care Excellence (NICE) (2006). *Nutrition support in adults: Oral nutrition support, enteral tube feeding and parenteral nutrition.* London: NICE.

National Patient Safety Agency (NPSA) (2005). *Reducing harm caused by the misplacement of nasogastric feeding tubes. Patient safety alert.* London: NPSA. http://www.nrls.npsa.nhs.uk/resources/type/alerts (accessed 21 August 2015).

National Patient Safety Agency (NPSA) (2011). *Patient Safety Alert NPSA/2011/PSA002. Reducing the Harm Caused by Misplaced Nasogastric Feeding Tubes in Adults, Children and Infants.* London: NPSA. http://www.nrls.npsa.nhs.uk/resources/type/alerts (accessed 21 August 2015).

National Patient Safety Agency (NPSA) (2012). *Harm from flushing of nasogastric tubes before confirmation of placement* NPSA/2012/RRR001 22/03/12. http://www.nrls.npsa.nhs.uk/resources/type/alerts/?entryid45=133441 (accessed 21 August 2015).

Nursing and Midwifery Council (2015). *The Code: Professional standards of practice and behaviour for nurses and midwives.* London: NMC. http://www.nmc.org.uk/standards/code/ (accessed 21 August 2015).

Windle, E.M., Beddow, D., Hall, E., Wright, J. & Sundar, N. (2010). Implementation of an electromagnetic imaging system to facilitate nasogastric and post-pyloric feeding tube placement in patients with and without critical illness. *Journal of Human Nutrition and Diet.* **23** (1), 61–68.

.ABCDE.

Exposure

41 Exposure, examination and evaluation

Karen E. Lumsden

This chapter focuses on the final part of the A–E mnemonic, encompassing the '4 Es' (exposure, environmental control, examination and evaluation of the patient) to ensure that no additional life-threatening factors have been overlooked, and that the safety of the patient remains central to care provision. Each of these key aspects should be considered by practitioners, bearing in mind that different areas may need to be emphasised, according to the individual patient's circumstances. As with each of the other chapters, these areas may have been considered and actioned during the A–D stages of patient management but should be revisited to ensure that no omissions have occurred.

By the end of this chapter, you should be able to put the 4 Es in the context of the other A–E assessment steps. You should also have an understanding of how to safely perform a spinal log roll, and appreciate the value of carrying out thorough examination and documentation of injuries. You will also understand the importance of continuous re-evaluation and be able to identify the post-resuscitation care that is required.

Background

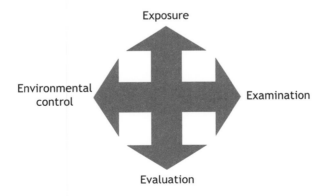

Figure 41.1 *The 4 Es.*

In most texts and journal resources, the 'E' part of the A–E assessment strategy tends to be covered briefly, with the primary focus on exposure and the environment. However, as will become evident in this chapter, there needs to be more emphasis on other aspects, such as examination and evaluation, so that all information regarding the patient's condition is captured and documented appropriately. This will enable healthcare staff to initiate any necessary additional investigations and management strategies in a timely and appropriate manner.

Exposure and spinal log rolling

During an initial assessment (particularly if this is for trauma in the emergency department), speed is of the essence in order to stabilise the patient. Most patients are managed in a supine position for the purpose of life-saving interventions, attachment of monitoring equipment and to facilitate radiological examination. Clothing is usually cut away to allow urgent vascular access and clinical assessment of the chest and abdomen.

However, this leaves a large proportion of the body initially unexamined, which could potentially result in untreated injuries being overlooked and affect the patient's overall clinical stability (Smith 2003). In order, therefore, to fully assess the patient and ensure visualisation of all body surfaces, it is essential to completely undress the patient, allowing a thorough examination to be facilitated, while maintaining and protecting the patient's dignity throughout.

When removing the garments, care must be taken to avoid any shards of glass, needles or weapons that may lie within the folds, as these objects may injure those caring for the patient and may also constitute valuable evidence that needs to be collected. If clothing has to be retained for forensic examination, local policy must be followed and any cutting of clothing must avoid the site of initial damage in order to preserve the available evidence, which should be stored correctly (in accordance with forensic requirements).

To remove the clothing, it may be necessary to roll the patient over, at the same time allowing for examination of the back of the head, body and lower limbs and to undertake assessment of sacral muscular tone through digital examination of the rectum (Evans & Tippins 2007). This also allows simultaneous removal of any spinal board from underneath the patient, as prolonged use of a spinal board may result in pressure injuries (Brohi 2002).

Box 41.1 Spinal log roll

For further guidance see Spinal Cord Injury Centres of the United Kingdom and Ireland (no date), p. 14

http://www.spinal.co.uk/userfiles/images/uploaded/pdf/288-709666.pdf

Personnel undertaking a spinal log roll for patients suspected of a spinal injury, should be formally trained before undertaking the procedure.

- The procedure used to maintain spinal alignment is the 'spinal log roll' and involves a minimum of five personnel – four to undertake the procedure and one to examine the patient fully.

- The person at the patient's head is responsible for coordinating the log roll and ensuring that cervical alignment is maintained by the team at all times (ENA 2014).

- Preparation is key to ensure that no further harm comes to the patient so this is the time to ensure that the brakes are applied on the trolley, and remove any earrings or necklaces left in situ. You should also assess crude neurological feeling by checking peripheral sensation in the patient's arms and legs prior to the roll. Ensure that the patient is given an adequate explanation regarding the procedure to be performed.

- Three other people are positioned alongside the patient in height order, starting with the tallest team member at the patient's shoulders and going down to the shortest person at the feet.

- Ensuring that appropriate manual handling techniques (such as posture and stance) are observed, the team members' hands are positioned at key points along the patient's body to prevent injury, both to the team and the patient.

- The tallest member of the team positions their hands on the shoulder and lower rib cage, the next member on the waist and under the thigh, and the next member under the lower leg.

- The two staff members at the chest/waistline borders should never cross hands, as this could affect their own health and safety by potentially twisting their backs. It could also impact on the alignment of the patient's spine as the manoeuvre is carried out, due to uneven manipulation by the team.

- Using appropriate commands by the team leader at the head ('ready, steady, roll'), the patient can be rolled smoothly onto their side.

- The fifth colleague should examine the posterior of the patient from the occiput to the sacrum, noting any pain, deformity, swelling and bruising (Harris & Sethi 2006) and remove any clothing or debris from underneath the patient.

- Once the examination has been completed, the roll technique is reversed and the patient's peripheral sensation is rechecked to ensure that the manoeuvre has done the patient no further harm (ENA 2014).

Patients on the ward will usually have already been identified as having an actual or potential spinal injury and staff should implement medical instructions. Although spinal log rolling is not usually required within the ward setting, it is still vital to expose and examine the patient (with consent) to detect other injuries and signs.

Environmental control

While fully exposing the patient allows identification of skin trauma, potential penetrating injuries, rashes and bleeding, it is vital to be aware of the risks this procedure can pose. One result of full exposure can be secondary hypothermia, due to low ambient surrounding temperatures and the stress of injury. Hypothermia combined with hypotension and acidosis can cause irreparable harm or even death (Søreide 2014). Therefore aggressive temperature management may be needed, by administering warmed intravenous fluids, using heat lamps to maintain a high ambient temperature and covering the patient with warmed blankets (ENA 2014).

Controlling the exposure of the patient for any further assessments or interventions will result in fewer fluctuations of body temperature and therefore have less adverse impact on clinical stability. Staff need to be aware of the operating guidance for any equipment used (such as warming blankets) to ensure they are effective.

Examination

The focus during the primary survey has been on life-saving interventions and responding to the patient's clinical presentation. However, it is essential that all clinical findings are accurately documented, with the level of assessment and examination being led by the relative clinical stability of the patient.

The use of a body map to record findings is helpful but you should always adhere to local policy. This should be an ongoing process that is continuously re-evaluated. If a process of examination is not followed systematically, it can result in some injuries being overlooked and have a negative impact on the patient's recovery and subsequent abilities. The information collected during the primary survey and exposure of the patient should be clear and succinct, and healthcare staff should use appropriate terminology to describe any additional injuries seen.

The 'look, listen and feel' approach helps to identify potential issues (Adam *et al.* 2010) and Table 41.1 outlines the aspects to assess.

Table 41.1 Aspects to look, listen and feel for during exposure

Look for:	Description
Contusion/bruises	Resulting from the application of blunt force trauma to the surface of the skin, where vessels rupture and blood infiltrates the tissues. Not always seen immediately after injury but can develop over hours or days.
Petechiae	Tiny haemorrhages on the skin surface, caused by constriction, suction or increased pressure.
Purpura	Larger, irregular haemorrhage shapes on the skin.
Haematoma/ haemorrhage	Blood collection under the skin or bleeding from wounds or drains.
Lacerations	Injuries due to direct blunt force trauma or shearing forces, resulting in a ragged-edged wound with associated bruising around the edges.
Incisions	Caused by the sharp edge of a cutting implement, such as a knife or tool, resulting in a straight-edged wound. If the incision is deep in origin, it can bleed profusely.
Wounds (such as stab wounds or pressure sores)	Wounds penetrate the skin and can lead to infection. Stab wounds can be misleading, as the surface appearance of the wound is a poor indicator of the depth of the injury.
Bite marks	Defined dentition appearance, with patterned bruises or abrasions.
Abrasions	Superficial injuries to the epidermal layer of the skin caused by simultaneous pressure and friction on the skin.
Avulsion	Involves the tearing of skin or tissue from the underlying body structures.
Inflammation	Look for redness and swelling.
Ischaemia/necrosis	Areas of dark purple or blackness, such as in limbs.

Rashes	There are numerous types of rashes and some can indicate allergy or sepsis.
Abnormalities	Some injuries, such as broken bones, should be considered if areas look misshapen.
Listen for:	
Pain	Ask the patient to describe the site and intensity of any pain; be alert for signs of pain when you examine the patient.
Feel for: (based on Adam *et al.* 2010)	
Swelling/distension/ oedema	Feel for lumps and swelling. An experienced practitioner should assess the abdomen. Look for excessive oedema (often in the legs).
Temperature	Inflammation may feel warm to touch and may cause pain (such as calf tenderness in deep vein thrombosis).
Surgical emphysema	This is air trapped in the subcutaneous tissue.

The 'look, listen and feel' approach, incorporating a full head-to-toe assessment, should be performed. It is essential to record all findings (such as wounds, bruises and rashes), including the anatomical position, size, shape, colour and any exudate/foreign matter as accurately as possible. Diagrams (such as a body map) or photographic records can be used to make these records, according to local policy.

Evaluation

It is imperative to evaluate the patient's clinical condition to ensure that primary interventions have been effective and that additional adjuncts and investigations are instigated appropriately. The Resuscitation Council (2005) recommends that these may include (but are not restricted to):

- Re-evaluation of vital signs (actual and trends)
- Recording of the patient's response to interventions on charts and patient notes
- Additional laboratory studies and review of test results (including blood glucose, full blood count and urea/electrolytes)
- Radiological imaging including x-rays, computerised tomography (CT) scans or magnetic resonance imaging (MRI) scans
- Splint or traction device application if indicated
- Wound care management and/or suturing
- Medication administration such as tetanus prophylaxis, antibiotic cover, sedation and pain control
- Preparation for transfer to the operating department or intensive care if required.

It is also appropriate at this stage to consider the patient holistically and ensure that fundamental nursing care is provided, to cover psychological and spiritual as well as physical needs. In addition, healthcare staff should recognise the importance of facilitating family attendance and collaboration with the multi-disciplinary team.

Conclusion

In conclusion, this chapter has given an overview of areas relating to 'E' aspects of assessment and the ongoing re-evaluation of the critically ill patient. While many practitioners would consider that some of these areas are usually undertaken during the secondary survey, it is important to acknowledge that care of the critically ill patient is dynamic and these actions may take place at any point during the patient's assessment, according to individual requirements.

References and further reading

Adam, S.K, Odell, M. & Welch, J. (2010). *Rapid Assessment of the Acutely Ill Patient.* Oxford: Wiley-Blackwell.

Brohi, K. (April 2002). *Spinal Stabilisation and Management.* **7**, 4.
http://www.trauma.org/archive/spine/cspine-stab.html (accessed 15 September 2015).

Emergency Nurses Association (ENA) (2014). *Trauma Nursing Core Course.* 7th edn. Illinois: ENA.
https://www.ena.org/education/ENPC-TNCC/tncc/Pages/aboutcourse.aspx (accessed 23 August 2015).

Evans, C. & Tippins, E. (2007). *The Foundations of Emergency Care.* Berkshire: Open University Press.

Harris, M. & Sethi, R. (2006). The initial assessment and management of the multiple trauma patient with an associated spine injury. *Spine.* **31** (11), S9–S15.

Jevon, P. (2012). *Monitoring the Critically Ill Patient.* 3rd edn. Oxford: Wiley-Blackwell.

Mulryan, C. (2011). *Acute Illness Management.* London: Sage

Resuscitation Council UK (2005). *A Systematic Approach to the Acutely Ill Patient.*
https://www.resus.org.uk/resuscitation-guidelines/a-systematic-approach-to-the-acutely-ill-patient-abcde/
(accessed 23 August 2015).

Smith, G. (2003). *ALERT Acute Life-threatening Events Recognition and Treatment.* 2nd edn. Portsmouth: University of Portsmouth.

Søreide, K (2014). Clinical and translational aspects of hypothermia in major trauma patients: From pathophysiology to prevention, prognosis and potential preservation. *Injury.* **45**, 647–54.
http://dx.doi:org/10.1016/j.injury.2012.12.027 (accessed 28 September 2015).

Spinal Cord Injury Centres of United Kingdom and Ireland (no date). *Moving and handling patients with actual or suspected spinal cord injuries.* Produced By Huntleigh.
http://www.spinal.co.uk/userfiles/images/uploaded/pdf/288-709666.pdf (accessed 4 April 2015).

Useful websites

Resusciation Council UK
http://www.resus.org.uk/
(Accessed 23 August 2015)

Trauma.org
http://www.trauma.org
(Accessed 23 August 2015)

42 Compartment syndrome

Ann M. Price

Compartment syndrome usually occurs when an injury leads to increased pressure within a body muscle compartment that affects the circulation (Singh *et al.* 2004), leading to tissue ischaemia. The decrease in circulation and damage to tissues can lead to deformity of the affected area, renal failure through muscle breakdown (rhabdomyolysis), amputation and, in severe cases, death. The area most commonly affected is the lower limbs (Singh *et al.* 2004, Mabvuure *et al.* 2012) but compartment syndrome can occur in any space within the body, including abdominal spaces. This chapter will concentrate on acute compartment syndrome but there are also sub-acute and chronic forms (Mabvuure *et al.* 2012).

By the end of this chapter, you should be able to define compartment syndrome and explain its basic pathophysiology; identify possible causes of compartment syndrome; recognise the signs and symptoms of compartment syndrome; and understand the initial treatment options.

Background and definitions

Matsen *et al.* (1980) defined compartment syndrome as 'a condition in which increased pressure within a limited space compromises the circulation and function of the tissues within that space' (p. 286). Kostler *et al.* (2004) stated that most cases of compartment syndrome occurred after a traumatic injury. Kostler *et al.* (2004) identified the following types of causes of compartment syndrome:

- Orthopaedic – both traumatic fractures and orthopaedic surgery can be implicated.
- Vascular – arterial and venous injuries, whether traumatic or secondary to surgery, can lead to compartment syndrome. Reperfusion injury and haemorrhage can deprive muscles and tissues of oxygen, thus leading to tissue swelling.
- Soft tissue damage – caused by conditions such as crush injuries, burns and prolonged limb compression, which may lead to compartment syndrome (Sahjian & Frakes 2007).
- Iatrogenic – accidental puncture in anticoagulated patients, use of pneumatic anti-shock garments and constricting casts or dressings.

- Rare causes – include snakebites and overuse of muscles.
- Abdominal – usually associated with severe abdominal injury, inflammatory processes (e.g. pancreatitis) or extensive surgery, where the abdominal contents swell, leading to tissue damage (Cresswell 2013).

Mabvuure *et al.* (2012) concur with these causes but note that young males, with traumatic limb injuries, are more likely to suffer acute compartment syndrome. Early recognition of the signs and symptoms of compartment syndrome is vital to prevent and reduce the possible serious effects on the patient.

Case scenario

A 28-year-old man was admitted after a motorcycle accident in which he sustained an open fracture of his tibia and fibula of his left leg. Surgery was undertaken and an external fixator frame inserted to support the bones while healing occurred. His calf became swollen and more painful over the following day and his toes became cool. Pedal pulses were difficult to palpate.

A diagnosis of compartment syndrome was made. Medial and lateral incision fasciotomies were performed to release the tissue pressure.

Pathophysiology, aetiology and mechanism of condition and therapy

The pathophysiology of acute compartment syndrome is not fully understood. However, we know that the increase in intra-compartmental pressure as a result of injury, either due to internal swelling or due to external pressure, is key (Mabvuure *et al.* 2012). Three possible mechanisms have been suggested for the development of compartment syndrome (Singh *et al.* 2004). These are:

1. The tissue swelling from the injury causes the arterioles to go into spasm and reduces blood flow.
2. The tissue swelling causes the arterioles to collapse and, thus, reduces blood flow.
3. The tissue swelling causes the venioles to collapse. As pressure rises from the arterial system, the veins slowly reopen. This affects the pressure gradient from veins to the tissues.

All the theories recognise that oxygen delivery to the affected area is restricted, and this causes tissue hypoxia. The affected tissue and muscles develop increased permeability, so allowing more fluid shifts within the compartment and increasing swelling further. This becomes a cycle of tissue damage that can be difficult to break (Singh *et al.* 2004).

Mabvuure *et al.* (2012) note that acute compartment syndrome can occur within 3 hours of injury and can cause irreversible effects within 12 hours. Compartment syndrome is therefore a medical emergency. It needs to be treated quickly to prevent serious and long-term effects such as contractures, amputation and disability.

Clinical diagnosis of compartment syndrome can be difficult, as the initial injury can mask the early signs. The '5 Ps' have been suggested as indicative of compartment syndrome (Singh *et al.* 2004). They are:

- **Pain**
- **Pallor**
- **Parasthesia**
- **Paralysis**
- **Pulselessness.**

Mabvuure *et al.* (2012) also include two more 'Ps':

- **P**ressure
- **P**oikilthermia (inability to regulate temperature).

However, pulselessness and paralysis are late signs and pain and pallor can be mistakenly related to the initial injury. Mabvuure *et al.* (2012) emphasise the need for a high degree of suspicion in at-risk patients, such as disproportionate pain, so that compartment syndrome is treated early. This is because as the number of signs increases, so does the risk of permanent damage (Mabvuure *et al.* 2012).

Dincer (2008) noted that these signs are not evident in the unconscious patient and suggests using addition tests such as serum creatinine, creatine phosphokinase (CPK), serum and urine myoglobulin levels to identify injury. Doppler and ultrasound can also be used to assess the extremity for poor blood flow (Dincer 2008).

Methods are available for measuring intra-compartment pressure (ICP), such as tonometers and ultrasound devices. The normal pressure is 0–15mmHg and pressures above 30mmHg, in conjunction with clinical signs, are diagnostic for compartment syndrome (Dincer 2008, Mabvuure *et al.* 2012). However, ICP measurements are not always reliable or easily available and they do not necessarily show a true picture of the pressure throughout the compartment. Thus clinical signs are vital and ICP measurement aids diagnosis (Mabvuure *et al.* 2012), particularly in unconscious patients.

Monitoring and management of compartment syndrome

As already noted, early detection and treatment of compartment syndrome are vital to reduce complications. Increasing pain is a key sign and some medics and surgeons may therefore avoid nerve blocks that might mask this symptom. Patients who are at risk of compartment syndrome should be monitored in a variety of ways, depending on the compartment/s likely to be affected.

- Limbs: at least hourly recording of temperature of the limb, pain, movement, feeling and pulses. Increasing pain, cooling of the limb, reduction in movement, feeling or pulses should be quickly reported to the relevant senior clinician. Pressure monitoring can be utilised where available.
- Abdominal: the '5 Ps' are difficult to apply to this compartment and measuring girth is an unreliable indicator of abdominal pressure. Therefore, abdominal pressure is usually measured using a urethral catheter and pressure transducer device. Pressures above 20mmHg are considered indicative of compartment syndrome (Cresswell 2013). However, in practice this is difficult to use on all susceptible patients and is generally confined to the intensive care patient.

Early decompression of the affected compartment is considered to be the treatment of choice (Singh *et al.* 2004, Mabvuure *et al.* 2012). The first-line treatment is to release or remove any restrictive bandaging or plaster casts. Supportive therapies of analgesia, fluids and mannitol should also be considered (Mabvuure *et al.* 2012). Second-line treatment is the use of fasciotomy for the affected compartments, moving on to amputation of limbs if needed (Mabvuure *et al.* 2012). Fasciotomies entail a risk of infection but, as already highlighted, early intervention is essential to limit tissue damage. The abdomen is often left open, with a sterile protective cover, until swelling has reduced.

The affected limb should be left at heart level to aid circulation and prevent further swelling (Mamaril *et al.* 2007, Mabvuure *et al.* 2012). Patients may need skin grafts or vacuum dressings to aid wound healing of the fasciotomy or open abdominal site.

Conclusion

This chapter has given an overview of the care of a patient with compartment syndrome. In general wards, these patients require close monitoring of vital signs, their limb (if a limb is affected) and their pain score. Staff should have a high suspicion of compartment syndrome if pain is higher than expected, or worsening, in relation to the aetiology.

Seek expert help quickly if deterioration occurs and ensure the hospital's pain team or anaesthetists are involved in the patient's management.

References and further reading

Cresswell, A.B. (2013). Recognition and management of intraabdominal hypertension and the abdominal compartment syndrome. *Surgery (Oxford)*. **31** (11), 582–87.

Dincer, H.E. (2008). Acute compartment syndrome: are we close to making an early diagnosis? *Critical Care Medicine*. **36** (6), 1962–63.

Kostler, W., Strohm, P.C. & Sudkamp, N.P. (2004). Acute compartment syndrome of the limb injury. *International Journal Care Injured*. **35**, 1221–27.

Mabvuure, N.T., Malahias, M., Hindocha, S., Khan, W. & Jumas, A. (2012). Acute Compartment Syndrome of the Limbs: current concepts and management. *The Open Orthopaedics Journal*. **6** (3: M7), 535–43. DOI: 10.2174/1874325001206010535

Mamaril, M.E., Childs, S.G. & Sortman, S. (2007). Care of the Orthopaedic Trauma Patient. *Journal of Perianesthesia Nursing*. **22** (3), 184–94.

Matsen, F., Winquist, R. & Krugmire, R. (1980). Diagnosis and management of compartmental syndromes. *Journal of Bone Joint Surgery*. **62** (2), 286–91.

Sahjian, M. & Frakes, M. (2007). Crush Injuries: Pathophysiology and Current Treatment. *The Nurse Practitioner*. **32** (9), 13–18.

Singh, S., Trikhab, S.P. & Lewis, J. (2004). Acute Compartment Syndrome. *Current Orthopaedics*. **18**, 468–76.

Useful websites

American Academy of Orthopaedic Surgeons
http://orthoinfo.aaos.org/topic.cfm?topic=a00204
(Accessed 23 August 2015)

Medline Plus
http://www.nlm.nih.gov/medlineplus/ency/article/001224.htm
(Accessed 23 August 2015)

Wheeless' Textbook of Orthopaedics
http://www.wheelessonline.com/ortho/compartment_syndrome
(Accessed 23 August 2015)

43 Organ and tissue donation

Tim Collins

Organ and tissue transplantation have been proven to be effective treatments for end-stage organ failure and have been shown to significantly improve the quality of life for patients awaiting a tissue transplant. Most solid organ donations come from donor patients following either Donation after Brainstem Death (DBD) or Donation after Circulatory Death (DCD) while in the intensive care unit (ICU) or emergency department, due to a sudden traumatic brain injury or cerebral insult.

Solid organs that can be donated include the kidneys, liver, heart, lungs and pancreas. These organs can be transplanted to replace a patient's failing organ, and they are often life-saving for the recipients. Solid organs need to have minimal interruptions in perfusion; otherwise the lack of oxygen delivered to the organs in a low-perfusion state will make them unviable. Solid organs can be retrieved from patients who have been declared dead following brainstem death testing or following DCD donation, previously referred to as non-heart-beating organ donation (NICE 2011).

By the end of this chapter, you will be able to identify the differences between organ and tissue donation, and will know which organs and tissues can be donated. You will also be able to describe the key concepts relating to the organ and tissue donation process, and discuss brainstem death testing as well as the differences between DBD and DCD. In addition, you will know the clinical criteria governing when to refer potential solid organ donors to the specialist nurse for organ donation (SNOD). You will know how to effectively approach families for tissue donation consent; and you will be able to analyse the role of the healthcare professional in identifying, managing, supporting and referring organ or tissue donors within the acute environment.

Background

DCD donation occurs when death is confirmed using cardio-respiratory criteria, often following withdrawal of treatment in the ICU or the emergency department. In this case, the retrieval of organs is undertaken promptly, following confirmation of asystole (NHSBT 2015a). Also, organs can be obtained from a living donor, who could donate a kidney to a patient in need of a transplant.

In addition to organs, tissues can be donated. These tissues include corneas, heart valves, bone, skin and tendons (HTA 2006). Most people who die can donate at least one tissue but, unlike organs, they can be retrieved from a patient up to 48 hours following death. Unlike organs, tissue donation is not life-saving but provides recipients with improvements in their quality of life – for instance, a corneal transplant can restore sight.

Currently there is a shortage of organs available for transplantation and the transplant waiting list continues to grow, as demand outstrips supply. Between April 2012 and 2013, a total of 3,509 solid organ transplants were undertaken in the United Kingdom, which were either life-saving or improved quality of life for recipients. However, there were still 7,026 people left on the transplant waiting list during the same year (NHSBT 2014). Through tissue donation, a further 3,313 people had their sight restored after transplant of corneas following the death of donor patients (NHSBT 2014).

Due to the significant benefits of organ and tissue donation, it is imperative that healthcare practitioners identify potential organ and tissue donors and refer to the specialist nurse for organ donation (SNOD) as per NICE guidance (2011). NICE (2011) have provided best practice guidance relating to organ donation and have stated that organ donation should be considered as a usual part of end of life care. This is further endorsed by the General Medical Council guidance, which states that consultant staff with clinical responsibility for patients who are potential donors have a duty to consider organ donation as part of end-of-life care (GMC 2010).

HOT TIP

In the UK, NHS Blood and Transplant (NHSBT) is the authority that oversees donation and transplantation. They have a very comprehensive website containing current resources and documents relating to the clinical management of organ and tissue donation:

http://www.odt.nhs.uk/

Differences between organ and tissue donation

Solid organs that can be donated include the heart, lungs, liver, kidneys, pancreas and small bowel. Solid organ retrieval within critical care can be undertaken by either DBD or DCD donation. During the donation process it is imperative that the organs do not sustain any major ischaemia before transplantation; otherwise they will not be salvageable (NHSBT 2015a). Therefore solid organ retrieval is normally undertaken after brainstem death certification or just after the patient becomes asystolic (DCD). The process is often more complicated than tissue donation, as the healthcare team have to manage a cardiovascularly unstable patient while trying to ensure maximum organ perfusion prior to retrieval.

In contrast, tissue donation can be undertaken up to 48 hours following cardio-respiratory cessation (NHSBT 2015 b). Tissues that can be donated following death include corneas, heart valves, skin, tendon and bone (HTA 2006). Studies have found that the majority of patients who die in hospitals may be eligible for tissue donation. However, relatives are infrequently asked for consent because nursing and medical staff are either unaware of tissue donation or they are inadequately prepared to obtain tissue donation consent (Collins 2005).

Box 43.1 Organs and tissues that can be donated

Tissues that can be donated following death include: corneas, heart valves, skin, tendon and bone (many up to 48 hours after death).

Solid organs that can be donated include: the heart, lungs, liver, kidneys, pancreas and small bowel.

Defining brainstem death

Managing the brainstem dead patient is one of the most challenging and demanding roles for the healthcare professional. Often these patients are young, having sustained a sudden and catastrophic insult that has left their family unprepared for them becoming unwell. The current position in UK law is that there is no statutory definition of death (Academy of Medical Royal Colleges 2008).

The definition of death recommended by the Academy of Medical Royal Colleges (2008) is as follows:

'death is the irreversible loss of essential characteristics which are necessary to the existence of a living human person. The definition should be regarded as the irreversible loss of the capacity to maintain consciousness, combined with the irreversible loss of capacity to breathe'.

Therefore death is not solely confirmed by the absence of a palpable pulse. A patient with irreversible damage to the brainstem can be declared dead, despite having a palpable pulse, and may have a sustained capacity to breathe via a mechanical ventilator.

The brainstem consists of the pons, medulla oblongata and midbrain (which contains the vital functions of life such as respiratory control). Brainstem death (BSD) occurs when the brainstem becomes irreversibly damaged and can no longer maintain life. Once the brainstem has died, it cannot recover and no treatment can reverse the damage. Brainstem death results in irreversible loss of consciousness and no independent capacity to breathe. These patients are normally intubated and ventilated so the function of breathing is maintained by means of a ventilator. BSD is caused by excessive raised intracranial pressure (ICP) that compresses the brainstem and subsequently causes ischaemia and hypoxia, resulting in irreversible brainstem damage that is incompatible with life.

Box 43.2 The causes of brainstem death

The causes of BSD can include (Bersten & Soni 2013):
- Intracerebral bleed (e.g. subarachnoid haemorrhage)
- Cerebral infarction
- Head trauma
- Cerebral hypoxia
- Cerebral tumour
- Drug overdose
- Intracerebral infection and meningitis.

However, if BSD occurs and the patient is being mechanically ventilated, the patient's respiratory function will be maintained. Following BSD, asystole usually occurs within 72 hours (Bersten & Soni 2013). This leaves two options – organ retrieval or discontinuing mechanical ventilation, which will terminate the patient's respiration.

Brainstem death testing

Brainstem death (BSD) testing is undertaken to determine whether the brainstem function is still intact and whether or not the patient is just suffering from a deep coma. In the UK there are three stages in the diagnosis of brainstem death: preconditions, exclusions and clinical tests. If the patient fails to show any response to the tests, it means the brainstem has been irreversibly damaged and death can be confirmed. The tests have to be undertaken by two doctors who have been registered for more than 5 years and are conversant with the tests. At least one has to be a consultant. Testing should be undertaken together and must be fully completed and successful on two occasions (Academy of Medical Royal Colleges 2008). The legal time of death is the time of completion of the first set of brainstem death tests.

All this needs to be explained to relatives by a practitioner with effective communication skills, who has built up a rapport with the relatives and has appropriate knowledge and understanding of the tests. If it is felt appropriate, consider allowing the relatives to observe the BSD tests themselves. In a small-scale study by Collins (2005), nurses found that relatives accepted the reality of their loved one's death more readily if they were effectively supported and given clear explanations of the tests being undertaken.

Box 43.3 Criteria diagnosing brainstem death

The criteria for the diagnosis of brainstem death from the Academy of Medical Royal Colleges (2008) consist of pre-conditions, exclusions and testing of the brainstem.

Pre-conditions:

- Patient is comatose and mechanically ventilated.
- Diagnosis of structural brain damage has been established or the immediate cause of coma is known.
- It is essential to have a period of observation.

Exclusions:

- Drugs (e.g. barbiturates) are not the cause if the patient is in a coma.
- Neuromuscular blockade has been demonstrably reversed.
- The patient is not suffering from hypothermia (>34° Celsius).
- There is no endocrine or metabolic disturbance.

Testing (using reflexes that involve brainstem function):

- No pupillary response to light
- No corneal reflex
- No vestibular ocular reflex
- No motor response to pain
- No gag reflex to suctioning through endotracheal tube or tracheostomy
- Apnoea persists despite a rise in $PaCO_2$ greater than 6.6Kpa against a background of a normal PaO_2.

For further information on BSD testing, please refer to the current guidance on brainstem death testing which can be obtained from your hospital's specialist nurse for organ donation (SNOD).

Identifying potential organ donors

It is essential to identify potential organ donors as early as possible and all hospitals have a SNOD who is contactable via the hospital switchboard or the hospital's ICU. SNODs have specialist knowledge and experience relating to donation and are employed and trained by NHSBT. They can offer healthcare practitioners valuable help and support relating to all issues concerning donation. NICE (2011) and NHSBT (2015) recommend that all patients who fulfil the following clinical triggers should be referred to the SNOD:

- Patients who have had a catastrophic brain injury: namely, the absence of one or more cranial nerve reflexes and a Glasgow Coma Scale (GCS) score of 4 or less that is not explained by sedation.
- Patients with a life-threatening or life-limiting condition that will, or is expected to, result in circulatory death (NICE 2011), and where it is the intention to withdraw life-sustaining treatment.

Gaining family consent for organ donation

A multi-professional approach is best practice when planning to ask a family for organ donation consent. The family should be approached by the SNOD as well as the patient's medical and nursing team (NICE 2011). Unless the family initiate discussions concerning donation, it is essential that the SNOD is present during the approach, as this will maximise the chances of gaining consent to organ donation. SNODs are experts in the field of donation and can provide professional advice for both medical and nursing staff, as well as offering valuable support to patients' relatives, even if the relatives decide not to consent to organ donation.

Management of the multiple organ donation patient is complex and is usually confined to the intensive care setting to ensure that the donation is successful.

Donation after circulatory death (DCD)

DCD donation is an option when it has been decided that further medical treatment is futile and there is to be a planned withdrawal of treatment. Unlike BSD patients (who are already declared dead but are mechanically ventilated and transferred to the operating theatre for donation with a beating heart), DCD takes place immediately after the patient has become asystolic (when their heartbeat stops). Ongoing treatment is considered futile and the decision has been made to withdraw treatment.

If the patient has no contraindications and meets the inclusion criteria, it is best practice (NICE 2011) to consider all patients as potential DCD donors when undertaking withdrawal of treatment. Prior to withdrawing treatment, discussions should take place with the SNOD to confirm eligibility for organ donation. In order to ensure that the organs are not affected by under-perfusion ischaemia, the patient needs to become asystolic within a short period of time after treatment is withdrawn. Long periods of hypotension will unfortunately exclude the patient from donation, as death needs to occur quickly.

Withdrawal of treatment is often undertaken in the anaesthetic room – to minimise delay before the patient enters surgery for organ retrieval. Family members can be present when their loved one's heart actually stops beating. (Some family members may want to be present when death occurs, which is not possible with brainstem death donation.) The patient is then certified dead in the anaesthetic room, the family members say their goodbyes and the patient is quickly moved into the operating theatre for prompt organ retrieval (to minimise the risk of organ ischaemia).

It is currently possible for kidneys, liver, lungs and the pancreas (for islet cells) to be donated following DCD at the onset of asystole (ICS 2004, HTA 2006). In the UK, an average of 2.6 transplantable organs are retrieved from DCD donors, compared to 4.0 from DBD donors. The biggest contribution of DCD donors is to kidney transplantation, with 38% of all deceased donor kidney transplants coming from this source in 2013–2014. The lower donation potential of DCD donors is largely due to the ischaemic injury suffered by solid organs in the time interval between treatment withdrawal and cold perfusion, with the liver and pancreas being particularly vulnerable (NHSBT 2015).

General criteria for organ donation

Any patient who meets the NICE (2011) criteria should be considered for organ donation and referred to the SNOD. There are no absolute age restrictions for solid organ donation. Each potential organ donor should therefore be individually assessed for suitability.

It is imperative that *all* patients who meet the NICE (2011) referral criteria are referred to the SNOD, who will assess suitability with reference to current transplant centre criteria, which are constantly changing as techniques improve. The Transplant Centre, rather than the local medical team, should decide whether a donor is to be excluded.

Tissue donation

Tissue donation is an option for many families following death in hospitals and palliative care settings. However, it has been documented that many nursing and medical staff are unaware of this option (Collins 2005, Cantwell & Clifford 2000). Tissues such as corneas, heart valves, skin, bone and tendons can be donated even if the patient has not been certified brainstem dead (NHSBT 2015b). Patients receiving a tissue transplant may not have their lives saved but they will experience significant improvements in the quality of their lives – for instance, regaining their eyesight following corneal transplant. It is recommended that healthcare staff routinely assess and approach relatives for tissue donation consent. This should ideally be done before the patient deteriorates so their wishes can be recorded (NHSBT 2015b).

General criteria for tissue donation

Tissue donation criteria regarding age and medical suitability will vary, depending on the tissue to be donated. Tissues can be retrieved up to 24 hours after circulatory cessation except for heart valves, which can be retrieved up to 48 hours after asystole (NHSBT 2015a). Individuals suffering from systemic malignancies are contraindicated in tissue donation except in the case of cornea donation.

There are some absolute contraindications for tissue donation. These include patients who have:

- Tested positive for HIV, hepatitis B and C, human T cell lymphotrophic virus (HTLV) or syphilis (or have high-risk behaviour for contracting these infections)
- Suffered from Creutzfeldt–Jacob disease or have a family history of it (ICS 2004)
- Progressive neurological disease of unknown pathophysiology (e.g. multiple sclerosis, Alzheimer's disease, Parkinson's disease or motor neurone disease)
- Leukaemia, lymphoma or myeloma
- Had a previous transplant requiring immunosuppressive treatment.

In addition to the above, there are contraindications for specific tissues. If in doubt, you are advised to contact your SNOD or specialist nurse for tissue donation (SNTD) to assess patient suitability.

Approaching families for organ and tissue donation consent

As previously discussed, NICE (2011) states that the planning of the approach for solid organ donation consent should be multi-professional and must involve a SNOD. The SNOD should be contacted early, as per the NICE (2011) clinical trigger referral criteria, so that potential organ donors can be identified at an early stage. This will enable a SNOD to be present in the ICU or ED to answer any questions from relatives and healthcare staff. Evidence suggests that having a SNOD present during the organ donation process may improve the chances of relatives giving consent (NHSBT 2015).

Tissue donation is slightly different. Due to the large number of tissue donation referrals, many SNODs do not have sufficient resources to offer a collaborative approach to tissue donation consent. This task is therefore usually undertaken by healthcare staff in the local hospital, even though many healthcare staff find it difficult to approach families for tissue donation consent. Following a systematic approach will aid the healthcare practitioner in this process (Bersten & Soni 2013, Cantwell & Clifford 2000). (See Box 43.4 for points to remember.)

Box 43.4 Key points to consider when approaching a family for tissue donation consent

When?
- When death is pronounced
- When the relatives are informed
- When the relatives understand the cause of death.

Where?
- Not at the bedside or a corridor
- In a private and quiet room.

Who?
- A practitioner who is familiar with the family
- A practitioner with sensitivity and effective interpersonal skills.
- It does not have to be a senior person or medical staff member, as long as they display the above skills.

Helpful phrases
- 'I know this is a very difficult time but I have some important information for you to consider…'
- 'Do you know if [name of patient] carried a donor card?'
- 'It may be possible for [name of patient] to donate if you think that is what s/he would have wanted to do.'
- 'Did you ever talk about organ donation as a family?'

Remember:
- It cannot get any worse for the family so there is no harm in asking. The relatives may gain some comfort in their bereavement by being given this option.
- If relatives refuse consent, respect their wishes and just say this was an option open to them to consider.
- If they do give consent, document this in the medical notes and get the relative to sign a consent form.
- Obtain the phone number for where the next of kin will be staying for the next few hours, as a transplant co-ordinator will personally ring to reconfirm consent and follow up any questions the relative may have.
- Once the family have consented, phone the SNOD (via the hospital switchboard), who will ask you some questions about the patient.

Role of the specialist nurse for organ donation (SNOD)

SNODs are nurses who have previously worked in critical care areas and have undergone additional training in organ transplantation. The role of the SNOD is varied and demanding and they facilitate the organ donation process by:

- Arranging the donor organ retrieval
- Communicating with and supporting the family of the patient before, during and after the donor organ retrieval
- Supporting and communicating with healthcare professionals at the donor hospital and liaising between different departments (e.g. operating theatres)
- Ensuring that appropriate medical investigations are undertaken and reviewing the patient's medical notes to ensure there are no contraindications that would exclude donation
- Coordinating the transplant retrieval team and liaising with the transplant centres
- Providing information and advice for both healthcare professionals and the public on all matters relating to donation and transplantation.

These are only some of the roles of a SNOD. SNODs provide a 24-hour service and are always available to give advice. Due to the shortage of available organs, they would always prefer patients to be referred, rather than potential donors to be missed. For this reason, healthcare professionals should never feel reluctant to contact them if they are unsure about a potential donor. Your hospital switchboard will have the number for your SNOD. There are also specialist nurses for tissue donation (SNTDs), who perform a similar role but specifically in relation to tissue donation.

Conclusion

Organ and tissue donation is an effective treatment for end-stage organ failure and has been shown to improve quality of life for patients awaiting organ and tissue transplants. It is imperative that healthcare staff respect the final wishes of their patients and ensure that the organ donation process is followed; otherwise the transplant waiting list will continue to get longer and the last wishes of our patients will be ignored.

Regional SNODs are always available to support and assist healthcare staff in the organ donation process and should be contacted early, as per NICE (2011) referral criteria, to enable a multi-professional approach to be used in the management of donor patients and their families. The NHS Blood and Transplant website should be consulted for current clinical aspects relating to organ and tissue donation.

References and further reading

Academy of Medical Royal Colleges (2008). *Code of Practice for the diagnosis and confirmation of death.* London: Millbank Media.

Adam, S. & Osborne, S. (2005). *Critical Care Nursing.* 2nd edn. London: Oxford University Press.

Bersten, A. & Soni, N. (2013). *Oh's Intensive Care Manual.* 7th edn. London: Butterworth Heinemann.

Cantwell, M. & Clifford, C. (2000). English nursing and medical students' attitudes towards organ donation. *Journal of Advanced Nursing.* **4,** 961–68.

Collins, T. (2005). Organ and tissue donation: a survey of nurses' knowledge and educational needs in an adult ITU. *Intensive and Critical Care Nursing.* **21,** 226–33.

General Medical Council (2010). *Treatment and care towards the end of life: good practice in decision making.* http://www.gmc-uk.org/guidance/ethical_guidance/end_of_life_care.asp (accessed 25 March 2015).

Human Tissue Authority (HTA) (2006). *Code of Practice – donation organs, tissues & cells for transplantation.* 2nd Code. London: DH.

Intensive Care Society (ICS) (2004). *Guidelines for adult organ and tissue donations.* London: ICS.

National Institute for Health and Care Excellence (NICE) (2011). *Organ Donation for Transplantation Clinical Guideline 135.* https://www.nice.org.uk/guidance/cg135/evidence/cg135-organ-donation-full-guideline3 (accessed 25 August 2015).

NHS Blood and Transplant (2015a). *Donation After Circulatory Death.* http://www.odt.nhs.uk/donation/deceased-donation/donation-after-circulatory-death/ (accessed 27 March 2015).

NHS Blood and Transplant (2015b). *Tissue donation.* http://www.nhsbt.nhs.uk/tissuedonation/how-to-become-a-donor/tissue-donation-after-death/ (accessed 27 March 2015).

NHS Blood and Transplant (2014). *Activity Report 2013/14.* http://www.odt.nhs.uk/uk-transplant-registry/annual-activity-report/ (accessed 23 March 2015).

Useful websites

British Transplantation Society
https://www.bts.org.uk/
(Accessed 25 August 2015)

Intensive Care Society
http://www.ics.ac.uk/
(Accessed 25 August 2015)

NHS Blood and Transplant
http://www.nhsbt.nhs.uk/
(Accessed 25 August 2015)

NHS Blood and Transplant clinical webiste
http://www.odt.nhs.uk/
(Accessed 25 August 2015)

44 Patient transport

Alistair Challiner

Transferring a patient between wards, departments or even hospitals can be a hazardous procedure. A patient may need to be moved around the hospital for various reasons.

For example, they may need to go:

- To theatre (for an operation)
- To a high dependency unit (for an escalated level of care)
- To the radiology department (for an x-ray or CT scan)
- From the high dependency unit to a ward (when they have improved)
- To a specialist ward.

The transfer of a critically ill patient (either within a hospital or between hospitals) requires a specialist team, including an anaesthetist or intensive care unit (ICU) doctor and an ICU trained nurse, as well as specialist equipment such as a ventilator. This type of transfer will not therefore be discussed here. At the other extreme, a relatively well patient may be transported by a porter and the risks are low. This type of transfer will not be discussed here either.

The aim of this chapter is to discuss the transfer of an unwell patient who is not unstable enough to need an ICU team. By the end of this chapter, you will know the key points to prepare for and undertake a patient transfer safely and efficiently.

When is a patient transfer necessary?

When a patient transfer is suggested, the first decision is whether or not they definitely need to be moved. For instance, if the patient needs an operation or they require imaging to give a diagnosis, then of course they do need to be moved. Likewise, if the patient is seriously unwell and needs maximal oxygen, with inotropes running via a central line, then they need to go to the high dependency unit (HDU), as additional monitoring is needed and escalation of care is likely. Think about these situations as you review the points in Box 44.1.

Preparing for patient transfer

Box 44.1 Potential safety problems to be considered

The problems that may occur during patient transfer include:

- Going to the wrong location
- Arriving at the wrong time
- An unstable patient deteriorating further while being moved down a corridor
- The transfer team not having the required skills
- Oxygen running out
- The battery running out on a monitor or pump
- A vital piece of equipment being unavailable
- Suction not being available to clear the patient's airway of vomit
- A drug or IV fluid being needed but unavailable
- Airway and breathing equipment being needed because the patient has deteriorated
- Vascular access being pulled out
- Arriving at the destination without any notes or test results.

We need to consider the following questions:

- How can the patient be stabilised before the transfer?
- Who is in charge of the transfer?
- What communication is needed before the transfer?
- What resources and expertise are required for the transfer?
- How should the patient be categorised?
- How should the patient be packaged for transfer?

Each of the questions in Box 44.1 will now be discussed in turn.

How can the patient be stabilised before the transfer?

The principle of patient transfer is to minimise risk. An unstable patient should never be moved unless they have a non-compressible haemorrhage requiring immediate surgery, such as a ruptured aortic aneurysm or a bleeding ectopic pregnancy. Think about the relative risk to the patient who is unstable in a ward area (with space, staff availability and gas and suction supply being readily available), compared to having the same patient in a corridor or lift and a sudden deterioration occurring. The patient must be stabilised using the principles covered in this book *before* transfer. If the patient is being monitored, the same level of monitoring must be continued during the transfer, including at least ECG, pulse oximetry and blood pressure (BP).

Who is in charge of the transfer?

Someone must take charge of the transfer, organise and delegate all the tasks required appropriately, before the transfer can be safely carried out – ideally this should be a practitioner who is experienced and trained in transfer procedures. Most importantly, they need to check that everything has been done; this can be aided by the use of a transfer checklist (your organisation may have one available to utilise).

What communication is needed before the transfer?

Prior to any move, everyone must be clear where the patient is going. Does the receiving location know they are coming? It is very important to telephone the destination beforehand so that they are ready to receive your patient. This avoids waiting in a corridor with your patient because another patient is in the scan room, or the theatre is not ready, or no bed is available on the ward. Remember to let relatives know about the move as well as the admitting team. If other resources are required, then help (including porters) and equipment must be sought.

What resources and expertise are required for the transfer?

In-hospital transfers usually require a trolley, which must be appropriately equipped with a full cylinder of oxygen and working suction. These items should be checked before the transfer takes place. The amount of oxygen required for the journey needs to be calculated, based on the oxygen required per minute by the patient and the anticipated transfer time. Consideration must also be given to the amount of oxygen stored in the available cylinder.

Box 44.2 Oxygen cylinder sizes

Standard oxygen cylinders are:

- D size – 340 litres
- E size – 680 litres
- F size – 1360 litres.

A D-size cylinder will last about 22 minutes, at 15 litres per minute oxygen flow. An E-size will last 45 minutes, and an F-size about 90 minutes. The time will be considerably shorter if the cylinder is not full. The cylinders should therefore always be checked – and changed if they are not full. Assume that maximum flow will be required if the patient deteriorates. Utilising wall supplies in ambulances or destinations (when available) can conserve oxygen.

Out-of-hospital transfers involve additional communication with the ambulance service. Most of these transfers will require a hospital nurse to attend with the patient, but will include at least an ambulance technician to help in the back of the vehicle. Many hospital staff are unfamiliar with the equipment in the back of an ambulance but the ambulance personnel are very helpful in this regard.

Ambulance equipment includes ECG, pulse oximetry and blood pressure monitors. Oxygen and suction have already been mentioned. Consider the worst that could happen, such as a cardiac arrest. Therefore at least a bag valve mask and defibrillator should be provided, as well as fluids and drugs.

There are strict regulations about carrying loose heavy equipment in an ambulance, as these items may become flying projectiles in case of an accident.

For higher-risk patients, the nurse should be trained in advanced life support (ALS), or a doctor may need to go as well. For ICU patients, a critical care team should be sent from the ICU.

How should the patient be categorised?

It is important to classify the personnel and equipment required for the transfer, according to the category of patient. Below are a number of patient categories and what each requires to undertake a transfer safely:

- Critical – extremely ill and at risk of deteriorating: Requires a rapid transfer, with medical staff and nursing staff with ALS skills.

- Intensive – requiring organ support and should be in ICU: Needs an ICU team in attendance who will assess the patient and usually provide monitoring and advanced treatment prior to transfer; they will consider the most appropriate time for the transfer to take place.
- Ill and unstable – such as acute myocardial infarction (MI), post convulsion, or patient with severe asthma: Requires at least a skilled nurse with ALS skills and a doctor may also be required.
- Ill and stable – such as post-operative patients or a stable MI: Requires at least a nurse with basic life support skills.

How should the patient be packaged for transfer?

Packaging the patient includes preparing the staff as well as the equipment.

Staff

For in-hospital transfers, there is a system for calling for help. If the nurse realises that assistance is required before the transfer, get extra help from outreach or medical staff before commencing the transfer. Otherwise, utilise the cardiac arrest call telephones in the hospital if urgent help is needed during the transfer. The most important factor is planning your route. Use the porter's knowledge of which lifts work and which corridors are unlocked at night.

For ambulance transfers, ensure that you have a mobile phone and a number to call for advice; this must be arranged before you go. Also bear in mind that the ambulance may break down. You need to consider what you are wearing. Ask yourself: is your clothing safe to be on the road in, and is it warm? Ideally, fluorescent yellow waterproof jackets should be provided. Footwear must be appropriate. Remember the ambulance may not be able to bring you home so take money or make arrangements for a taxi before you go.

Always be clear on where you are going (e.g. precisely which inner-city hospital you are going to and via which entrance) and check that the ambulance crew has the same information.

Equipment

Consider the following ABC principles, as covered in this book. Also consider specifics for the patient.

Make sure electronic equipment (such as monitors, defibrillators and pumps) are charged and ideally have spare batteries. When at your destination (such as CT scan), plug everything in to save batteries for the return journey. Remember oxygen, full cylinders and suction, including spare catheters and yankauer. A bag valve mask is invaluable, as it can work without an oxygen supply and is truly portable. The same equipment is usually required for most transfers so it is very useful to keep it all in a bag. This must be checked and replenished after every transfer and staff should be familiar with its contents.

The patient must be transferred on to a trolley for the transfer. This is best achieved using a device such as a 'pat slide' to avoid injury by lifting. All equipment must be secure and accounted for before moving the patient so that nothing gets pulled out. If the patient is on oxygen, this must be continued at all times. In order to conserve the trolley supply, only switch over when you are almost ready to move the patient. All intravenous (IV) lines must be secured well. For any patient worse than 'ill stable', at least two IV lines should be placed in case of emergency.

Chest drains should be well secured to the patient and the bottles kept below the patient. Chest drains should not be clamped, as there is a risk of tension pneumothorax – especially if the clamp gets forgotten. If the bottle has to be lifted up, level with or above the patient, transiently on moving, there will be a risk of fluid going back into the thorax (but it will drain out again as soon as the bottle is placed below the patient). The bottles can be tied under the trolley for transfer.

It is good practice to check all around the patient before sliding them on or off the trolley to ensure that nothing gets caught and pulled out. It is important to keep the patient warm during transfer down corridors, and this can be achieved by wrapping warm blankets around the patient (while ensuring that there is easy access to cannula sites). If it is very cold on the journey, consider providing a hat of some sort for the patient, as the scalp blood vessels do not vasoconstrict and tend to lose heat easily.

Preventing problems during transfer

Before setting off, check that everything is ready and safe by following an ABCDE approach. Think about the common problems that may occur; they include the list (see Box 44.3) below:

Box 44.3 Potential problems during transfer

- Something may run out: e.g. oxygen, fluids, drug infusions or batteries.
- Something may happen: e.g. ABCD problems, cardiac arrest, respiratory arrest or convulsions. Do you have the skills and equipment needed to deal with a predictable or unpredictable event?
- Something may be forgotten: e.g. notes and x-rays or equipment as described above. Do you have a special transfer equipment bag that is checked regularly?
- Something may stop working: e.g. monitors or drips. Have you got a spare or a back-up?

Monitoring during transfer

This should follow the same standards as before the transfer. For in-hospital transfers, vital signs should at least be measured immediately before the journey and immediately afterwards at the destination. For longer journeys, they should be taken at least every 10 minutes, to ensure that any deterioration is picked up early.

Handover

The person performing the transfer needs to hand over the patient at the destination if the patient is to be left there. This should be a familiar practice but in the case of transfers it is important to hand over all notes and x-rays as well as retrieving any equipment.

Documentation

Many critical care networks have devised a specific form to be used for transfers. This includes space for observations and has checklists as well. Such forms provide a useful basis for audit of transfers.

Training of staff for transfers

It is important to delegate the job of transferring patients to experienced staff who have ideally had some specialist training. For inter-hospital transfers where the team is remote from the hospital, ALS is a good start, but in-house training or courses such as Safe Retrieval and Transfer (Advanced Life Support Group) are appropriate. Intensive care transfers should always be performed by doctors and nurses trained in ICU or anaesthetics.

HOT TIP

Preparation: Preparation is key – to fail to prepare is to prepare to fail!

Safety: Maintain patient safety at all times.

Equipment: Check all equipment before moving the patient. Check all medical devices and their battery life before moving the patient. Calculate and ensure oxygen supplies are adequate. Do not remove monitoring – if it is on already, they need it!

People: Ensure that you have the right people and the right equipment (and enough of both). Communicate with key personnel.

Conclusion

Moving a patient is potentially a dangerous task. However, by following the guidance in this chapter, the risks of moving sick patients can be minimised. It is essential to think ahead about possible problems and be prepared to deal with them. Patient safety is always paramount when transferring unwell ward patients either within or between hospitals.

References and further reading

Intensive Care Society (2011). *Guidelines for the transport of the critically ill adult.* 3rd edn. http://www.ics.ac.uk/ (accessed 27 August 2015).

Useful websites

Advanced Life Support Group – Safe Transfer and Retrieval Course (STaR)
http://www.alsg.org/uk/STaR (Accessed 27 August 2015)

Psychosocial aspects of acute illness

45 The post-ICU patient

Catherine Plowright

Admission to an intensive care or high dependency unit (ICU/HDU) has been described as a traumatic and frightening experience for patients and their families, and many highlight the fear, anxiety and psychological distress induced by critical illness (McGonigal 1986, Quinn *et al.* 1996, Viney 1996, Jones 2002, Skirrow 2002) as well as the physiological problems induced by critical illness on leaving the intensive care unit (Jones & Griffiths 2002, Kennedy *et al.* 2002, Waldmann 2002). This phenomenon is defined in a number of ways – for example, as transfer anxiety, relocation anxiety and translocation anxiety. It is recognised as a Diagnostic and Statistical Manual of Mental Disorders (DSM) diagnosis (American Psychiatric Association 2013).

This chapter offers practical guidance on how to care for patients recently relocated to a ward environment from the critical care area, enabling healthcare professionals to care for these patients with understanding. By the end of this chapter, you should understand the physical care needs of patients following a spell in the intensive care or high dependency unit, understand the psychological effects of critical illness, and know how to assess and deliver holistic care to this patient group.

Background

Patients who have been critically ill not only suffer from the effects of their critical illness but can also find that the transfer to a ward environment poses problems for them, despite their improved health status (Whittaker & Ball 2000). Healthcare professionals need to remember that critical illness affects each patient differently, regardless of the length of time they have spent in the intensive care unit. Whether or not the patient was intubated and ventilated will also have a bearing on how they experience the transition.

Evidence from patients has shown that many of them experience physiological, psychological and emotional effects following critical care (Herridge 2007, Desai *et al.* 2011, Harvey & Davidson 2011). ICU survivors and their families often face wide-ranging challenges. These can include, for example, a lower health-related quality of life (Myhren *et al.* 2010) and ICU-acquired weaknesses (e.g. neuromuscular dysfunction) (Herridge 2009, Griffiths & Hall 2010) and their effects on normal everyday activities such as walking and brushing one's hair or teeth.

There are also emotional and cognitive consequences of ICU treatment (Rattray *et al.* 2010, Jackson *et al.* 2012), from making sense of delirium experiences in the ICU (Samuelsona 2011) to the need to rebuild one's life after critical illness (Deacon 2012). 'Surviving a critical illness does come at a cost for patients and their families and nurses ... at different times' (Kean 2013, p. 603) during the critical illness experience journey.

HOT TIP

Misak (2011, p. 845) experienced a stay in intensive care as a patient and she states, 'it is hard to convey just how debilitated one is after an insult of ICU magnitude'.

Handover from intensive care or the high dependency unit

Handover from the intensive care or high dependency unit to the general ward is of paramount importance. The National Institute of Health and Care Excellence guidance (NICE 2007) states that the handover of care from these areas should include:

- A summary of the critical care stay, including diagnosis and treatment
- A monitoring and investigation plan
- A plan for on-going treatment, including drugs and therapies, nutrition plan, infection status and any agreed limitations of treatment
- Physical and rehabilitation needs
- Psychological and emotional needs
- Specific communication and language needs.

The guidance also states that the critical care team and the ward multidisciplinary team should take shared responsibility for the care of the patient being transferred. The handover should be formal, structured and supported by a written plan. It is important for the critical care team caring for the patient to ensure that the receiving ward can deliver the agreed plan. This ensures that continuity of care is maximised and that the ward staff (including nursing, medical and allied healthcare professionals) have adequate and relevant information about the patient's condition and needs.

Specific needs of patients

The post-intensive care needs of patients fall into two broad categories: physical and non-physical (NICE 2009). Physical issues include muscle loss, muscle weakness, musculoskeletal problems (such as contractures), respiratory problems, sensory problems, pain, and swallowing and communication problems. Non-physical problems may include psychological, emotional and psychiatric problems, and cognitive dysfunction (NICE 2009).

Evidence shows that mortality rates are higher when patients are discharged from critical care units in the evening or at night-time and at weekends (Elliot *et al.* 2012, Bramma *et al.* 2012, Gantner *et al.* 2012). It is advisable for patient safety and continuity of care to ensure that the transfer to a ward from the ICU or HDU takes place before 22.00 hours at night and not before 07.00 in the morning (NICE 2007). Bramma, Allan & Sundaram (2012) suggest that the discharge from intensive care should occur before 17.00 and Elliot, Worral-Carter & Page (2012) imply that weekend discharges should be avoided. It has been suggested that all ICU or HDU discharges that occur outside these times should be recorded as untoward incidents.

Box 45.1: Physical and non-physical problems after intensive care (NICE 2009)

Physical issues include:

- Muscle loss
- Muscle weakness
- Musculoskeletal problems (including contractures)
- Respiratory problems
- Sensory problems
- Pain
- Swallowing problems
- Communication problems.

Non-physical problems include:

- Psychological
- Emotional
- Psychiatric
- Cognitive dysfunctional.

Regardless of what time of day or night the patient is transferred to a ward, the multidisciplinary team must be available to care for all the patient's needs.

This step down can be a difficult time for patients who have been critically ill, and for their visitors. They are moving from a very highly staffed and complex area to a general ward area, where there are fewer nurses per patient. Patients who have had a long stay in intensive care sometimes experience a sense of abandonment when transferred to the ward. This is in addition to the other physical and psychological problems they may have.

The physical and non-physical psychological problems this creates, and ways to resolve them, are now discussed.

Physical problems

Muscle weakness is probably the most obvious and incapacitating feature of recovery from critical illness that patients and healthcare professionals are presented with. It would have contributed to the overall recovery of the patient while on intensive care, and will continue to do so on return to the ward. Critically ill patients can develop critical illness polyneuropathies, myopathies or a combination of both (Kennedy *et al.* 2002). They can also develop drug-induced neuropathies or generalised demyelination caused by infections (Kennedy *et al.* 2002).

Whatever the cause, muscle wasting will occur, as well as wastage of lean tissue and skeletal muscle. Critically ill patients can lose 1% of their lean body mass per day of their critical illness (Griffiths 2002). The consequences of this are often manifested on the intensive care unit, especially if the patient has been intubated and ventilated for any significant period of time, and during what is often a prolonged weaning phase from the ventilator. Prolonged weaning from a ventilator in intensive care is necessary because the diaphragm and other respiratory muscles are among the muscles affected by the wastage. They need to build up strength over the weaning period.

Respiratory problems

Patients who have respiratory muscle weakness often endure prolonged weaning from mechanical ventilation. Less obvious may be their inability to cough and clear secretions adequately because they need to have respiratory muscle power and cough power to perform this simple task. A tracheostomy is often required during admission to intensive care and this may remain in place when the patient returns to the ward environment, for secretion control (see Chapter 7 on tracheostomies and also Dawson 2014).

The multidisciplinary healthcare team (especially physiotherapists and nurses) need to work together with the patient to maintain respiratory function and remove the tracheostomy as soon as possible (see Chapter 4 on physiotherapy). The nurse should encourage the patient to undertake the breathing exercises that the physiotherapist has given them, and to use any adjuncts that they were given (such as inspirometers).

Eating and drinking problems

Patients should have received nutrition when on the intensive care or high dependency unit, and yet they will lose weight. It is important for their nutrition to continue when they leave the unit; yet this can be challenging to ward staff (see Chapter 39 on feeding patients). Patients who are recovering from critical illness present a number of challenges that need to be overcome, including lack of desire, opportunity and physical ability to eat and drink.

The desire to eat is limited by many factors such as pain, tiredness, psychological issues and taste problems. Changes reported by patients include food tasting metallic or salty, or having no taste at all. Merriweather, Smith & Walsh (2014) reviewed post-intensive care patients from a nutritional perspective and found that their nutritional needs were not met. Some of the reasons for this included the ward culture, service-centred delivery of care and disjointed discharge planning.

Patients who do not experience the desire to eat and drink pose specific challenges to healthcare professionals, for whom achieving adequate nutritional status is of paramount importance. The physical ability to eat and drink can be affected by general muscle weakness, which limits their use of their arms when bringing food from the plate to their mouths. In addition, they may not be able to sit up or hold their heads up. These problems are easily identified by healthcare professionals, as they can be visualised, but the effects of muscle weakness that cannot be seen are often not appreciated, such as difficulty in swallowing and chewing.

Eating, drinking and swallowing are complex mechanisms that require control and timing because breathing is interrupted as part of the process. A number of swallowing difficulties (including aspiration, regurgitation and avoidance of food and drink) can also be presented and healthcare professionals must be aware of these (Griffiths 2002). It is important to involve dieticians and speech and language therapists in the care of these patients. This will ensure that they are able to swallow and that all their nutrition needs are being met.

Information about nutrition on discharge from hospital may help patients who are still experiencing some of the difficulties noted above. General advice would consist of having small and frequent meals, and a broad, balanced diet. Healthy eating and exercise should be encouraged to promote muscle growth and fat distribution and improve pulmonary and cardiovascular function (Griffiths 2002).

Mobility

Mobility is often reduced when patients are discharged from the intensive care or high dependency unit, as a direct result of muscle weakness. The longer the length of stay in critical care areas and the greater the number of days spent ventilated, the higher the chance of mobility problems (Jones & Griffiths 2002). The extent of the problem is clear when patients have difficultiy getting in and out of bed, moving themselves up in the bed, walking to the toilet, and balancing.

Teams need to work together to improve the recovery of these patients, and it is vital that physiotherapists and occupational therapists are involved at an early stage. Patients need encouragement to mobilise within their limits. By working together with the patient, teams can agree a plan that will enable the patient to recover strength and independence. For example, if the physiotherapist assists the patient to sit out in a chair, the nurse should agree with the patient and the physiotherapist the length of time the patient should remain there. The patient should also be encouraged to do exercises that the physiotherapist has prescribed for them.

Caring for patients with physical problems after intensive care

Significant numbers of patients surviving critical illness have continuing physical problems. For many, being discharged from the ICU or HDU is the start of an unknown journey. Rehabilitation of these patients should commence in intensive care and be followed up when they are on a ward, and should continue through to discharge from hospital and into the community (NICE 2009). Healthcare professionals in ward environments should continue to ensure that any rehabilitation initiated during the stay on the ICU or HDU is continued on the ward.

It is essential that all healthcare teams work together to improve the recovery of these patients, and it is vital that nurses, doctors, physiotherapists, speech and language therapists and occupational therapists are involved in the needs of the patients. The physical rehabilitation of these patients must be specific and individualised.

There is limited evidence on the clinical effectiveness of rehabilitation strategies when these patients are in ward environments (NICE 2009). Jones *et al.* (2003) devised a 6-week structured and supported self-help rehabilitation programme, which has been shown to improve the physical recovery of patients. This programme is based on the individual physical and cognitive capacity of patients at different stages in their recovery. The rehabilitation manual includes information on the types of exercise that patients should be undertaking, including leg and arm strengthening exercises, as well as providing information about what to expect during the journey to recovery, about eating and drinking and sex after serious illness.

Some hospitals have employed generic rehabilitation assistants to promote recovery after a critical illness (Salisbury, Merriweather & Walsh 2010). Work currently being undertaken in Scotland is looking at how a complex rehabilitation intervention programme, with generic rehabilitation assistants, can promote physical recovery following critical illness (Ramsay, Salisbury, Merriweather *et al.* 2014).

Non-physical (psychological) problems

There has been increasing awareness of the psychological problems encountered by patients following admission to the ICU or HDU over recent years. Non-physical problems identified include anxiety, depression, and post-traumatic stress (Cuthbertson *et al.* 2004, Myhren *et al.* 2010, Rattray Johnston *et al.* 2005), as well as hallucinations, sleep disorders, memory disturbances, confusion and cognitive impairment (Jones *et al.* 2000, Jones *et al.* 2001, Jones 2002).

It is important for all healthcare professionals caring for patients following discharge from intensive care to understand that they may have psychological problems. Patients often have little or no memory of the time they spent in the critical care area, or of how critically ill they were. For this reason, they may have difficulty understanding the slowness of their recovery and feel hopeless, which can lead on to psychological problems (Jones 2002). These patients often cannot recall the events that occurred before their admission to hospital (Jones *et al.* 2000).

Some healthcare professionals take the view that not remembering may be helpful. However, this is not the case (Griffiths *et al.* 1996). Staff should ensure that patients have a full understanding of what happened to them and how ill they were. These patients often have delusional memories, such as hallucinations, which they find very frightening and very real. In addition, they often suffer from anxiety and depression and demonstrate symptoms of post-traumatic stress disorder (Griffiths *et al.* 1994, Jones & Griffiths 2000, Scragg *et al.* 2001). Post-traumatic stress is more likely to occur if the only memories that patients have are delusional (Jones *et al.* 2001). Patients experiencing sleep difficulties often have nightmares and it can be the fear of the nightmares that causes the sleep difficulty. Remember that night sedation may not help the situation, as the nightmares will still be present.

Evidence suggests that non-physical symptomatology is increased by pre-illness factors, such as previous psychiatric history (Cuthbertson *et al.* 2004, Jones *et al.* 2001). In addition to non-physical issues, significant cognitive decline in many patients has been found following critical illness, including impaired memory and executive function (Pandharipande *et al.* 2013, Wolters *et al.* 2013).

Caring for post-intensive care patients with psychological problems

The anxiety and depression experienced by recently discharged intensive care unit patients often resolve with time, but if prolonged psychological problems are evident then formal help must be obtained. You need to talk to these patients, using simple techniques such as breathing control to help with any panic attacks, and have an understanding of the experiences they had while on the unit. If you are unable to give them this type of help, perhaps the critical care outreach nurses, intensive care unit nurses or nurse consultants for critical care, if available, will be able to assist you. In addition, it is essential to seek out whatever specialist help is available within the organisation to assist with this aspect of a patient's care. Although they are alarming, these types of post-intensive care unit problems are not uncommon and should resolve in time with appropriate help.

Some intensive care units use patient diaries as a tool to explain to patients what happened to them when they were so sick that they were not aware of anything (Backman 2002, Backman & Walther 2005, Coombe 2005, Aitken *et al.* 2013, Akerman *et al.* 2013). These diaries can assist with any gaps in their memory and give the facts of what happened while the patient was on the unit. There are two types of diaries: prospective and retrospective.

Retrospective diaries involve a healthcare professional examining the patient's health records after discharge from intensive care, and writing a record of the significant events and care and treatment received. Patients can find this type of diary impersonal and difficult to relate to, and they are time-consuming for staff to complete (Coombe 2005).

Prospective diaries are written by all healthcare professionals involved in the care of the patient and the family, and are added to on a daily basis, recording the all-important milestones. They might also include photographs (Backman 2002, Backman & Walther 2005) and serve to give the patient a realistic picture of how unwell they were. The diary is then given to the patient, following discharge from the unit, when it is considered that they are psychologically ready to read about the extent of their illness. It requires time from the critical care nurse to explain about the diary to the patient. In some organisations, this role is shared between the intensive care staff and critical care outreach nurses.

The efficacy of this initiative has yet to be robustly evaluated, but testimony from patients and their families is that the diary helps to fill memory gaps and helps patients understand what happened. Garrouste-Orgeas *et al.* (2012) have shown that the use of diaries can reduce post-traumatic stress-related symptoms in patients and their families.

Case scenario

A 25-year-old woman is admitted to your ward following a 2-week stay in intensive care and a 6-day stay in the high dependency unit. She was admitted to hospital with community-acquired pneumonia and Type 1 respiratory failure and in septic shock. She was previously fit and healthy and worked full-time as a schoolteacher. She lives with her partner. You are the registered nurse caring for her.

Describe how you would plan this patient's critical care rehabilitation up to the time of her discharge from hospital. What other healthcare professionals would you involve?

Conclusion

Patients who have been discharged from intensive care and high dependency units may experience significant physical and non-physical effects of their critical illness, which will affect their care when on a ward. An understanding of why this occurs enables the healthcare professional to care for these patients in a way that minimises these effects.

The latest National Institute for Health and Care Excellence (NICE) clinical guidelines concerning critical care were published on 25 March 2009 (NICE 2009). These are for critical illness rehabilitation (rehabilitation after critical care). The guidelines look at the care and rehabilitation of patients after critical illness, and they apply to patients in both England and Wales.

References and further reading

Aitken, L.M., Rattray, J., Hull, A., Kenardy, J.A., Le Brocque, R. & Ullman, A. J. (2013). The use of diaries in psychological recovery from intensive care. *Critical Care.* **17** (6), 253–60.

Akerman, E., Ersson, A., Fridlund, B. & Samuelson, K. (2103). Preferred content and usefulness of a photodiary as described by ICU-patients: A mixed method analysis. *Australian Critical Care.* **26** (1), 29–35.

American Psychiatric Association (2013). *Diagnostic and Statistical Manual of Mental Disorders* 5th edn. Washington DC: American Psychiatric Association.

Backman, C. (2002). 'Patient diaries in ICU' in R.D. Griffiths & C. Jones (eds) *Intensive Care Aftercare.* Oxford: Butterworth Heinemann.

Backman, C. & Walther, S.M. (2005). 'The photo-dairy and follow-up appointment on ICU: Giving back time to patients and relatives' in S. Ridley (ed.) *Critical Care Focus: The Psychological Challenges of Intensive Care.* Oxford: Blackwell Publishing.

Brett, S. (2005). 'Cognitive impairment and consequences for recovery' in S. Ridley (ed.) *Critical Care Focus: The Psychological Challenges of Intensive Care.* Oxford: Blackwell Publishing.

Coombe, D. (2005). The use of patient diaries in an intensive care unit. *Nursing in Critical Care.* **10** (1), 3–4.

Cotton, K. (2012). NICE CG83 – rehabilitation after critical illness: implementation across a network. *Nursing in Critical Care.* **18** (1), 32–42.

Cuthbertson, B.H., Hull, A., Strachan, M. & Scott, J. (2004). Post-traumatic stress disorder after critical illness requiring general intensive care. *Intensive Care Medicine*. **30** (3), 450–55.

Dawson, D. (2014). Essential principles: tracheostomy care in the adult patient. *Nursing in Critical Care*. **19** (2), 63–72.

Deacon, K. (2012). Re-building life after ICU: a qualitative study of the patients' perspective. *Intensive and Critical Care Nursing*. **28** (2), 114–122.

Desai, S., Law, T. & Needham, D. (2011). Long-term complications of critical care. *Critical Care Medicine*. **39** (12), 371–79.

Elliot, M., Worral-Carter, L. & Page, K. (2012). Factors associated with in-hospital mortality following ICU discharge: a comprehensive review. *British Journal of Intensive Care*. **22** (4), 120–25.

Garrouste-Orgeas, M., Coquet, I., Perier, A., Timsit. J. F., Pochard, F., Lancrin, F., Philippart, F., Vesin, A., Bruel, C., Blel, Y., Angeli, S., Cousin, N., Carlet, J. & Misset, B. (2012). Impact of an intensive care unit diary on psychological distress in patients and relatives. *Critical Care Medicine*. **40** (7), 2033–40.

Griffiths, R.D. (2002). 'Nutrition after intensive care' in R.D. Griffiths & C. Jones (eds) *Intensive Care Aftercare*. Oxford: Butterworth Heinemann.

Griffiths, R.D., Jones, C. & Macmillan, R.R. (1996). Where is the harm in not knowing? Care after intensive care. *Clinical Intensive Care*. **7**, 14–45.

Griffiths, R.D., Jones, C., Macmillan, R.R. & Palmer, T.E.A. (1994). Psychological problems occurring after intensive care. *British Journal of Intensive Care*. **4**, 46–53.

Griffiths, R., & Hall, J. (2010). Intensive care unit-acquired weakness. *Critical Care Medicine*. 38 (3), 779–87.

Harvey, M. & Davidson, J. (2011). Long-term consequences of critical illness: a new opportunity for high-impact critical care nurses. *Critical Care Nurse*. **31** (5), 12–15.

Herridge, M. (2007). Long-term outcomes after critical illness: past, present, future. *Current Opinion in Critical Care*. **13** (5), 473–75.

Herridge, M. (2009). Legacy of intensive care unit-acquired weakness. *Critical Care Medicine*. **37**, S457–461.

Jackson, J., Ely, W., Morey, M., Anderson, V., Denne, L., Clune, J., Siebert, C., Archer, K., Torres, R., Janz, D., Schiro, E., Jones, J., Shintani, A., Levine, B., Pun, B., Thompson, J., Brummel, N. & Hoenig, H. (2012). Cognitive and physical rehabilitation of intensive care unit survivors: results of the RETURN randomized controlled pilot investigation. *Critical Care Medicine*. **40** (4), 1088–97.

Jones, C., Griffiths, R.D. & Humphris, G.M. (2000). Disturbed memory and amnesia related to intensive care. *Memory*. **8** (2), 79–94.

Jones, C., Griffiths, R.D., Humphris, G.M. & Skirrow, P. (2001). Memory, delusions and the development of post-traumatic stress disorder-related symptoms after intensive care. *Critical Care Medicine*. **29** (3), 57–80.

Jones, C. (2002). 'Acute psychological problems' in R.D. Griffiths & C. Jones (eds) *Intensive Care Aftercare*. Oxford: Butterworth Heinemann.

Jones, C. & Griffiths, R.D. (2002). Identifying post intensive care patients who may need physical rehabilitation. *Clinical Intensive Care*. **11**, 3–8.

Jones, C., Skirrow, P., Griffiths, R.D., Humphris, G.H., Ingleby, S., Eddleston, J., Waldmann, C. & Gager, M. (2003). Rehabilitation after critical illness: a randomized, controlled trial. *Critical Care Medicine*. **31**, 2456–61.

Kean, K. (2013) Surviving critical illness: Intensive care and beyond. *Journal of Clinical Nursing*. **23** (5–6), 603–604.

Kennedy, D.D., Coakley, J. & Griffiths, R.D. (2002). 'Neuromuscular problems and physical weakness' in R.D. Griffiths & C. Jones (eds) *Intensive Care Aftercare*. Oxford: Butterworth Heinemann.

McGonigal, K.S. (1986). The importance of sleep and the sensory environment to critically ill patients. *Intensive Care Nursing*. 2(2), 73–83.

Merriweather, J., Smith, P. & Walsh, T. (2014). Nutritional rehabilitation after ICU – does it happen: a qualitative interview and observational study. *Journal of Clinical Nursing*. 23 (5–6), 654–62.

Misak, C.J. (2011). ICU-acquired weakness: obstacles and interventions for rehabilitation. *American Journal of Respiratory Critical Care Medicine*. **183** (7), 845–46.

Myhren, H., Ekeberg, Ø. & Stokland, O. (2010). Health-related quality of life and return to work after critical illness in general intensive care unit patients: a 1-year follow-up study. *Critical Care Medicine*. **38** (7), 1554–61.

Myhren, H., Ekeberg, O., Toien, K., Karlsson, S. & Stokland, O. (2010). Posttraumatic stress, anxiety and depression symptoms in patients during the first year post intensive care discharge. *Critical Care*. **14** (1), R14.

National Institute of Health and Care Excellence. (2007). *Acutely ill patients in hospital: Recognition of and response to acute illness in adults in hospital.* http://www.nice.org.uk/guidance/CG50 (accessed 31 August 2015).

National Institute of Health and Care Excellence (2009). *Critical illness rehabilitation – rehabilitation after critical care.* http://www.nice.org.uk/Guidance/CG83 (accessed 31 August 2015).

Pandharipande, P.P., Girard, T.D., Jackson, J.C., Morandi, A., Thompson, J.L., Pun, B.T., Brummel, N.E., Hughes, C.G., Vasilevskis, E.E., Shintani, A.K., Moons, K.G., Geevarghese, S.K., Canonico, A., Hopkins, R.O., Bernard, G.R., Dittus, R.S. & Ely, E.W.; for the BRAIN-ICU Study Investigators (2013). Long-term cognitive impairment after critical illness. *New England Journal of Medicine.* **369**, 1306–16.

Quinn, S., Redmond K. & Begley, C. (1996). The needs of relatives visiting adult intensive care units as perceived by relatives and nurses. *Intensive and Critical Care Nursing.* **12** (3), 16–72.

Ramsay, P., Salisbury, L.G., Merriweather, J.L., Huby, G., Rattray, J. E., Hull, A.M., Brett, S.J., Mackenzie, S.L.,Murray, G.D., Forbes, J.F. & Walsh, T.S., on behalf of the RECOVER trial collaboration (2014). A rehabilitation intervention to promote physical recovery following intensive care: a detailed description of construct development, rationale and content together with proposed taxonomy to capture processes in a randomised controlled trial. *Trials.* **15**, 38.

Rattray, J. (2014). Life after critical illness: an overview. *Journal of Clinical Nursing.* **23** (5–6), 623–33.

Rattray, J.E., Johnston, M. & Wildsmith, J.A. (2005). Predictors of emotional outcomes of intensive care. *Anaesthesia.* **60** (11), 1085–92.

Rattray, J., Crocker, C., Jones, M. & Connaghan, J. (2010). Patients' perceptions of and emotional outcome after intensive care: results from a multicentre study. *Nursing in Critical Care.* **15** (2), 86–93.

Samuelsona, K. (2011). Unpleasant and pleasant memories of intensive care in adult mechanically ventilated patients – findings from 250 interviews. *Intensive and Critical Care Nursing.* **27** (2), 76–84.

Salisbury, L.G., Merriweather, J.L. & Walsh, T. (2010). Rehabilitation after critical illness: could a ward-based generic rehabilitation assistant promote recovery? *Nursing in Critical Care.* **15** (2), 57–65.

Scragg, P., Jones, A. & Fauvel, N. (2001). Psychological problems following intensive care unit treatment. *Anaesthesia.* **56**, 9–14.

Skirrow, P. (2001). 'Delusional memories of intensive care unit' in R.D. Griffiths & C. Jones (eds). *Intensive Care Aftercare.* Oxford: Butterworth Heinemann.

Viney, C. (ed.) (1996). 'Pain and sedation needs' in *Nursing the Critically Ill.* London: Bailliere Tindall.

Waldmann, C. (2002). 'Sexual problems and their treatments' in R.D. Griffiths, & C. Jones (eds). *Intensive Care Aftercare.* Oxford: Butterworth Heinemann.

Wolters, A.E., Slooter, A.J.C., van der Kooi, A.W. & van Dijk, D. (2013). Cognitive impairment after intensive care unit admission: a systematic review. *Intensive Care Medicine.* 39 (3), 376–86.

Whittaker, J. & Ball, C. (2000). Discharge from intensive care: a view from the ward. *Intensive and Critical Care Nursing.* **16** (3), 13–43.

Ullman, A.J., Aitken, L.M., Rattray, J., Kenardy, J., Le Brocque, R., MacGillivray, S. & Hull, A.M. (2014). Diaries for recovery from critical illness. *Cochrane Database Systematic Review.* **9**, 12.

Useful websites

ICU Diary
http://www.icu-diary.org/diary/start.html
(Accessed 31 August 2015)

ICUSteps
http://www.icusteps.org/
(Accessed 31 August 2015)

National Institute for Health and Care Excellence (NICE)
http://www.nice.org.uk
(Accessed 31 August 2015)

NHS Choices
http://www.nhs.uk/Conditions/Intensive-care/Pages/Recovery.aspx
(Accessed 31 August 2015)

Society of Critical Care Medicine
http://www.myicucare.org/Adult-Support/Pages/Post-intensive-Care-Syndrome.aspx
(Accessed 31 August 2015)

46 Ethics of acute care

Victor Nebbiolo and Sally A. Smith

The ethics of acute care is a vast, controversial and complex topic. With the advancement in medical science over recent years, it is has become more so, and the situation is further complicated by the multicultural and ethnic backgrounds of patients, their relatives, and staff who live and work in our society. Today's healthcare system truly knows no cultural or ethnic boundaries for its staff or clients.

Access to information via the media, television and Internet means people are better informed (accurately or otherwise), about options and alternatives that may be available nationally and internationally. In today's society, expectations of healthcare have changed, and will continue to do so.

By the end of this chapter, you should have an understanding of ethical principles, human rights, 'do not resuscitate' decisions, consent and resuscitation in acute care; and be more aware of your own personal, social, cultural, ethnic and political background, which may influence the decision-making process.

Background

Today's modern healthcare system has changed and continues to do so. Gone are the days when patients and their relatives did as healthcare professionals told them because 'they knew best'. Today, people are more prepared to challenge decisions about care options, and patients have a legal right to be involved in the decision-making process (BMA 2013). Decisions taken by doctors are likely to be compliant with the Human Rights Act 1998, which covers issues such as human dignity, communication and consultation, and best interests (Mason & Laurie 2013, Herring 2014, BMA 2013). All are central to good clinical practice (see Table 46.1).

Table 46.1 The Human Rights Act 1998

Convention rights with particular relevance to the practice of medicine	
Article 2	Right to life
Article 3	Right to freedom from torture or inhuman or degrading treatment or punishment

Article 5	Right to liberty and security
Article 6	Right to a fair trial
Article 8	Right to respect for private and family life
Article 9	Freedom of thought, conscience and religion
Article 10	Freedom of expression
Article 12	Right to marry and found a family
Article 14	Enjoyment of these rights to be secured without discrimination

For all professionals, practice must always entail ethical decision-making within our professional codes of conduct as laid down by our professional bodies, such as the General Medical Council, and the Nursing and Midwifery Council. In addition, caring for patients and decisions made about care must take into account the patient's rights under the Mental Capacity Act: Making Decisions (2014). This poses particular challenges with the acutely unwell patient, who may not be competent to understand or agree to treatment options. Box 46.1 outlines the five principles that underpin this Act.

Box 46.1
The five principles underpinning the Mental Capacity Act 2014

1. **A presumption of capacity**: every adult has the right to make their own decisions and must be assumed to have capacity to do so unless it is proved otherwise.

2. **Individuals being supported to make their own decisions**: a person must be given all practicable help before anyone treats them as not being able to make their own decisions.

3. **Unwise decisions**: just because an individual makes what might be seen as an unwise decision, they should not be treated as lacking capacity to make that decision.

4. **Best interests**: an act done or decision made under the Act for or on behalf of a person who lacks capacity must be done in their best interests.

5. **Less restrictive option**: anything done for or on behalf of a person who lacks capacity should be considerate of options that are less restrictive of their basic rights and freedoms if they are as effective as the proposed option.

In addition, there can be some very challenging situations when there is a difference in the perceived care pathways and the likely benefit of the chosen pathway for all concerned. Discussions will include the patient, their relatives, carers and the wider establishment that is charged with providing and managing resources to provide optimum care. In order to try and address some of these complex moral and ethical dilemmas, some simple fundamental rules should be applied to the situations that we may find ourselves in. Ideally, we should be doing what the patient wants, with an underlying principle of always doing what is best for the patient.

In the simplest terms, all care pathways should be guided by:

- Beneficence
- Nonmaleficence
- Respect for autonomy
- The principle of justice.

Beneficence

This means that the care and decisions made by all concerned should benefit the patient: not only in their short-term care, but ultimately in their holistic management (both physical and psychological), during the long-term disease process. In the past, this has often been perceived as prolonging life to its maximum.

The principle of beneficence relates to the notions of 'do no harm' and 'maximise possible benefits, and minimise possible harms' (National Commission for the Protection of Human Subjects of Biomedical and Behavioural Research 2003). It means nurses and doctors doing what will benefit the patient 'according to their best judgement'.

In today's modern health service, it is sometimes possible to maintain and preserve functionality of the physical body with no perceived benefit to the person as a whole. Different cultural, religious and personal values can be encountered, depending on the priority given to the preservation of physical life versus quality of the person's life. Wherever possible, the wishes of the patient need to be ascertained and considered, thinking about their view of beneficial treatment. Healthcare staff also have values and different views of 'benefit' that they need to acknowledge and discuss when dealing with complex situations.

Non-maleficence

This requires all concerned to look at their motives during the decision-making process and ensure they are always following the principle of 'doing the patient no harm' (Seedhouse 2002).

Respect for autonomy and the principle of justice

Linked with the patient's ability to understand and make decisions, as stated in the Mental Capacity Act 2005, these principles require us to respect the patient's choices and to ensure that all care prescribed and given is just and fair (Cribb 2002).

Resuscitation issues

These days, resuscitation no longer means 'blowing and bashing', although this is still a misperception commonly held by the public – and some healthcare professionals. In fact resuscitation today covers a vast array of treatments, from simple oxygen and fluid therapy to full intensive-care-unit therapy with its multi-organ support facilities.

Any discussion of issues surrounding resuscitation must be very specific to the patient in question. There must also be very clear parameters for the decisions being made, and the discussion must be an intrinsic part of the patient's care pathway, following the principles of beneficence and non-maleficence. Ideally, these decisions should be made in advance, as part of the overall planning of care and treatment (BMA 2014, Resuscitation Council 2015).

These issues can be expanded to cover some of the legal aspects and practicality of attempting resuscitation. Consider the following case scenario.

Case scenario

A 71-year-old man has been admitted to a medical ward with pneumonia. He is very short of breath and requires high-flow oxygen to maintain his oxygen saturations at above 90%. His respiratory rate is 34 breaths per minute, his heart rate is 110 beats per minute, and his blood pressure is 98/54mmHg. He is drowsy and responds to verbal commands by opening his eyes. He appears to be tiring.

His past medical history is that he has chronic obstructive pulmonary disease and uses home oxygen. He cannot get out of the house, and sleeps and stays in his armchair at home. His family care for him by doing his shopping, cooking for him and helping him with his hygiene needs.

His family reports that he has requested that he be left to die peacefully should he become unwell. They too do not want him to suffer unduly. Staff on the ward assess his condition as deteriorating and they have called the medical team to review him and agree a treatment plan.

Taking into consideration the principles outlined above, the healthcare teams, along with the patient and his family, will consider the following ethical questions in order to agree a treatment plan:

1. *What does the patient want? If possible, when addressing these issues, it should be with consideration of the patient's known or obtainable wishes.*

2. *What is the likely outcome for the patient, both in the short and long term, and would that be acceptable to him?*

3. *What are the legal implications, including the European Court of Human Rights Act 1998 (implemented in the UK in October 2000), 'The right to life and the right to be free from degrading treatment'? Have all reasonable treatments and treatment options been considered, with beneficence and non-maleficence in mind?*

When taking the patient's known or obtainable wishes into consideration, some criteria need to be followed. According to the Mental Capacity Act 2014 and the principle of promoting patient autonomy, the patient should be:

1. Of sound mind
2. Free from duress
3. Fully informed.

However, issues relating to resuscitation pathways most commonly arise when the patient is acutely unwell. In the above case scenario, the patient was drowsy and unable to communicate clearly. That being the case, some serious consideration needs to be given to these basic questions. If the patient is acutely unwell, are they really:

1. Of sound mind
2. Free from duress
3. Fully informed (in an unbiased manner)?

With patients like the man in the case scenario (who lack capacity, which is common in emergency care), it is necessary to determine the patient's best interests and act in accordance with whatever they are deemed to be (BMA 2014). Discussion with the patient's family about the patient's previously expressed wishes and opinions may help, although this has no standing in law (BMA 2013). Ultimately, the clinician in charge must make the decision, and it would be reasonable to assume that most people would want any intervention likely to save a life or prevent disability (BMA 2013).

In this case scenario, the family were in agreement that escalating the patient's care to support his respiratory function through ventilation, or resuscitating him should he die, would not be in accordance with his wishes, nor in his best interests – given his comorbidities.

Patient consent

Consent should be sought before starting a patient on an agreed pathway of care. It should include a full explanation of the risks, benefits and possible alternatives available. However, in reality, when patients become acutely unwell, the validity and practicality of gaining consent with these criteria fully met is dubious and is certainly open to being challenged. Failure to obtain valid consent could lead to criminal charges of assault or negligence.

When formal consent is not available, healthcare professionals may act with implied consent (that being what they think the patient would want and with the patient's best interest in mind, and in the absence of a clear refusal). All consent gained or implied must be clearly documented in the patient's notes, without ambiguity, for future reference. Other professionals may scrutinise these documents very thoroughly at a later date. It would have been very difficult to gain consent from the patient in the above case scenario. Fortunately, his wishes were known and could therefore be respected. A 'Do not resuscitate' order was agreed and a form was completed and filed in his notes.

Do Not Attempt Resuscitation (DNAR) orders

There are a number of terms used for this inaction when a patient has a full cardiac arrest, defined by no breathing and no effective circulation (Resuscitation Council 2015):

- DNAR – Do Not Attempt Resuscitation
- DNR – Do Not Resuscitate
- NFACPR – Not For Attempted Cardio Pulmonary Resuscitation
- DNACPR – Do Not Attempt Cardio Pulmonary Resuscitation.

There is often a misperception of what such a decision means in relation to patient treatment options. It should mean that if a patient stops breathing and their heart does not pump blood around the body with sufficient pressure to provide organ perfusion, artificial ventilation and external cardiac compressions will not be started. This does not mean withholding other forms of resuscitation action (such as oxygen and intravenous fluids) or treatments such as inotropic drugs, antibiotics and analgesia. Decisions to withhold some of these might be classified as 'non-escalation of treatment'. Once treatment has been started, removing said treatment might be classified as 'withdrawal of treatment' – sometimes because the patient is improving and no longer requires that treatment, or because the treatment is having no beneficial effect on their recovery.

In order for an NFACPR order to be valid, it should (whenever possible) be discussed with the patient using the above criteria. It should be written, signed, and dated and, if possible, witnessed by an independent party. Most, but not all, will have a review date. This is to allow for the patient's condition to improve, and also for the patient to change their mind. The decision should be clearly documented in all patient notes, and staff involved in the care of the patient should be informed.

The patient in the above case scenario continued to receive his oxygen, fluids, nutrition and drugs, as the ceiling of his medical treatment. However, it was essential that he was also kept comfortable.

Decision makers

Who has ultimate responsibility for deciding on a patient's care pathway and treatment options? It should be the most senior doctor in charge of that patient's care (BMA 2013). This would normally be the patient's GP in the community or their consultant (if they are under hospital care). It may be delegated to someone more junior (i.e. a registrar), but ultimate responsibility is with the GP or consultant.

When making these decisions, the criteria of beneficence, non-maleficence and 'what the patient wants' should be employed. It is considered best practice to seek input from other members of the team involved in the patient's care, including the relatives if appropriate, but at present there is no legal obligation to do this. Delays and controversies are more likely to arise when there is a large and diverse group contributing to the decision-making process. All decisions made should be very clearly documented and it should be ensured that all personnel responsible for, or involved in, delivering care to the patient are aware of the specific treatment pathway for that patient. This will prevent confusion and stop inappropriate resuscitation attempts.

Post-cardiac arrest

Patients who have survived a cardiac arrest will require some form of acute care. This may range from simple monitoring to full multi-organ support. There have been various studies on survival outcome predictors, but to date none are sufficiently accurate to be relied upon. The available resources and the abilities of the staff in the location of the patient may raise some dilemmas for those involved in managing and providing for that patient's optimum care. In today's stretched healthcare system the resources available often govern the optimum treatment.

Accessing more advanced treatment options may require transfer of the patient, which in itself could be detrimental. Therefore all the options need to be considered and then the optimum course of action for that patient, in that specific situation, can be decided upon. When sub-optimal decisions have to be made, they should be clearly documented, stating the exact reason for the decision, with the options explored and reasons given for not choosing these, always following the principles of beneficence and non-maleficence and ethical decision-making in professional codes of conduct.

Confidentiality

All patients have a right to confidentiality, and this is essential in all forms of clinical consultations. This principle is vital when working in the field of acute care and is governed in law by the European Convention on Human Rights, Respect for Privacy and Family Life (Article 8) Act 1998 (Data Protection Act 1998). Disclosures required by law or made in connection with legal proceedings are exempt from the non-disclosure provisions by virtue of section 35 of the Act. Also, all NHS Trusts and private sector establishments should have some form of policy covering or incorporating aspects on confidentiality.

The 1998 Act aims to protect and control the flow of patient information (data) while ensuring that confidentiality is not undermined. More recently, the Caldicott Information Governance Review (2013) addressed concerns about the ease with which data can be disseminated. Patient confidentiality must be maintained, and the patient's best interest must be ensured when sharing and passing on information between professionals. This can be very difficult in the ward environment, where highly sensitive decisions may sometimes need to be made at the bedside.

For discussion and further thought, consider the following case scenario. It may be helpful to discuss this with your colleagues.

Case scenario

A 65-year-old woman has breast cancer and is receiving chemotherapy treatment for this. She is admitted to the accident and emergency department with a one-week history of chest pain and shortness of breath and is now in what appears to be a moribund state. A chest x-ray shows bilateral lower lobe pneumonia, pleural effusion and what appear to be multiple skeletal metastatic growths.

The relatives say that she has been complaining of 'excruciating pain' prior to admission. Her husband says, 'I want everything done to save her.' Her daughter says, 'Mum wanted to go in her sleep with no pain.'

How would you address this situation?

What concepts of beneficence need to be addressed?

What principles of non-maleficence need to be considered before planning a care pathway for this patient?

How would you maintain this patient's confidentiality?

Conclusion

Ethical decision-making while caring for the critically ill patient poses a huge challenge for healthcare professionals. Following the four ethical principles of beneficence, non-maleficence, justice and autonomy, as well as adhering to professional codes of conduct, the patient's best interests will be kept at the heart of the decision and management plan. Good teamwork, open communication and consideration of the patient's known wishes are central to caring for the sick ward patient.

References and further reading

British Medical Association Ethics Department (BMA) (2013). *Medical Ethics Today.* 3rd edn. London. British Medical Association.

British Medical Association (BMA) (2014). *Decisions relating to cardiopulmonary resuscitation, 2014. A joint statement from the British Medical Association, The Resuscitation Council (UK) and the Royal College of Nursing.* BMA House, Tavistock Square, London. https://www.resus.org.uk/pages/dnacpr.htm (accessed 31 August 2015).

Caldicott Committee (1997). *Report on the Review of patient-identifiable information.* http://webarchive.nationalarchives.gov.uk/20130107105354/http://www.dh.gov.uk/en/Publicationsandstatistics/Publications/PublicationsPolicyAndGuidance/DH_4068403 (accessed 31 August 2015).

Calicott, F. (2013). *The Information Governance Review.* https://www.gov.uk/government/uploads/system/uploads/attachment_data/file/192572/2900774_InfoGovernance_accv2.pdf (accesssed 17 September 2015).

Cribb, A. (2002). 'The Ethical Dimension: Nursing Practice, Nursing Philosophy and Nursing Ethics' in J. Tingle & A. Cribb (eds) *Nursing Law and Ethics.* 2nd edn. Oxford: Blackwell Publishing.

Department of Health (1998). *The Data Protection Act.* London: Department of Health.

Department of Health (2014). *The Mental Capacity Act: Making Decisions.* https://www.gov.uk/government/collections/mental-capacity-act-making-decisions (accessed 31 August 2015).

Herring, J. (2014). *Medical Law and Ethics.* 5th edn. Oxford: Oxford University Press.

Mason, J.K. & Laurie, G.T. (2013). *Mason & McCall Smith's Law & Medical Ethics.* 9th edn. Oxford: Oxford University Press.

National Commission for the Protection of Human Subjects of Biomedical and Behavioural Research (2003). 'The Belmont Report: Ethical Principles and Guidelines for the Protection of Human Subjects of Research' in S. Eckstein (ed.) *Manual for Research Ethics Committees.* 6th edn. Centre of Medical Law and Ethics, Kings College London. Cambridge University Press.

Resuscitation Council UK (2015). *Resuscitation Guidelines.* London: Resuscitation Council UK (accessed 29 Novemebr 2015).

Seedhouse, D. (2002). 'An Ethical Perspective – How to Do the Right Thing' in J. Tingle & A. Cribb (eds) *Nursing Law and Ethics.* 2nd edn. Oxford: Blackwell Publishing.

Useful websites

Resuscitation Council UK
https://www.resus.org.uk/pages/dnacpr.htm
(Accessed 31 August 2015)

British Medical Association
http://bma.org.uk/practical-support-at-work/ethics
(Accessed 31 August 2015)

Mental Capacity Act: making decisions
https://www.gov.uk/government/collections/mental-capacity-act-making-decisions
(Accessed 31 August 2015)

47 Communication

Julie Cook

This chapter considers the key principles of communication and how they apply when caring for critically ill patients, especially in the ward environment. It critiques a number of ways in which communication takes place and suggests a framework for practice.

By the end of this chapter, you will be able to apply the principles of good communication to your clinical practice.

The importance of effective communication

As a healthcare professional, high-quality communication with patients, their families and the multidisciplinary team (MDT) is not an optional extra; it is not a choice about whether or not you wish to participate. The practice of communication should be considered as a professional tool. In order for the multidisciplinary team to work together effectively, it is essential that everyone interacts successfully in working towards a shared goal. This is particularly important when patients are critically ill and based in a ward environment where additional support is required.

There is documented evidence that improved communication and teamwork leads to improved patient outcomes (Dutton *et al.* 2003, National Patient Safety Agency 2007, Shrader *et al.* 2013). Assessment is essential when caring for critically ill patients, and communication with everyone involved is considered to be vital (Alasad & Ahmad 2005). Happ *et al.* (2011) note that communication difficulty is extremely frustrating for critically ill patients and, even when patients are sedated or unconscious, it may still be possible for them to hear and understand what is being said (Alasad & Ahmad 2005).

Background and definitions

The topic of communication is vast and includes numerous different aspects. The following will be considered in this chapter in relation to the cases described:

- Verbal and non-verbal communication
- Active listening
- Styles of questioning
- The provision of information

- Collaboration
- Documentation
- Barriers to communication
- The effects of anger and frustration.

A number of factors relevant to the critically ill ward patient can influence communication. These are:

- The variety of individuals involved (including patients, relatives, and medical and nursing staff)
- The physical environment (the ward environment can be a very busy and noisy place; just because you pull the curtains around a patient's bed does not mean that nobody else can hear you)
- The high levels of stress and anxiety for everyone involved
- The complexity of the information to be communicated.

Communication in the critical care environment

When patients are critically ill, they usually have to undergo a significant number of clinical investigations that can be both invasive and intimate. Communication (in an accessible form) is therefore essential – to reduce anxiety and stress and to ensure that you elicit as much information as possible about your patient and their condition at an early stage.

When communicating with critically ill patients, closed questions (which elicit a simple 'yes' or 'no' answer) may be appropriate because less effort is required to answer them. However, it is important to acknowledge that closed questions yield less information than open questions. Through the use of semi-structured interviews Sutcliffe *et al.* (2004) investigated the role that communication played in adverse clinical events. They found that in 91% of adverse events, failures in communication were either a contributory or an associated cause. They highlighted three factors that affect the effectiveness of communication:

- The hierarchy, power or social structure
- A lack of information
- The mode of communication or misinterpretation.

Because we know that failures in communication adversely affect patient safety and are commonly highlighted when undertaking analysis of adverse events or clinical incidents (National Patient Safety Agency 2007, Royal College of Nursing 2015), it is imperative to ensure effective communication at all times. This is especially important in the care of the acutely unwell patient where the information that has to be imparted may be complex and detailed, as well as being uncomfortable and difficult to express clearly, gently, appropriately and properly. This relates to communication between teams and with the patient and their visitors.

Communicating with a patient's family and friends

When patients are acutely unwell, they may be unable to communicate due to exhaustion, or because of intrusive invasive monitoring or equipment. Where appropriate, communication with a patient's family and friends can assist in maintaining confidence and helping to clarify a patient's wishes.

Communication by telephone

When patients are critically ill, a significant amount of communication and coordination of care takes place over the telephone. This can include keeping members of the multidisciplinary team up to date about any changes in a patient's health. Consider the following scenario in which a nurse calls a doctor about a patient she is worried about.

Case scenario

Nurse: I'm calling you about Mrs Simpson. Will you come and see her?

Doctor: I'm really tied up with another patient at the moment. Could you tell me a bit more about her?

Nurse: Well, she came into hospital a number of days ago with a chest infection and she doesn't look right to me.

Doctor: What are her vital signs? What medication is she on?

Nurse: Hang on a minute and I'll go and get her charts.

Doctor: Don't bother. I'll be down when I've finished here.

In this situation it is important to consider the person at the other end of the phone. They may be involved in caring for a number of patients who are acutely unwell. It is important to provide them with enough information to prioritise their workload. At the end of this conversation the nurse is unsure quite when the doctor is going to arrive, and the doctor is unaware of just how ill Mrs Simpson really is.

Evidence has shown that medical staff find it more helpful if nurses use concrete information, such as trends of observations, and say exactly what these vital signs are (Andrews & Waterman 2005). Indeed, in this scenario it would have helped the doctor if the nurse had been better prepared with the relevant information.

When communicating with colleagues about a critically ill patient over the telephone, consider the following points:

- Take a few seconds to think about what you want to say, and what you want. This ensures that you include the salient points.
- Be as concise as possible, while including all the relevant information.
- Ensure that you have all the necessary information to hand.
- Consider the people you are communicating with and use jargon appropriately.

Form and style of communication

Regardless of who you are communicating with, it is essential to communicate in a calm and respectful manner. It is not necessarily the person who shouts loudest who gets the most attention – often the complete opposite is true. If you become agitated with someone, the information is often lost among the negative messages that you are sending out. Generally the only thing the person will remember from such an encounter is that they were shouted at – not what they were told! This also occurs when people are afraid to ask for help and it can apply to colleagues as well as patients. Amon (2002) describes a 'failure to communicate syndrome' whereby other members of the team are reluctant to provide timely updates on a patient's progress. Consider the following case scenario.

Case scenario

Mr Brown has just returned to the ward following an elective total knee replacement. Morphine has been prescribed as part of his post-operative analgesia regimen. Naloxone has also been prescribed, with the additional note 'to be given if respirations low'.

During the review the following morning, it is noticed that Mr Brown had what the team considered to be a low respiratory rate overnight and the ward staff were asked why the naloxone had not been given.

You cannot expect your colleagues to be mind-readers. When patients are critically ill, a number of different healthcare professionals can be involved in their care. In this situation, the documentation becomes vital to ensure continuity of care and to keep all members of the multidisciplinary team up to date with appropriate information regarding the patient's progress. Documented information about a patient's care must contain precise information about when further assistance should be sought.

Guidance from the National Institute for Health and Care Excellence (NICE 2007) on recognising and responding to acute illness in adults in hospital states that this should include 'prescribing' exactly how frequently a patient's vital signs should be taken, and what to do if these signs either improve or deteriorate. The following is a typical example of what is commonly seen in a patient's notes:

- Continue with regular observations.
- Contact team if respiratory rate low.

But this information requires further clarification. How frequently are the observations to be recorded? Vital signs could be measured twice a day and still be 'regular'.

Furthermore, just how low is a 'low' respiratory rate? These sorts of instructions place extra stress on the other healthcare professionals involved in the patient's care, as they have to 'second guess' precisely what is required. An alternative way to phrase the information might be:

- Continue recording vital signs 4 hourly.
- Contact primary team if respiratory rate less than 8 breaths per minute.

This removes all ambiguity and ensures that everyone involved in the patient's care is aware of what has been requested. It is also important to ensure that sufficient contact details are available, and to meet the standards of the Department of Health (NICE 2007, National Patient Safety Agency 2007).

When documenting information about a patient, the following details should be considered for inclusion:

- The date and time
- A signature, name and designation
- The frequency of monitoring
- Further investigations that are required
- When to contact the primary team and how to contact them.

The writing should of course be legible.

Active listening

An important part of communication is listening. This is even more vital if you are communicating with someone over the telephone. The most effective way to do this is through active listening, which involves:

- Giving the person who is talking your full attention
- Making sure they know you are listening, either by giving visual cues (e.g. nodding) or auditory cues (e.g. by saying 'Yes' or 'I see')
- Repeating the key points about what you have been told.

Boyle *et al.* (2005) stress the importance of active listening and summarising what you have said in their patient-centred communication technique. If you are communicating face to face, this can be facilitated by leaning slightly forward towards the person who is speaking, which shows interest and encourages them to continue talking.

Medical jargon

As healthcare professionals, we are all guilty of using 'in-house' jargon to speed up our communication – and in many situations this is a useful and time-saving tool. However, we must beware of using jargon in inappropriate situations, such as talking to patients and their families or talking to colleagues within earshot of patients. For example, when we say 'Patient X is normotensive and apyrexial' the patient thinks it means 'I am in a very bad way with lots wrong with me … I may not pull through'. Many patients will not feel confident enough to ask you to clarify what you have said, and will sit and draw their own conclusions instead.

Managing anger and frustration

Experiencing a critical illness can be very stressful for all involved, especially the patients and their relatives. This can manifest itself as anger and frustration. The following case scenario is an example of how this situation can be managed in a positive manner. Families and patients may well focus on any comments or aspects of care that appear to be different between healthcare professionals. It is therefore important to ensure consistency between different teams, and this can be greatly assisted by thorough documentation. Clearly document all meetings, who the meeting was with, who was present, what was said and what was agreed in the patient's notes.

Case scenario

Relative: What is happening to [patient's name]? They have been waiting for ages to see someone. They just don't seem to be getting any better!

Nurse: I appreciate that this situation must be very distressing for you. If you would like to speak to someone I will contact them for you. In the meantime, we are caring for [patient's name] in the following way...

The SBAR framework for communication

The National Patient Safety Agency (2007) proposed a simple framework that enables staff to communicate their concerns simply and effectively to each other. Its use and effectiveness have been demonstrated in a variety of different clinical settings (Leonard *et al.* 2004, Carroll 2006, Denham 2008, Shannon *et al.* 2011). The SBAR tool is based on the principle of ensuring that salient points are made and it comprises the following:

S – Situation

B – Background

A – Assessment

R – Recommendations.

Table 47.1 SBAR

S – Situation	Describe what is actually happening at the time you are calling. For example, the patient may have become confused or aggressive. What is your main concern?
B – Background	Explain briefly what has led to the situation. This might be a summary of why they were admitted and how they have been today so far, or their diagnosis.
A – Assessment	Give an overview of your assessment of the patient, such as their vital signs and what you think is wrong with them (if possible).
R –Recommendations	Explain what you wish this person to do and, if possible, what you think needs to be done. It may be that they need to review the patient or need to prescribe something, or they need to come and speak to the family.

Table 47.1 explains how each of these factors relates to your practice. It may also be helpful to talk to the person you are seeking advice from, and agree a time when you will call them again, and what you will call them about, if they have given you telephone instructions to carry out. For example, you could say that if the blood pressure is still below 90mmHg in 30 minutes' time you will call again. They may ask you to inform them in half an hour's time of the patient's progress. Setting these communication parameters helps reduce pressure among staff, and enables planned care to be delivered using a team approach.

Recently a system called **RSVP** has been devised. This is specifically intended to help with communicating about patients who are deteriorating while in hospital (Featherstone *et al.* 2008). RSVP stands for:

R – Reason

S – Story

V – Vital signs

P – Plan.

The RSVP acronym may be easier to remember than SBAR. The method is becoming more popular in addition to the current tools available for staff to use. Table 47.2 shows how it relates to your practice.

Table 47.2 RSVP

R – Reason	The nurse calling usually has an overview of the patient and has a reason for the call. They should say who they are and why they are calling for help.
S – Story	The nurse usually knows the story about the patient and should relate the events that have led to their concerns.
V – Vital signs	The vital signs are important for the person receiving the call, along with any other pertinent information (such as the early warning score).
P – Plan	The nurse may describe the plan or what actions have been implemented so far, or they may request that the recipient comes and helps to develop a plan of care for the patient following their review of the patient's condition.

The power of timing

Finally, it is worth remembering that a mis-timed comment regarding a patient or their condition can significantly affect their care or others' perceptions of that patient.

Conclusion

When communication works well, it is a tool that allows all members of the multidisciplinary team, the patient and the patient's relatives to cooperate in the effective provision and acceptance of care given to that patient. It links and integrates the various elements that must work together if the best-quality care is to be given. But getting it wrong causes problems. People begin to argue about the form of communication – rather than taking on board the message that is being given – and that can only lead to a reduction in the quality of care provided, and an increase in the anxiety levels of all concerned. Using a structured communication tool (such as the SBAR or RSVP) may aid communication between teams and team members, as well as among patients and their families.

References and further reading

Alasad, A. & Ahmad, M. (2005). Communication with critically ill patients. *Journal of Advanced Nursing.* **50**, 356–62.

Amon, E. (2002). A guest editorial: Communication strategies for reducing hospital error and professional liability. *Obstetrical and Gynaecological Survey.* **57**, 713–14.

Andrews, T. & Waterman, H. (2005). Packaging: a grounded theory of how to report physiological deterioration effectively. *Journal of Advanced Nursing.* **52** (5), 473–81.

Boyle, D., Dwinnell, B. & Platt, F. (2005). Invite, listen, and summarize: A patient-centered communication technique. *Academic Medicine.* **80**, 29–32.

Carroll, T.L. (2006). SBAR and nurse physician communication: pilot testing an educational intervention. *Nursing Administration Quarterly.* **30** (3), 295–99.

Denham, C.R. (2008). SBAR for patients. *Journal of Patient Safety.* **4** (1), 38–48.

Dutton, R.P., Cooper, C., Jones, A., Leone, S., Kramer, M.E. & Scalea, T.M. (2003). Daily multidisciplinary rounds shorten length of stay for trauma patients. *The Journal of Trauma, Infection, and Critical Care.* **55**, 913–19.

Featherstone, P., Chalmers, T. & Smith, G.B. (2008). RSVP: a system for communication of deterioration in hospital patients. *British Journal of Nursing.* **17** (13), 860–64.

Happ, M.B., Garrett, K., Thomas, D.D., George, E., Houze, M., Radtke, J. & Sereika, S. (2011). Nurse-patient communication interactions in the intensive care unit. *American Journal of Critical Care.* **20** (2): e28-40 doi: 10.4037/ajcc2011433.

Leonard, M., Graham, S. & Bonacum, D. (2004). The human factor: the critical importance of effective teamwork and communication in providing safe care. *Quality and Safety in Health Care.* **13**, i85–90.

National Institute for Health and Care Excellence (2007). *Guideline 50. Acutely ill patients in hospital: Recognition and response to acute illness in adults in hospital.* London: NICE.

National Patient Safety Agency (2007). *Safer care for the acutely ill patient: Learning from serious incidents. Fifth Report from the Patient Safety Observatory.* London: National Patient Safety Agency.

Royal College of Nursing (2015). *Patient Safety and Human Factors: human factors – communication.* http://www.rcn.org.uk/development/practice/patient_safety/human_factors_communication (accessed 31 August 2015).

Shannon, S., Long-Sutehall, T. & Coombs, M. (2011). Conversations in end-of-life care: communication tools for critical care practitioners. *Nursing in Critical Care.* 16 (3), 124–30.

Shrader, S., Kem, D., Zoller, J. & Blue, A. (2013). Interprofessional teamwork skills as predictors of clinical outcomes in a simulated healthcare setting. *Journal of Allied Health.* **42** (1), e1–6.

Sutcliffe, K.M., Lewton, E. & Rosenthal, M.M. (2004). Communication failures: an insidious contributor to medical mishaps. *Academic Medicine.* **79**, 186–94.

48 Family care

Catherine Plowright

Admission to an intensive care unit or high dependency unit has been described as a traumatic and frightening experience for patients and their families. Over the last 30 years, authors have highlighted the fear, anxiety and psychological distress induced by critical illness (McGonigal 1986, Quinn *et al.* 1999, Jones 2002, Skirrow 2002), as well as the physiological problems induced by critical illness on leaving the intensive care unit (Cochran 1984, Chew 1986, Booth 1991).

A number of useful websites have been designed for families of critically ill patients and healthcare professionals will find these resources helpful when caring for these families. These websites include those run by the Intensive Care Society, Healthtalk and ICUSteps (Intensive Care Unit Support Team for Ex-Patients). Healthtalk has video clips with patients (or their relatives) experiencing a particular illness or health problems and includes a section on intensive care. ICUSteps is a support group set up by former intensive care patients and family members based in Milton Keynes, UK. They hold regular drop-in sessions and offer support for other ex-patients or family members who may wish to come along and talk about their experiences and rehabilitation. The website includes ex-patients' and family members' own experiences. It is worth checking this website to see if your local hospital has a support group available.

The terms 'family', 'families' and 'relatives' include everyone who is significant to the patient. Families need to be cared for by all healthcare professionals before, during and after their loved one's stay on the intensive care unit. The responsibilities of healthcare professionals extend both before and after admission to intensive care.

By the end of this chapter, you will have an understanding of the care that families of patients on the intensive care unit require within the ward environment.

Before admission to intensive care

Many admissions to intensive care are emergencies and cannot, therefore, be planned. It is important that families are informed as soon as possible about the deteriorating condition of their relative. Communication must be timely and appropriate, and delivered by someone who has been trained to deliver bad news (see Chapter 49 on caring for the suddenly bereaved in the acute care setting). If the admission is an elective one, then the family (as well as the patient) should be involved and fully informed. The effect of good preoperative information is well documented with respect to preparing patients psychologically for operations and providing information (Cochran 1984, Chew 1986, Booth 1991, Scott 2004).

Care while in intensive care

Families need to be cared for as much as the critically ill patient in the intensive care unit. Family members suffer from the physical, social and psychological effects of their loved one's critical illness. Nursing research exploring the care received by relatives of critically ill patients has generally focused on the relatives' self-perceived needs and satisfaction levels around those needs (Molter 1979, Plowright 1995, Engstrom & Soderberg 2004, Kinrade *et al.* 2009, Hughes *et al.* 2005). The seminal work of Molter (1979) was significant in identifying the needs of relatives of critically ill patients. Molter developed a tool known as the 'critical care family needs inventory' (the CCFNI), which has been used widely over the last two decades for analysing the needs of family members while the patient is in intensive care. Such relatives always have a tendency to prioritise their needs around the patient, rather than themselves (Plowright 1995) and this can be seen in various studies where they often rank their personal needs as the lowest (Molter 1979, Daley 1984, Farrell & Frost 1992, Dyer 1991). Research carried out over the years has clearly identified the need categories of families when a patient is in intensive care.

The needs of relatives in intensive care

1 The need for relief of anxiety

- To know what the expected outcome may be
- To know what treatments the patient is receiving
- To have someone explain the equipment being used
- To be called at home if the patient's condition changes
- To know the nurses are giving the best care possible
- To be told about transfers ahead of time
- To be told there is hope.

2 The need for information

- To know what is wrong with the patient
- To be able to talk to a doctor
- To be able to talk to a nurse
- To have questions answered honestly
- To be informed if the patient's condition changes
- To be called at home every morning
- To have understandable explanations
- To know the qualifications of the staff caring for the patient
- To be allowed to call at any time.

3 The need to be with the patient

- To be able to stay with the patient
- To be able to stay nearby

- To be allowed to visit at any time
- To have visiting start on time
- To be able to have friends visit.

4 The need to be helpful

- To be able to help with the care of the patient
- To be told how to help by a healthcare professional.

5 The need for support

- To be reassured that the patient is doing all right
- To have the chaplain visit
- To have friends nearby
- To be able to talk to others who have a family member in intensive care
- To be able to talk to the same nurse every day
- To have a nurse nearby
- To be able to talk to someone about feelings
- To be accepted by staff.

6 Personal needs

- To have a toilet nearby
- To have food and drinks nearby
- To be alone
- To have a private room to sit in
- To have a place to rest when visiting
- To have a place to take care of personal needs.

The greatest need that families have when their family member is in an intensive care unit is the need for relief of anxiety. The cultural and spiritual needs of families must also be met when patients are in critical care (Davidson *et al.* 2007). The American College of Critical Care Medicine has developed clinical practice guidelines for the support of families in the high dependency unit (Davidson *et al.* 2007).

Although there has been little research on the needs of families following discharge of the patient from intensive care, it follows that their needs may not be very different from what they were when the patient was in intensive care.

After discharge from the intensive care unit

A family's perception of discharge to the ward environment often involves dread and fear. There can be anxiety about transferring to another location, rather than appreciating the improving health status of the patient (Russell 1999, Jones *et al.* 1999). Paul *et al.* (2004) identified relatives' information needs around the time of transfer; they designed an information booklet that improved relatives' satisfaction with information and enhanced the communication between intensive care, the wards and families at this stressful time in the patient journey. It may also be helpful to give relatives diaries written for patients (see Chapter 45 on post-ICU patient support). These diaries are written to help patients understand their stay on intensive care and come to terms with their illness, and they can also help relatives (Roulin *et al.* 2007).

Bench & Day (2010) and Bench *et al.* (2011) examined the information given at critical care discharge and found that there needed to be improvements. Wong and Wickham (2013) showed that 60 intensive care units in the UK used 'in-hospital' discharge communication that appeared superficially good. However, they also showed that inadequacies in communication with patients, relatives and General Practitioners still needed to be addressed. These studies tell us that critical care discharge information can be improved.

Physical effects of the critical illness on families

Once patients are discharged from intensive care, families continue to experience difficulties. A study of 2,129 families of patients who had been seriously ill, and were no longer in hospital, found that the families experienced burdens of care when the patient was discharged (Covinsky *et al.* 1994). These burdens included direct physical care of the patient, loss of employment as a result of the care-giving, and financial implications. Studies in cancer patients (Siegel *et al.* 1991), cardiac patients (Stanley & Frantz 1998) and paediatric cancer patients (Bodkin *et al.* 1982) found similar burdens existed in families caring for patients following their illness. If they continue to have these physical burdens of care, then they may be reminded about the seriousness of the illness that the patient experienced, which may have psychological effects.

Even when patients are not discharged from hospital, their families will be experiencing physical burdens of care which, as healthcare professionals, we must recognise and understand. These could be simple things, like the relative who needs to visit outside the ward's usual visiting hours for various reasons – because they cannot afford the taxi to take them home after an evening visit, because there is no longer a suitable bus service, or because they can only visit when their children are at school. Visiting hours have now been restricted in many hospitals, citing infection control as the reason; this may need to be reconsidered when caring for families of critically ill patients who have been in intensive care.

Psychological effects of the critical illness on families

There are also psychological burdens when family members become ill, whether the illness is an acute event or a chronic illness. Studies on the families of patients with a diagnosis of cancer revealed that a substantial number experienced psychological problems up to 12 months after the diagnosis (Ell *et al.* 1988; Kazak *et al.* 2004).

Family members of critically ill patients are affected psychologically by the illness; they can clearly recall events that occurred during the time spent in intensive care, and these events may still have a profound effect on them several months later (Russell 1999, Adamson *et al.* 2004). One relative remembered: 'It was said in front of me that Kathy was not going to be alright and that we may as well pull the plug … I was sitting beside Kathy' (Russell 1999, p. 786). Families who have such recall 6 months after the critical care experience are angry and afraid (Jones *et al.* 1999).

However, these studies identified these families' memories but did not investigate the effects their memories were having on them. Several other studies have investigated the psychological state of families of critically ill patients (Jones *et al.* 1999, Jones *et al.* 2000a, Azoulay *et al.* 2001, Pochard *et al.* 2001, Young *et al.* 2005). They all used the Hospital Anxiety and Depression Score (HADS) questionnaire and administered it when the families still had patients in the critical care unit or who were recovering within the hospital. All the studies reported that significant numbers of these families had symptoms of anxiety and depression.

One study continued their investigation of critical care relatives and found that at 2 months and 6 months post-discharge a third of relatives in their sample remained very anxious (Jones *et al.* 2000b). A study comparing cardiac and critically ill patients and their relatives (Young *et al.* 2005) collated data from patients and relatives in both groups: all participants completed a HADS questionnaire at a follow-up clinic 3 months after the patients had been discharged home. They found that critical care relatives had a significantly higher number of anxiety symptoms and greater indicators of depression than the relatives of the cardiac surgery relatives; they also had more worrying and life-altering experiences than the relatives of cardiac surgery patients. Critical care relatives have significant memories of what they witnessed when the patient was critically ill, and this may have been traumatic for them.

Transfer anxiety

These families need to be cared for by all members of the healthcare team when the patient is transferred to the ward from the intensive care unit. It is vital, therefore, that the families are prepared for the patient's transfer. Transfer anxiety can be seen when people display some or all of the following symptoms:

- Insecurity
- A lack of trust
- A need for excessive reassurance
- An unfavourable comparison of staff on the ward with those on the intensive care unit
- Anger or outbursts.

Healthcare professionals caring for relatives and patients following discharge from an intensive care unit may see any of these emotional symptoms displayed by patients or their families. The staff in the intensive care unit should therefore prepare the families for the transfer with appropriate planning, explanation and education (Jones & O'Donnell 1994, Hall-Smith *et al.* 1997, Coyle 2001). However, discharge planning often has a low priority in critical care units (Coyle 2001). If families do not know what to expect when the patient is transferred, they will be understandably frightened. Healthcare professionals must remember that, although the patient is perceived to be physically ready for discharge to a ward, neither the patient nor their family may be psychologically ready. The patient and the family often perceive the patient as still being critically ill. Meanwhile, for the ward staff, the discharged patient may be the sickest patient in their care, which adds to the level of anxiety both for the ward staff and the patient and their family.

Preparing families before discharge to a ward is obviously vital, but sometimes patients are discharged quickly to accommodate emergency admissions, often at night or in the late evening, or to accommodate planned elective surgery. As a result, many families are not prepared psychologically for the change. Their anxiety may be reduced when there is a follow-up visit from a critical care nurse (Hall-Smith *et al.* 1997), or if a ward nurse visits the patient and family on the intensive care unit before discharge.

If your hospital has a critical care outreach team, their role is not only to facilitate admission to critical care units, but also to enable safe discharge back to the wards (Intensive Care Society 2002). This can greatly improve the discharge process. Many critical care units produce booklets to give to patients and families before or on discharge. These booklets explain the differences between the intensive care unit and wards in terms of staffing, what is to be expected, and what to expect during the patient's recovery.

Conclusion

The families of critically ill patients must be cared for within ward environments – as well as the patients. The family's needs must be met because the family will probably be the main caregivers when the patient is discharged from hospital.

References and further reading

Adamson, H., Murgo, M., Boyle, M., Kerr, S., Crawford, M. & Elliot. D. (2004). Memories of intensive care and experiences of survivors of a critical illness: an interview study. *Intensive and Critical Care Nursing.* **20**, 257–63.

Azoulay, E., Pochard, F., Chevret, S. *et al.* (2001). Meeting the needs of intensive care unit patient families. *American Journal of Respiratory and Critical Care Medicine.* **163**, 135–39.

Bench, S. & Day, T. (2010). The user experience of critical care discharge: A meta-synthesis of qualitative research. *International Journal of Nursing Studies.* **47**(4), 487–99.

Bench, S.D., Day, T. & Griffiths, (2011). Involving users in the development of effective critical care discharge information: A focus group study. *American Journal of Critical Care.* **20** (6), 443–52.

Bodkin, C.M., Pigott, T.J. & Mann, J.R. (1982). Financial burden of childhood cancer. *British Journal of Medicine.* **284**, 1542–44.

Booth, J. (1991). Preoperative visiting: a step by step guide. *British Journal of Theatre Nursing.* **7**, 30–31.

Chew, S.L. (1986). Psychological reactions of intensive care patients. *Care of the Critically Ill.* **2**, 62–65.

Cochran, T.M. (1984). Psychological preparation of patients for surgical procedures. *Patient Education and Counselling.* **5**, 153–58.

Covinsky, K.E., Goldman, L., Cook, F. *et al.* (1994). The impact of serious illness on patient's families. *Journal of the American Medical Association.* **272** (23), 1839–44.

Coyle, M.A. (2001). Transfer anxiety: preparing to leave intensive care. *Intensive and Critical Care Nursing.* **17**, 138–43.

Daley, L. (1984). The perceived immediate needs of families with relatives in the intensive care unit. *Heart and Lung.* **13**, 231–37.

Davidson, J. E., Powers, K., Hedayat, K.M. *et al.* (2007). Clinical practice guidelines for support of the family in the patient-centred intensive care unit: American College of Critical Care Medicine Task Force 2004–2005. *Critical Care Medicine.* **35** (2), 605–22.

Dyer, I.D. (1991). Meeting the needs of visitors – a practical approach. *Intensive Care Nursing.* **7**, 135–44.

Ell, K., Nishimoto, R., Mantell, J. & Hamovitch, M. (1988). Longitudinal analysis of psychological adaptation among family members of patients with cancer. *Journal of Psychosomatic Research.* **32**, 429–38.

Engstrom, A. & Soderberg, S. (2004). The experiences of partners of critically ill persons in an intensive care unit. *Intensive and Critical Care Nursing.* **20**, 299–08.

Farrell, M.F. & Frost, C. (1992). The most important needs of parents of critically ill children: parents' perception. *Intensive and Critical Care Nursing.* **8**, 130–39.

Hall-Smith, J., Ball, C. & Coakley, J. (1997). Follow-up services and the development of a clinical nurse specialist in intensive care. *Intensive and Critical Care Nursing.* **13**, 243–48.

Hughes, F., Bryan, K. & Robbins, I. (2005). Relatives' experiences of critical care. *Nursing in Critical Care.* **10**, 23–30.

Intensive Care Society (2002). *Guidelines for the Introduction of Outreach Services.* London: Intensive Care Society.

Jones, C. (2002). 'Acute psychological problems' in R.D. Griffiths & C. Jones (eds). *Intensive Care Aftercare.* Oxford: Butterworth Heinemann.

Jones, C. & O'Donnell, C. (1994). After intensive care – what then? *Intensive and Critical Care Nursing.* **10**, 89–92.293

Jones, C., Griffiths, R.D. & Humphris, G. (1999). Relatives are still very anxious 2 weeks after patient's intensive care discharge. *British Journal of Anaesthesia.* **82**, 97–98.

Jones, C., Griffiths, R.D. & Humphris, G.M. (2000a). Disturbed memory and amnesia related to intensive care. *Memory.* **8**, 79–94.

Jones, C., Skirrow, P., Griffiths, R.D., Humphris, G., Dawson, S. & Eddleston, J. (2000b). Predicting intensive care relatives at risk of post traumatic stress disorder. *British Journal of Anaesthesia.* **84**, 666–67.

Kazak, A.E., Alderfer, M., Rourke, M.T., Simms, S., Striesand, R. & Grossman, J.R. (2004). Post-traumatic stress disorder and post-traumatic stress symptoms in families of adolescent childhood cancer survivors. *Journal of Pediatric Psychology.* **29**, 211–19.

Kinrade, T., Jackson, A.C., & Tomnay, J.E. (2009). The psychosocial needs of families during critical illness: comparison of nurses' and family members' perspectives. *Australian Journal of Advanced Nursing.* **27** (1), 82–88.

McGonigal, K.S. (1986). The importance of sleep and the sensory environment to critically ill patients. *Intensive Care Nursing.* **2** (2), 73–83.

Molter, N.C. (1979). Needs of relatives of critically ill patients: A descriptive study. *Heart and Lung.* **8**, 332–39.

Paul, F., Hendry, C. & Cabrelli, L. (2004). Meeting patient and relatives' information needs upon transfer from an intensive care unit: the development and evaluation of an information booklet. *Journal of Clinical Nursing.* **13** (3), 396–405.

Plowright, C.I. (1995). Needs of visitors in the intensive care unit. *British Journal of Nursing.* **4** (18), 1081–83.

Pochard, F., Azoulay, E., Chevret, S. *et al.* (2001). Symptoms of anxiety and depression in family members of intensive care unit patients: Ethical hypothesis regarding decision-making capacity. *Critical Care Medicine.* **29**, 1893–97.

Quinn, S., Redmond K. & Begley, C. (1996). The needs of relatives visiting adult intensive care units as perceived by relatives and nurses. *Intensive and Critical Care Nursing.* **12** (3), 168–72.

Roulin, M.J., Hurst, S. & Sririg, R. (2007). Diaries written for ICU patients. *Qualitative Health Research.* **17** (7), 893–901.

Russell, S. (1999). An exploratory study of patient's perceptions, memories and experiences of an intensive care unit. *Journal of Advanced Nursing.* **29**, 783–91.

Scott, A. (2004). Managing anxiety in ICU patients: the role of pre-operative information provision. *Nursing in Critical Care.* **9** (2), 72–79.

Siegel, K., Raveis, V.H., Houts, P. & Mor, V. (1991). Caregiver burden and unmet patient needs. *Cancer.* **68**, 1131–40.

Skirrow, P. (2002). 'Delusional memories of ICU' in R.D. Griffiths & C. Jones (eds). *Intensive Care Aftercare.* Oxford: Butterworth Heinemann.

Stanley, M. & Frantz, R. (1998). Adjustment problems of spouses of patients undergoing coronary bypass graft surgery during early convalescence. *Heart Lung.* **17**, 677–82.

Thompson, T.L. (1985). Discharge planning for critical care. *Critical Care Nurse.* **5**, 48–51.

Waldmann, C. (2002). 'Sexual problems and their treatments' in R.D. Griffiths & C. Jones (eds). *Intensive Care Aftercare.* Oxford: Butterworth Heinemann.

Wong, D. & Wickham, A. (2013). A survey of intensive care unit discharge communication practices in the UK. *Journal of Intensive Care Society.* **14** (4), 330–33.

Young, E., Eddleston, J., Ingleby, S. *et al.* (2005). Returning home after intensive care: A comparison of symptoms of anxiety and depression in intensive care unit and elective cardiac surgery patients and their relatives. *Intensive Care Medicine.* **31**, 86–91.

Useful websites

HealthTalk.org
Intensive care: experiences of family and friends
http://www.healthtalk.org/peoples-experiences/intensive-care/intensive-care-experiences-family-friends/emotional-impact-relatives-friends-icu
(Accessed 2 September 2015)

ICUSteps (Intensive Care Unit Support Team for Ex-Patients)
http://icusteps.org/
(Accessed 2 September 2015)

Intensive Care Foundation – Patient and Relative Information
http://www.ics.ac.uk/icf/patients-and-relatives/further-information/
(Accessed 2 September 2015)

Intensive Care Society
http://www.ics.ac.uk/
(Accessed 2 September 2015)

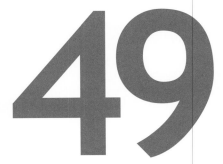

Caring for the suddenly bereaved in the acute care setting

Sally A. Smith and Catherine Plowright

The sudden death of a patient in acute care is not uncommon. For healthcare workers, this can be challenging on both a professional and a personal level. At these times they may feel out of their depth and inept (Ferrand *et al*. 2008, Dolan 2013). It is not uncommon to feel that there is little to offer the bereaved at this time.

The sudden death of a close person is always traumatic and has the potential to result in many ongoing problems for the bereaved (Li *et al*. 2002). The importance of some initial interventions after sudden death and their impact on the bereaved cannot be over-emphasised (Antonacci 1990, McLauchlan 1990, Hall & Smith 1999, Li *et al*. 2002, DH 2005, DH 2011, Dolan 2013, Doka 2014). It is a time that the relatives will always remember, and – if undertaken incompetently – it may result in complicated and protracted grief reactions. Knowing how to deal with these situations will therefore help build greater confidence and competence among healthcare workers.

This chapter offers practical guidance, based on current evidence on how to manage the bereavement of a patient who has died suddenly. It outlines some theories of bereavement, and describes the special needs and challenges that unexpected death brings. We hope it will enable healthcare workers to care effectively for the suddenly bereaved in acute care settings.

By the end of this chapter, you should understand the needs of the suddenly bereaved; have greater confidence that you can provide care that helps the bereaved to begin to come to terms with the death of a loved one; know what strategies to use in order to break bad news kindly and effectively; and be able to act helpfully when dealing with different reactions from those who have been bereaved.

Specific needs with sudden death

Loss is a universal experience, common to all people of all ages, and it is an inevitable part of life. It is painful for the bereaved person, and for some it can be catastrophic and paralysing. Evidence suggests that the impact of a sudden death on relatives is often more pronounced than death after a long illness. It has the capacity to leave people damaged and disabled (Wright 1996, Kendrick 1997). It involves intense feelings of distress and disorder, creating a sense of powerlessness, whereby the bereaved person has neither control nor autonomy and is robbed of a preparatory grief time (Wright 2007). One reason for this is that sudden death gives no-one time prior to the death to prepare for it. This lack of preparation can lead to two kinds of grief – firstly, for what is lost, and secondly, for what might have been (Kendrick 1997). Unfinished business can be difficult to come to terms with for the suddenly bereaved.

The implication, therefore, is that sudden death is more painful than an expected death, and that having time to prepare and begin the grieving process prior to the death of the patient makes the death easier to cope with. Certainly, foreknowledge of the death of someone allows for planning, preparation and farewells. However, it could be argued that no matter how well prepared the family is, the death itself is almost always unexpected, and the family may have needs that are not met.

Box 49.1 The work of grieving

A theory of grief and work (Freud 1917)
'Each single one of the memories and situations of expectancy which demonstrate the libido's attachment to the lost object is met by the verdict of reality that the object no longer exists. When the work of mourning is completed the ego becomes free and uninhibited again.'

Four tasks of grieving (Worden 1991)
- Accepting the reality of loss
- Experiencing the pain of grief
- Adjusting to an environment without the deceased
- Withdrawing emotional energy and re-investing in another relationship.

Recovery tasks (Scrutton 1995)
- Intellectual acceptance of bereavement
- Emotional acceptance of bereavement
- Adjusting to loss
- Social re-investment.

Syndrome of grief (Stroebe *et al.* 1993)
- Shock
- Protest
- Despair
- Reorganisation.

The normal course of grief (Parkes 1996, Parkes 1998)
- Numbness
- Pining and anxiety (pangs of grief)
- Disorganisation and despair
- Reorganisation.

Grief theories

Many responses to grief have been described and debated over time, from the work of Freud (1917) to Parkes (1996) and that of Wright (2007). Bearing in mind the additional difficulties a sudden death may bring, grief can be considered as work – work that needs to be undertaken and completed prior to moving on in one's life (Wright 2007).

Some theorists believe this work can be described as stages or tasks. It is not a passive process but requires the bereaved person to work hard in order to move on. Box 49.1 describes these theories. The diversity of grief responses needs to be respected because reactions vary enormously. The active processes involved need to be understood and supported. Box 49.1 presents responses and stages in a certain order, but people undergoing grief oscillate among the reactions and can go through them in any order. Improved understanding of the grieving process and what influences it helps inform the way health professionals deal with the bereaved. Certainly, training, end-of-life protocols and attending to the needs of families have enhanced the perception of staff that the person who died was cared for in an acceptable way (Ferrand *et al.* 2008).

Grief reactions

Due to the catastrophic nature of sudden bereavement, people in grief are quite likely to experience a sense of unreality and helplessness, and heightened feelings of guilt about having failed to avert the death. Some may have a strong need to blame someone in order to make sense of their loss. The possible reactions are many and varied, and may manifest at different times and for varying durations. Common grief reactions (Wright 1999, Wright 2007) include:

- **Feelings**: shock, disbelief, fear and anxiety, numbness, anger and hostility, denial, guilt, physical symptoms (e.g. chest pain) and regret
- **Behaviours**: anxiety attacks and panic, crying and sobbing, inappropriate behaviour (e.g. laughing), withdrawing, bargaining, aggression, searching for the deceased.

Therapeutic interventions

Now consider the case scenario below. It often feels as if there is very little staff can do to help the suddenly bereaved in an acute care setting. The bereaved are in shock and a state of disbelief. Their need for hope has been dashed and they often struggle to assimilate any information given to them. Because there has been no opportunity to build a trusting relationship with the staff, it can be difficult to assess the needs of family and friends. However, there are many helpful actions that can help bereaved people, even in such a tragic situation as the one described in the following case scenario.

Case scenario

A 55-year-old woman is admitted to accident and emergency, having collapsed at home. She had been complaining of feeling 'odd' over the past week. She had been to the GP, who said she was suffering from stress and that she should rest. She was found by her daughter unconscious on the floor.

On arrival, she was intubated and attached to a ventilator. The ambulance crew had assessed her Glasgow Coma Score as 3. She remained unresponsive. Following a CT scan, she was diagnosed as having had an extensive cerebral bleed. Her prognosis was hopeless and the decision was made to withdraw treatment.

Her husband and three children arrived, along with her brother and sister-in-law. Her children were aged 20, 15 and 10. Her disabled father was telephoned and collected. The sister-in-law was tearful, but remained calm and in control throughout. She seemed to have accepted that death was imminent.

The patient's husband and the youngest son (aged 10) were very withdrawn, not responding and remaining silent. The 20-year-old son was crying, hugging his mother and calling her to wake up. The middle child, the 15-year-old daughter, displayed a range of reactions, from denial and bargaining (with the accident and emergency and critical care outreach staff to make her better and do anything to ensure this), to hysteria (screaming, running round the car park shouting) and anger (directed at the GP) as well as sobbing and guilt (for not making her mother go back to the GP).

Goals of care

The goals of care include enabling the bereaved person to understand events so that they can begin the grieving process in as healthy way as is possible. Bereaved families and healthcare providers have identified a number of helpful actions such as:

- Providing privacy for bereaved family members
- Offering them emotional support
- Allowing them to verbalise their anxieties and concerns
- Letting them know that all appropriate treatment had been given to their loved one
- Providing them with the opportunity for them to view the deceased's body (Li *et al.* 2002) and allowing them to be with the deceased.

Giving clear, unambiguous, honest information at the earliest available point at least allows relatives to begin to come to terms with the death. Townsend (1995) states that relatives who are aware that the death will occur, even within hours, may have time to collect their thoughts and memories together in order to prepare themselves. This may help them cope better than having no warning. Lautrette *et al.* (2007) evaluated the use of an information booklet for bereaved relatives and found a significant reduction in signs of depression after the death.

The family in the current case scenario did not respond well to the news of the imminent death. They continued to display a range of distressing grief reactions to the news, which was painful for them to experience and for the healthcare team to witness.

Breaking bad news

Suddenly bereaved people are often so overwhelmed that they are, for a time, incapable of the level of functioning required for grief work; mourning is simply postponed. The efforts of healthcare professionals will relate to enhancing the perception, reality and understanding of the event. In the acute setting, we cannot be responsible for their long-term care, so our aims are to:

- Give the facts
- Confirm reality
- Acknowledge feelings
- Identify support (Wright 1999).

Supporting and comforting the bereaved

Staff sometimes perceive a difficulty in developing a rapport with relatives. This has been cited as affecting the relatives' perception of the quality of care delivered (Ferrand *et al.* 2008). Researchers found that a close relationship can be developed in a short timespan if the nurses showed understanding and support towards the relatives (Jackson 1998). This is particularly so if the same nurse caring for the patient also deals with the relatives.

An essential aspect of supporting and comforting the bereaved is knowing how to manage their emotional responses. Wright (1996) studied 100 sudden deaths and found that it was the bereaved person who became withdrawn who posed the most difficulty for nurses. Crying, sobbing, weeping and acceptance were the easiest for them to manage. Whatever the profession, caring for the suddenly bereaved can quickly leave healthcare staff feeling as if they are not in control and are ineffective in their care. It is therefore imperative for staff members to receive training and education on how best to deal with emotional responses. Guidance regarding this is available in the literature and should be integral in the knowledge and skill acquisition training that healthcare professionals undertake. Some of this evidence is described below, particularly in regard to enabling staff to care for themselves while caring for the bereaved.

Given the helplessness and overwhelming pain the healthcare worker witnesses (and sometimes experiences themselves), there may be a tendency to 'rush in' and attempt to offer comfort (Bowman 1999). When people are shocked and disorientated, it can be destabilising. The goal should be to focus on helping them accept that the death has occurred and to foster and promote autonomy and control. Sometimes it is necessary to guide the relatives because they may not know how to grieve (Wright 1996). Anticipating their needs and implementing a proactive approach is important. This may involve simply providing certain conditions for the relatives, such as refreshments, or more complex issues (like creating a safe open environment in which they are able to ask questions and respond) or making suggestions about what may be helpful to do. This helps to promote a sense of control and choice. A useful tool for actively caring for the bereaved is the 'Four Es' (see Box 49.2).

Box 49.2 The four Es (McLauchlan 1990)

E – Empathise

E – Enable relatives to accept reality and to experience the pain

E – Encourage in an appropriate way, offering help for example

E – Encounter your own feelings and express them later, perhaps as part of a debriefing.

Continuous assessment of how each person is coping allows specific interventions and care to be planned and delivered, maximising coping strengths and strategies.

Preparation of the bereaved

Consideration must be given to where the news is to be broken and by whom. The best person to tell the family is someone who has the skills to do so, who knows the patient, who has the correct information, and who is able to answer their questions. The setting needs to be private, peaceful and free from interruption.

In the above case scenario, the team ensured that the sister-in-law, who appeared to be coping the best, was present with the family and was the main point of liaison for the nurses and doctors. The news was broken in a quiet room, away from the main resuscitation room.

Preparation is vital, including ensuring that staff have adequate time. Simple measures are important, such as ensuring that bleeps and telephones are silenced. If there are any communication issues – such as English not being understood, or deafness – these need to be addressed.

Begin by getting a feel from the family about what they already know and understand – this is a good starting place. Remember, all efforts are focused on facts, reality and helping the bereaved to fully understand the situation. Misunderstandings and misinterpretations occur easily with someone who is upset, so avoid euphemisms and instead use the words 'dead' and 'died'. Using phrases like 'I am sorry we have lost her' are open to misunderstanding and may feed denial (Wright 2007). Families value honest, direct information. There is an overwhelming need for them to know the 'bottom line'.

Be aware of your posture, and the tone and pace of your voice. Be aware of your facial expressions and the amount of eye contact you make. Consider which of your mannerisms may put people off, but bear in mind that mannerisms are a feature of your personality and that these families will appreciate a glimpse of the real you. Being comfortable with silences is also important, although this can be very challenging. If the bereaved person becomes very distressed while you are caring for them, remember that it is the information being imparted that is causing the distress – not you personally.

Dealing with grief reactions

The way bereaved people display their grief can be challenging. However, there are certain ways in which staff can manage tricky situations and help them.

Denial

When the reality becomes too much to bear, the relative or friend may begin to deny the facts. Some families will ask the same question repeatedly, hoping that subsequent answers will become more favourable. Try not to be swayed or allow any other member of the family or your colleagues to do so either. Continue repeating the same statements of fact in a gentle but assertive way.

Bargaining

Sometimes families may try bargaining with the person breaking the news. Again, you should continue to give the facts, confirming the reality of the death. Sometimes a remark about life being of inestimable value may help them regain insight into what can be realistically achieved.

In the above case scenario, the teenage daughter was oscillating between several grief reactions; bargaining with the team was just one. She was able to move on from it by seeing her mother and hearing again that there was nothing that could be done, even though this was very painful and distressing for her.

Anger

Anger can pose problems for the doctor or nurse. It can be frightening to witness and sometimes feel threatening. Remembering that anger is a feeling and acknowledging it as such can often help to diffuse it.

Withdrawing and isolation

Some people withdraw and need time to assimilate all the information given to them. If someone reacts like this, it may be enough simply to be with them and show them support. Similarly, some bereaved people may feel a great sense of isolation, despite being surrounded by their close family. When they express this feeling, the rest of the family may feel rejected. It may be worth pointing out that this is because the bereaved person is concentrating on their specific relationship with the dead person who has gone, leaving them alone. Again, acknowledge this feeling, but ensure that they are not left alone, because the fear this feeling brings will be compounded by the physical reality of being isolated.

The husband in our case scenario displayed these grief reactions. He spent some time with his wife, with a nurse nearby. He did request solitude, during which time he hugged her and sobbed, finally reaching a point where he could accept she was not going to live.

Guilt

Many people feel guilty even when they have no reason to feel guilt. They will not stop feeling guilty until they have gained insight into the reality. Again, acknowledge the feeling and just listen to them.

Inappropriate behaviour

Inappropriate behaviour, such as telling jokes or laughing, arises because focusing on the death is just too painful for some people (Wright 1996). It is a common response in children and adolescents, who often have little or no experience of grief and have no idea how to react. Remain non-judgemental; the person may well become embarrassed about such responses later on.

Crying

Crying is a very common response and one that healthcare professionals find the easiest to deal with. Bear in mind that men may need permission to cry, and that some people are distressed by a normal early reaction of not being able to cry. Reassurance and comforting often help. Staff who feel they do not know how to react or manage the situation can fall back on basic humanity and on what feels right and natural – these are often helpful.

Resuscitation

On some occasions, relatives arrive when resuscitation attempts are still in progress. It is important not to exclude relatives from the proceedings. Giving regular updates, and informing them that every effort is being made to save the patient, are sensible measures to take. Some relatives may wish to be present during resuscitation. This does have identified benefits and allows them to be present at the time of death (Wright 1999, Royal College of Nursing 2002, Baskett *et al.* 2005, Fulbrook *et al.* 2007). Make sure a member of staff stays with the relative. The staff member should be able to provide support and explain procedures as well as to assess and act if the relative becomes very distressed (and accompany them if they need to leave) (see Chapter 46 on ethics in acute care).

Culture and religion

Religion and culture are important when a person dies. Ensure this aspect of a family's lifestyle is addressed, consulting them about their wishes and specific requirements so that appropriate religious and cultural interventions are found that are spiritually and culturally acceptable. In certain circumstances, organ donation may be discussed, which may provide some comfort or meaning to the death they are experiencing (see Chapter 43 on organ and tissue donation).

Closure and viewing the body

Closure is an important aspect of accepting the reality of the death and it should be actively promoted. Viewing the body and taking the opportunity to say goodbye is a positive intervention that staff can encourage, no matter how young, old or frail the relatives are. Reality, although painful, is more manageable than fantasy, which can become intrusive and uncomfortable – especially in children. Telling people what to expect when they see the body will help them.

Talking to and touching the dead person allows some of the unfinished business to be addressed. In fact there is little doubt that time and effort spent with the deceased is tremendously valuable. However, because of the disordered thought processes associated with loss, many people are unsure about what is 'allowed' or considered normal. It is therefore helpful if they are told that it is all right to touch, hold and speak to their loved one. Family members should be allowed to decide for themselves whether or not they want to see the dead person (Haas 2003). If they act on someone else's advice, they may risk profound regrets later. Point this out to well-meaning family members who try to decide who should see or not see the body.

Sadly, as previously discussed, suddenly bereaved people remain numb and shocked for some time. Despite their insatiable need for highly detailed information, they may later realise they have not understood or remembered very much. There may be no formal way in which to rectify this. A common perception by families is of abrupt withdrawal of care. Many relatives express a wish to retain contact with staff, and it has been recommended for the use of support programmes for relatives. Aftercare can help fulfil the long-term needs of families in terms of obtaining information and clarifying issues surrounding the death of their loved one. Support programmes also provide a vehicle through which reassurance and support can be sought, with the opportunity to make referrals to specialist bereavement groups where applicable.

Conclusion

Although it feels as if there is nothing one can do to minimise the pain and distress of sudden death when dealing with the bereaved, aiming for simple goals (such as giving the facts and confirming reality so that the person accepts that the death has happened) can be beneficial later, when they begin their journey of grief work. By taking these simple steps, the healthcare professional can ensure that the last moments with a loved one are meaningful and precious.

A greater awareness of the grieving process and ways in which the suddenly bereaved can be helped will improve practice; the essence of bereavement care is about intervening in order to facilitate a healthy grieving process.

References and further reading

Antonacci, M. (1990). Sudden death: helping bereaved parents in the PICU. *Critical Care Nurse.* **10**(4), 65–70.

Baskett, P.J.F., Steen, P.A. & Bossaert, L. (2005). European Council Guidelines for resuscitation 2005: Section 8: The ethics of resuscitation and end of life decisions. *Resuscitation.* **67**(1), S171–80.

Bowman, T. (1999). *Promoting resiliency in those who do bereavement work. National Association of Bereavement Services.* London: National Association of Bereavement Services.

Chapple, H.S. (1999). Changing the game in the intensive care unit: letting nature take its course. *Critical Care Nurse.* **19** (3), 25–34.

Department of Health (DH) (2005). *When a Patient Dies – Advice on Developing Bereavement Services in the NHS.* London: DH.

Department of Health (DH) (2011). *Bereavement Care Services: A Synthesis of the Literature.* London: DH.

Doka, K.J. (ed.) (2014). *Living with Grief: After Sudden Loss, Suicide, Homicide, Accident, Heart Attack, Stroke.* London: Taylor & Francis.

Dolan, B. (2013). 'Care of the Bereaved' in B. Dolan & L. Holt, L. (eds). *Accident and Emergency: Theory and Practice.* 3rd edn. Elsevier Health Sciences.

Ferrand, E., Jabre, P., Vincent-Genod, C. *et al.* (2008). Circumstances of death in hospitalized patients and nurses' perceptions: French multicenter mort à l'hôpital survey. *Archives of Internal Medicine.* **168**, 867–75.

Freud, S. (1917). *Mourning and Melancholia. Volume XIV.* London: Hogarth.

Fulbrook, P., Latour, J., Albarran, J. *et al.* (2007). The presence of family members during cardiopulmonary resuscitation: European Federation of Critical Care Nursing Associations, European and Neonatal Intensive Care and European Society of Cardiology Council on Cardiovascular Nursing and Allied Professions Joint position statement. *CONNECT: The World of Critical Care Nursing.* **5** (4), 86–88.

Haas, F. (2003). Bereavement care: Seeing the body. *Nursing Standard.* **17** (28), 33–37.

Hall, S.J. & Smith, G.B. (1999). Breaking bad news to the friends, family and partners of intensive care unit patients: A practical guide. *Care of the Critically Ill.* **15** (3), 101–04.

Jackson, I. (1998). A study of bereavement in an intensive therapy unit. *Nursing in Critical Care.* **3** (3), 141–50.

Kendrick, K. (1997). Sudden death: walking in a moral minefield. *Emergency Nurse.* **5** (1), 17–19.

Kubler-Ross, E. (1969). *On Death and Dying.* New York: Springer.

Lautrette, A., Darmon, M., Megarbane, B. *et al.* (2007). A communication strategy and brochure for relatives of patients dying in the ICU. *New England Journal of Medicine.* **356**, 469–78.

Lewis, C.S. (1961). *A Grief Observed.* London: Faber.

Li, S.P., Chan, C. & Lee, D. (2002). Helpfulness of nursing actions to suddenly bereaved family members in an accident and emergency setting in Hong Kong. *Journal of Advanced Nursing.* **40** (2), 170–80.

McLauchlan, C.A.J. (1990). Handling distressed relatives and breaking bad news. *British Medical Journal.* **301**, 1145–49.

Parkes, C. (1996). *Bereavement: Studies of Grief in Adult Life.* 3rd edn. London: Routledge.

Parkes, C.M. (1998). Coping with loss: Bereavement in adult life. *British Medical Journal.* **316** (7134), 856–59.

Royal College of Nursing (2002). *Witnessing Resuscitation: Guidance for Nursing Staff.* London: Royal College of Nursing.

Russell, P. & Sander, R. (1998). Palliative care: promoting the concept of a healthy death. *British Journal of Nursing.* 7 (5), 255–61.

Scrutton, S. (1995). *Bereavement and Grief: Supporting Older People Through Loss.* London: Edward Arnold.

Stroebe, M.S., Stroebe, W. & Hansson, R.O. (1993). *Handbook of Bereavement: Theory, Research and Intervention.* Cambridge: Cambridge University Press.

Townsend, A. (1995). Sudden death in critical care units. *Care of the Critically Ill.* **11** (3), 126–28.

Weston, R., Martin, T. & Anderson, Y. (1998). *Loss and Bereavement: Managing Change.* Oxford: Blackwell Science.

Worden, J. (1991). *Grief Counselling and Grief Therapy.* London: Tavistock Publications.

Wright, B. (1996). *Sudden Death – A Research Base for Practice.* London: Churchill Livingstone.

Wright, B. (1999). Responding to autonomy and disempowerment at the time of a sudden death. *Accident and Emergency Nursing.* **7**, 154–57.

Wright, B. (2007). *Loss and Grief.* Keswick: M&K Update.

Useful websites

The British Psychological Society
http://www.bps.org.uk/ Search the site with 'caring for the suddenly bereaved'.
(Accessed 2 September 2015)

Cruse Bereavement Care
http://www.cruse.org.uk/
(Accessed 2 September 2015)

Department of Health
https://www.gov.uk/government/publications
(Accessed 2 September 2015)

Dying Matters
http://www.dyingmatters.org/
(Accessed 2 September 2015)

Index